BEDSIDE CARDIOLOGY

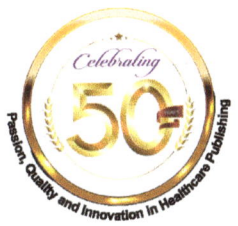

BEDSIDE CARDIOLOGY

Second Edition

Achyut Sarkar MD DM (Cardiology) FACC
Professor of Cardiology
Institute of Postgraduate Medical Education and Research (IPGME&R)
Senior Interventional Cardiologist
BM Birla Heart Research Center
Kolkata, West Bengal, India

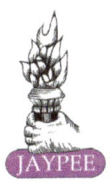

JAYPEE BROTHERS MEDICAL PUBLISHERS
The Health Sciences Publisher
New Delhi | London

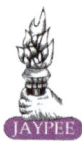 **Jaypee Brothers Medical Publishers (P) Ltd**

Headquarters
Jaypee Brothers Medical Publishers (P) Ltd
4838/24, Ansari Road, Daryaganj
New Delhi 110 002, India
Phone: +91-11-43574357
Fax: +91-11-43574314
Email: jaypee@jaypeebrothers.com

Overseas Offices
J.P. Medical Ltd
83 Victoria Street, London
SW1H 0HW (UK)
Phone: +44 20 3170 8910
Fax: +44 (0)20 3008 6180
Email: info@jpmedpub.com

Website: www.jaypeebrothers.com
Website: www.jaypeedigital.com

© 2020, Jaypee Brothers Medical Publishers

The views and opinions expressed in this book are solely those of the original contributor(s)/author(s) and do not necessarily represent those of editor(s) of the book.

All rights reserved. No part of this publication may be reproduced, stored or transmitted in any form or by any means, electronic, mechanical, photocopying, recording or otherwise, without the prior permission in writing of the publishers.

All brand names and product names used in this book are trade names, service marks, trademarks or registered trademarks of their respective owners. The publisher is not associated with any product or vendor mentioned in this book.

Medical knowledge and practice change constantly. This book is designed to provide accurate, authoritative information about the subject matter in question. However, readers are advised to check the most current information available on procedures included and check information from the manufacturer of each product to be administered, to verify the recommended dose, formula, method and duration of administration, adverse effects and contraindications. It is the responsibility of the practitioner to take all appropriate safety precautions. Neither the publisher nor the author(s)/editor(s) assume any liability for any injury and/or damage to persons or property arising from or related to use of material in this book.

This book is sold on the understanding that the publisher is not engaged in providing professional medical services. If such advice or services are required, the services of a competent medical professional should be sought.

Every effort has been made where necessary to contact holders of copyright to obtain permission to reproduce copyright material. If any have been inadvertently overlooked, the publisher will be pleased to make the necessary arrangements at the first opportunity. The **CD/DVD-ROM** (if any) provided in the sealed envelope with this book is complimentary and free of cost. **Not meant for sale.**

Inquiries for bulk sales may be solicited at: jaypee@jaypeebrothers.com

Bedside Cardiology / Achyut Sarkar

First Edition: **2012**

Second Edition: **2020**

ISBN: 978-93-89587-57-9

Dedicated to
My students—past, present, and future

Preface to the Second Edition

I am excited to bring you the second edition of "*Bedside Cardiology*". This is because in its first edition, I expressed my concern that clinical cardiology would be relegated in the history of medicine! That hasn't happened.

As quoted by Silas Weir Mitchell at Transaction of the Congress of American Physicians and Surgeons held at Washington DC in 1892, "How useful, how simple, it seemed to count the pulse and respiration, or to put a thermometer under the tongue, and yet it took in one case a century, and in another far more, before the mass of the profession learned to profit by the wisdom of the few". We love to forget those few, because we love only our present.

I will remind you Clark HG, who, in his article on "Execution of Magee: Post-mortem appearance" in 1858, reported that in a criminal, a single heart sound was audible for 90 minutes following execution! On opening the chest, "the ventricles were seen to be inert, but the right auricle was contracting regularly at 80 beats/min", and was evidently responsible for the sound. And that was S4!

Clark auscultated a dead person for 90 minutes. Let us auscultate a living person for a few minutes!

Achyut Sarkar

Preface to the First Edition

For the sake of stethoscope, please read this preface!

Why another one? Why another one, when *Bedside Cardiology*, as a science, has been relegated in the History of Medicine and as an art, has been described an art of artifact!

There is no noble intention. This is only for stethoscope, for which I have a romantic nostalgia. Still, I cannot accept the image that a cardiologist is giving round in the ward or seeing patient in his chamber, with the echo Doppler probe of his palmtop echocardiogram machine hanging from his neck and no stethoscope!

Newer investigating tools, newer interventions are evolving almost every day and replacing the new ones. We are appreciating those. Even then, are we not thrilled when we detect an Austin Flint murmur or Graham Steell murmur, described two centuries back? Are we not thrilled when we detect a continuous murmur on the back of any patient?

May not be that useful, we all, still enjoy *Bedside Cardiology*. We completely agree to Dr Basil M RuDsky–"This is one of the few pleasures that can be derived from the ever-changing practice of medicine. It stimulates acquisition of a good doctor–patient relationship and provides a satisfying alternative to many of the idiopathic inconsistencies and inadequacies of medical practice. It is unquestionably an art and skill that must not be allowed to succumb to the way of the impossible dream of Don Quixote".

Achyut Sarkar

Acknowledgments

I wish to thank M/S Jaypee Brothers Medical Publishers (P) Ltd New Delhi for whom the creation of this book has become possible. I thank my late mother and father. Their memories are still great inspiration. I thank my daughter Parnisha, my son Arjab, and my son-in-law Baishakh. Their academic aptitude has always been encouraging to me. And Dr Asima Sarkar, my wife who is a great blessing in my life. She has sacrificed her invaluable professional time and supported my academic activities. I thank her with immense gratitude.

Contents

1. Bedside Cardiology: Is it Evidence-based? 1
2. Functional Classification 6
3. A Triad: Cardinal Symptoms in Cardiovascular System 17
4. A Triad: Minor Symptoms in Cardiovascular System 34
5. A Triad: Cardinal Symptoms in Left-to-Right Shunt 41
6. A Triad: Cardinal Symptoms in Congenital Cyanotic Heart Disease 44
7. Syndrome and Measurements 50
8. Clinical Instruments 68
9. A Triad: Cardinal Signs in Congenital Cyanotic Heart Disease 77
10. Jugular Venous Pulse 87
11. Arterial Pulse 106
12. Blood Pressure 127
13. Precordium: Inspection, Palpation, and Percussion 140
14. First Heart Sound 164
15. Second Heart Sound 173
16. Third Heart Sound 185
17. Fourth Heart Sound 190
18. Ejection Sound 195
19. Nonejection Sound 200
20. Murmur 212
21. Continuous Murmur 239
22. Innocent Murmur and Sound 247

23.	Dynamic Auscultation	251
24.	Clinical Assessment: Congestion and Perfusion	262
25.	Clinical Assessment: Pulmonary Hypertension	272
26.	Segmental Approach in Congenital Heart Disease	281
27.	Clinical Approach: Congenital Cyanotic Heart Disease	303
28.	Clinical Approach: Tetralogy Physiology	315
29.	Clinical Approach: Left-to-Right Shunt and Eisenmenger Physiology	330

Index   *345*

CHAPTER 1

Bedside Cardiology: Is it Evidence-based?

INTRODUCTION

"There is already plenty of evidence to show that we are in danger of losing our clinical heritage, and of pinning too much faith in figures thrown up by machines. Medicine must suffer if this tendency is not checked."[1]

Paul Wood expressed this apprehension in 1950. Since then, around seven decades have passed. And now, justifying his apprehension, bedside cardiology has become a heritage science! Most importantly, evidence-based medicine is asking and demanding evidences in favor of bedside cardiology.

DYSPNEA

In a study[2] to evaluate symptoms as predictor of heart failure or chronic obstructive pulmonary disease (COPD), dyspnea on effort predicted depressed left ventricular systolic function with a sensitivity of 100% and specificity of 20%. Orthopnea predicted heart failure with a sensitivity and specificity of 71% and 65% and paroxysmal nocturnal dyspnea (PND) with the sensitivity and specificity of 47% and 75%, respectively. All these symptoms had a likeli hood ratio (LR) of 2 or less. In Evaluation Study of Congestive Heart Failure and Pulmonary Artery Catheterization Effectiveness (ESCAPE) trial, orthopnea requiring two or more pillows independently predicted pulmonary capillary wedge pressure (PCWP) >30 mm Hg with an odd ratio of 3.6.[3]

In acute heart failure, exertional dyspnea is a poor predictor for diagnosis with a LR+ of 1.3 and LR– of 0.48. Orthopnea and PND are better predictors. The former has a LR+ of 2.2 and LR– of 0.65. The later has a LR+ of 2.6 and LR– of 0.7.[4] In chronic heart failure, dyspnea on exertion is more sensitive (72-100%) and less specific (17-44%) symptom to diagnose heart failure. PND and orthopnea are less sensitive (27-40%) and more specific (80-99%).

CHEST PAIN[4]

In acute coronary syndrome (ACS), nature of chest pain has mixed predictive value. Pressure-type chest pain has LR+ of 1.3 only. Radiation down to arm has a better predictive value with LR+ of 2.3-4.7. A stabbing or pleuritic chest pain, with tenderness has lesser predictive value with LR− of 0.2-0.3. Chest pain responding to nitrate is not a predictive feature for chest pain in ACS. For stable patient, typical angina bears a high predictive value for coronary artery disease (CAD) with LR+ of 5.8, whereas nonanginal chest pain shows least predictive value for CAD, with a LR of 0.1.

PALPITATION

From history of palpitation, arrhythmic palpitation is more likely, when the age of the patient is >60 years with a LR+ of 1.70, male gender with a LR+ of 1.70, and sleep disturbances due to palpitation with a LR+ of 2.29.

JUGULAR VENOUS PRESSURE

In one study,[5] central venous pressure was determined clinically from jugular venous pressure (JVP) and by central venous catheter. The sensitivity of JVP at identifying low (<0 mm Hg), normal (0-7 mm Hg), or high (>7 mm Hg) central venous pressure was 33%, 33%, and 49%, respectively. The specificity was 73%, 62%, and 76%, respectively. In another study,[6] clinically detected central venous pressure was compared to pulmonary artery pressure by catheter. Clinical prediction was correct in 55% cases. It has been shown[7] that a raised JVP increases the probability, that the monitored central venous pressure will be four times higher.

When the clinically measured JVP is low, there is least possibility (LR 0.2) of a higher monitored central venous pressure. A normal JVP (LR 1), however, does not increase or decrease the probability of abnormal central venous pressure. Hepatojugular reflux[8] is a more specific test. It is suggestive of increased right atrial and ventricular end-diastolic pressure and increased PCWP of >15 mm Hg with a LR+ of 6.7 and LR− of 0.08.

PULSE

"Is the pulse in atrial fibrillation irregularly irregular?"[9] In this excellent study, it has been shown that nonrandom sequence of R-R interval is found in 30% cases and pulsus alternans in 46% cases of atrial fibrillation. Thus, a particular pattern of regularity is common in atrial fibrillation, rather than irregular irregularity. Detection of transient pulse irregularity has a LR+ of 3.3 of atrial fibrillation in ECG, whereas persistent pulse irregularity has a LR+ of 24.1. Absence of any irregularity in pulse indicates a negative LR of 0.1 for having atrial fibrillation.

Hill sign recently has been challenged.[10] Intra-arterial pressure tracing has shown that there is no major difference between upper and lower limb pressure in aortic regurgitation and Hill sign is a sphygmomanometric artifact! Pulse pressure has a good predictive value on severity of aortic regurgitation and a pulse pressure >80 mm Hg has a LR+ of 10.9 for the presence of moderate to severe aortic regurgitation.

Presence of femoral bruit, even in asymptomatic patient, bears a good predictive value for the presence of peripheral artery disease with a LR+ of 4.80. Presence of renal bruit with both systolic and diastolic component enhances the likelihood of renal artery stenosis with a sensitivity of 39% and specificity of 99%. Similarly, a carotid bruit increases the likelihood of significant carotid artery stenosis with a sensitivity of 53% and specificity of 83%.

APICAL IMPULSE

In one study,[11] left ventricular enlargement, as determined by the site of the impulse and its diameter, was compared with echocardiographic left ventricular enlargement. Sensitivity and specificity of apical impulse outside left midclavicular line as an indicator of left ventricular enlargement was 100% and 18%, respectively with a LR of 1.2. When midsternal line was taken as reference point in place of midclavicular line, apical impulse situated >10 cm outside, indicated left ventricular enlargement with a sensitivity of 100% and specificity of 33%. An increased diameter of apical impulse was a good indicator of left ventricular enlargement with a sensitivity of 92% and specificity of 75%.

HEART SOUND

A loud S2 (P2) is a strong predictor of pulmonary hypertension. When P2 is audible at the apex, systolic pulmonary artery pressure may be assumed >50 mm Hg.[12]

The S3 was first described, long back, in 1856. It is taken as a hallmark of left ventricular dysfunction. Its predictive value was studied, which quantitated the interobserver variability of S3.[13] In that study, it was found that if one observer heard S3, the probability that a second observer would, was between 34-38%. When, on the other hand, one observer found S3, the chance that a second observer would agree was between 69 and 79%. Auscultatory findings were verified by phonocardiogram and the positive and negative predictive value to identify S3 was 71% and 64%, respectively. When this and few other studies cast doubt about the clinical usefulness of S3, Studies of Left Ventricular Dysfunction (SOLVD) trial[14] strongly established its usefulness. In patients with heart failure, clinical detection of S3 increased the risk of hospitalization or death due to pump failure by 50%.

MURMUR

Clinical skill to detect murmur was compared with echocardiogram in several studies. Murmur of mitral regurgitation is detected clinically in 13-56% cases and that of tricuspid regurgitations in 28-33% cases.[15,16] Aortic stenosis murmur can be identified clinically better than other murmurs, ranging from 20% to 88%.[17] Clinical identification of aortic regurgitation and mitral stenosis murmur are poorer. Sensitivity to diagnose diastolic murmur was only in 5-24% cases.[18] The sensitivity and specificity to detect a functional murmur are 67% and 91%,

> **BOX 1** **Bedside cardiology: Limitations.**
> - To identify low-frequency sound
> - To identify murmur of low-frequency like, mitral stenosis and murmur of lower grade like aortic regurgitation
> - To appreciate the gap between sounds (such as, S2-OS, S1-EC, S1-NEC)
> - Bedside diagnosis of some common cardiac conditions such as pericardial effusion, early ventricular dysfunction, early cardiomyopathy, silent valvular disease, and mass lesions is a difficult task, but can be diagnosed comprehensively by echocardiogram
> - Early and presymptomatic diagnosis of disease, which can alter the eventual prognosis

respectively and for an organic murmur, the sensitivity and specificity are raised to 79% and 93%.

CONCLUSION (BOX 1)

May evidence-based medicine is casting shadow on bedside cardiology, its survival as a science depends upon the process of its filtration through the stringent criteria of evidence-based medicine. Clinician should remember that the paradigm is shifting from "intuition, unsystemic clinical experiences, and pathophysiologic rationale as sufficient grounds for clinical decision making" to evidence from clinical research.[19]

REFERENCES

1. Wood PH. Disease of the Heart and Circulation. Philadelphia, PA: Lippincott; 1950.
2. Zema MJ, Masters AP, Margouleff D. Dyspnoea: the heart or the lungs? Differentiation at bedside by use of the simple valsalva maneuver. Chest. 1984;85: 59.
3. Drazner MH, Hellkamp AS, Leier CV, et al. Value of clinician assessment of hemodynamics in advanced heart failure: the ESCAPE trial. Circ Heart Fail. 2008;1:170-7.
4. Japp AG, Sumpson L, Pettit S, et al. Chapter 1.2 Cardiovascular symptom. In: Camm AJ, Serruys PW, Maurer G. The ESC Textbook of Cardiovascular Medicine. Oxford University Press; 2019. p. 11.
5. Connors AF, McCaffree DR, Gray BA. Evaluation of right heart catheterization in the critically ill patient without acute myocardial infarction. N Eng J Med. 1983;308:263.
6. Eisenberg PR, Jaffe AS, Schuster DP. Clinical evaluation compared to pulmonary artery catheterization in the hemodynamic assessment of critically ill patients. Crit Care Med. 1984;12:549.
7. Cook DJ. The clinical assessment of central venous pressure. Am J Med Sci. 1990;299:175.
8. Cook DJ, Simel DL. Does this patient have abnormal central venous pressure? JAMA. 1996;275:630.
9. Rawles JM, Rowland E. Is the pulse in atrial fibrillation irregularly irregular? Br Heart J. 1986;56:4.
10. Kutryk M, Fitchett D. Hill's sign in aortic regurgitation: enhanced pressure wave transmission or artifact? Can J Cardiol. 1997;13(3):237.
11. Eilen SD, Crawford MH, O'Rourke RA. Accuracy of precordial palpation for detecting increased left ventricular volume. Ann Intern Med. 1983;99:628.
12. Gaine SP, Rubin LJ. Primary pulmonary hypertension. Lancet. 1998;352(9129):719.
13. Lock CE, Morgan CD, Ranganathan N. The accuracy and interobserver agreement in detecting the "gallop sound" by cardiac auscultation. Chest. 1998;114:128.

14. Drazner MH, Rame JE, Phil M, et al. Prognostic importance of elevated jugular venous pressure and a third heart sound in patients with heart failure. N Engl J Med. 1983;308:263.
15. Mangione S, Nieman LZ, Gracely E. The teaching and practice of cardiac auscultation during internal medicine and cardiology training. Ann Intern Med. 1993;119:47.
16. Attenhofer Jost CH, Turina J, Mayer K, et al. Echocardiography in the evaluation of systolic murmurs of unknown cause. Am J Med. 2000;108:614.
17. Spencer KT, Allen S, Anderson AS, et al. Physician-performed point-of-care echocardiography using a laptop platform compared with physical examination in the cardiovascular patient. J Am Coll Cardiol. 2001;37:2013.
18. Roldan CA, Shively BK, Crawford MH. Value of the cardiovascular physical examination for detecting valvular heart disease in asymptomatic subjects. Am J Cardiol. 1996;77:1327.
19. Evidence-based medicine working group. Evidence-based medicine, a new approach to teaching the practice of medicine. JAMA. 1992;268:2420.

FURTHER READING

1. McGee S. Evidence-based Physical Diagnosis, 3rd edition. Philadelphia, PA: Elsevier Saunders; 2012.
2. Yusuf S, Cairns JA, Camm AJ, et al. Evidence-based Cardiology, 2nd edition. London: BMJ Books; 2003.

CHAPTER 2

Functional Classification

INTRODUCTION

The most important part of clinical examination of a patient suffering from cardiac disease is to assess the functional impairment based on the degree of physical activity. There are several methodologies for this assessment, of which, New York Heart Association (NYHA) and Canadian Cardiovascular Society System (CCSS) are most popular.

NYHA FUNCTIONAL CLASSIFICATION

In 1928, the New York Heart Association (NYHA) published a classification of patients with cardiac disease, based on clinical severity and prognosis. This classification has been updated in seven subsequent editions of Nomenclature and Criteria for Diagnosis of Diseases of the Heart and Great Vessels. In 1964 edition,[1] the committee described NYHA functional classification as "only approximate" and representative of "an opinion of the physician's opinion." The ninth edition,[2] revised by the Criteria Committee of the American Heart Association, New York City Affiliate, was released on 1994.

Changes

In the initial editions, the terms functional capacity and therapeutic classifications were used. In the subsequent editions in 1973 and 1979, the terms cardiac status and prognosis were used. In the last edition, functional classes, which depend upon subjective symptoms, and objective assessment, based on investigations were included. Anginal symptoms were also included in the functional class, from this edition.

The classifications are summarized in **Table 1**.

Thus a complete diagnosis, according to this classification, is:
- Etiology
- Anatomic lesions
- Physiologic disturbances
- Functional capacity
- Objective assessment

TABLE 1: New York Heart Association functional classifications.[1]

Functional capacity	Objective assessment
Class I: Patients have cardiac disease but without the resulting limitation of physical activity. Ordinary physical activity does not cause undue fatigue, palpitation, dyspnea, or anginal pain	No objective evidence of cardiovascular disease
Class II: Patients have cardiac disease resulting in slight limitation of physical activity. They are comfortable at rest. Ordinary physical activity results in fatigue, palpitation, dyspnea, or anginal pain	Objective evidence of minimal cardiovascular disease
Class III: Patients have cardiac disease resulting in marked limitation of physical activity. They are comfortable at rest. Less than ordinary physical activity causes fatigue, palpitation, dyspnea, or anginal pain	Objective evidence of moderately severe cardiovascular disease
Class IV: Patients have cardiac disease resulting in inability to carry on any physical activity without discomfort. Symptoms of cardiac insufficiency or of the anginal syndrome may be present even at rest. If any physical activity is undertaken, discomfort is increased	Objective evidence of severe cardiovascular disease

Thus, a patient with minimal or no symptom with severe obstruction at right ventricular outflow tract or severe regurgitation across mitral valve may be classified as:
- Functional capacity I and objective assessment D

On the other hand, a patient with severe symptom and only a moderate gradient across aortic valve may be classified as:
- Functional capacity IV and objective assessment B

The 1994 classification also includes the following as described here.

Uncertain Diagnosis

No Heart Disease: Predisposing Etiologic Factor
This category includes patients in whom no apparent cardiac disease, but there is a history of etiologic factor that might cause heart disease. These patients need periodic follow-up.

No Heart Disease: Unexplained Manifestation
This category includes patients with symptoms or signs referable to the heart but in whom a diagnosis of cardiac disease is uncertain at the time of examination. These patients need re-examination after a stated interval.

No Heart Disease
When there is a reasonable uncertainty that the symptoms or signs are not of cardiac origin, the diagnosis should be no heart disease.

Uniqueness of NYHA Classification System

- Clinician can assess patient's functional status very quickly by this classification, during the clinical assessment.
- The classification is the best available prognostic marker. This is because NYHA functional classification assesses the patient pertaining to exercise. All other parameters, including clinical examination, ECG, X-ray, and echocardiogram are assessed in resting status. This edge over other factors makes this system a very important prognostic factor.

Limitation of NYHA Functional Classification

- Reproducibility and validity are 56% and 51%, respectively.[3]
- In one study,[4] "Limitations of the New York Heart Association functional classification system and self-reported walking distances in chronic heart failure," it was shown that "54% concordance between cardiologists even when assessing the same patient on the same day". There was a poor agreement between "cardiologists in differentiating between patients belonging to class II and class III", which is most important issue, because of the fact that to classify a patient in class I or class IV is easy and indication of spironolactone and resynchronization therapy depend on whether patient belongs to class II or class III.
- Research papers using the NYHA classification, either as an inclusion and/or outcome measure, should record the criteria or questions used to ascertain a patient's functional class.
- Use of specific questions can markedly improve the reproducibility of this classification system.
- Many clinicians ask patients with heart failure, how far they can walk. Walking distance does not measure exercise capacity or correlate with a known measure of exercise capacity. Even the poor ability of patients to estimate distance does not explain the lack of correlation with objectively measured exercise capacity.

CANADIAN CARDIOVASCULAR SOCIETY FUNCTIONAL CLASSIFICATION OF ANGINA PECTORIS

The Canadian Cardiovascular Society Angina (CCSA) functional classification[5] is based on the functional class in relation to angina only (**Table 2**). CCSA class showed an excellent linier relation with angiographic findings, revascularization rates, mortality, and nonfatal myocardial infarction in ACRE study.[6] To assess the validity, CCSA classification was compared to DASI (Duke Activity Status Index) in another study.[7] In this study CCSA class I to III showed an inverse relation to DASI score and linearly related to mortality. Class IV showed a similar outcome to class III, which may be explained by the confounding effect of the stability of the patient's symptoms.

TABLE 2: The Canadian Cardiovascular Society functional class of angina.

Class	
Class I	Ordinary physical activity does not cause angina, such as walking and climbing stairs. Angina with strenuous or rapid or prolonged exertion at work or recreation
Class II	Slight limitation of ordinary activity. Walking or climbing stairs rapidly, walking uphill, walking or stair climbing after meals, or in cold, or in wind, or under emotional stress or only during the few hours after awakening. Walking more than two blocks on the level and climbing more than one flight of stairs at a normal pace and in normal condition
Class III	Marked limitation of ordinary physical activity. Walking one or two blocks on the level and climbing one flight of stairs in normal condition and at normal pace
Class IV	Inability to carry on any physical activity without discomfort; anginal syndrome may be present at rest.

SPECIFIC ACTIVITY SCALE

The SAS (Specific Activity Scale) denotes the activity in relation to usual daily life (**Table 3**). Goldman et al. proposed this functional classification in 1981 (**Table 4**).[3]

TABLE 3: Goldman specific activity scales.

Class I	Patient can perform to complete any activity requiring >7 metabolic equivalent (MET)
Class II	Patient can perform to complete any activity requiring >5 METs but cannot perform to complete activity requiring >7 METs
Class III	Patient can perform to complete any activity requiring >2 METs but cannot perform to complete activity requiring >5 METs
Class IV	Patient cannot perform to complete any activity requiring >2 METs

TABLE 4: Criteria for determination of Goldman-specific activity scale.

Activities	METs	Any yes	No
Can you walk down a flight of steps without stopping	4.5–5.2	Go to 2	Go to 4
Can you carry anything up to a flight of eight steps without stopping or can you: • Have sexual intercourse without stooping (5–5.5 METs) • Garden, rake, weeds (5.6 METs) • Roller skate, dance foxtrot (5–6 METs) • Walk at a 4 miles-per-hour rate on level ground (5–6 METs)	5–5.5		

Continued

Continued

Activities	METs	Any yes	No
Can you carry at least 24 pounds up eight steps or can you: • Carry objects that are at least 80 pounds (8 METs) • Do outdoor work-shovel snow, spade soil (7 METs) • Do recreational activities such as skiing, basketball, touch football, squash, handball (7–10 METs) • Jog/walk 5 miles/h (9 METs)	10	Class I	Class II
Can you shower without stopping or can you: • Strip and make bed (3.9–5 METs) • Mop floors (4.2 METs) • Hang washed cloths (4.4 METs) • Clean windows (3.7 METs) • Walk 2.5 miles per hour (3–3.5 METs) • Bowl (3–4.4 METs) • Play golf (4.5 METs) • Push power lawn mower (4 METs)	3.6–4.2	Class III	Go to 5
Can you dress without stopping because of symptoms	2–2.3	Class III	Class IV

(METs: metabolic equivalents)

DUKE ACTIVITY STATUS INDEX

Duke Activity Status Index is a self-administered questionnaire that measures the ability to perform a set of 12 common activities of daily living. Each activity is scored as 1 point, whereas the weighted score is calculated by adding together the "MET units" for each activity. Metabolic equivalents (METs) units are a measure of the metabolic cost of the activity and were derived in the original study by Hlatky (**Table 5**).[8]

After its first description, DASI has been used to monitor progress in patients with coronary artery disease, to do prognostication in patients with chronic heart failure and to determine long-term survival after cardiac surgery. A reduced version of DASI was developed, in which item 1 and 10 were excluded and 3 items were clubbed together, making all together 8 items.[9] Reduced DASI is reliable, valid, and responsive to clinical changes (**Table 6**).

NYHA VERSUS SPECIFIC ACTIVITY SCALE VERSUS DASI

How the three functional classifications, NYHA, Goldman specific activity scale, and DASI being comparable to each other was examined in a study,[10] which included 2,353 patients with congestive heart failure. About 700 cardiologists took part in this study. Heart failure was of an ischemic origin in 37% of cases, idiopathic in 25%, and due to hypertension in 25%. Symptomatology was left sided in most cases. The study showed the following observation—"Among NYHA class IV patients, 75% belonged to class IV of the SAS (23% class III, 1%

TABLE 5: Duke Activity Status Index (Hlatky).

Can you	METs: Yes	METs: No
Take care of yourself?	2.75	0
Walk indoor?	1.75	0
Walk a block or two on level ground?	2.75	0
Climb up a flight of stairs?	5.50	0
Run a short distance?	8.00	0
Do light work around the house like dusting or washing dishes?	2.70	0
Do moderate work around the house like vacuuming, sweeping floor, or carrying the groceries?	3.50	0
Do heavy work around the house like scrubbing floor or lifting heavy furniture?	8.00	0
Do yard work like raking leaves, weeding or pushing a power mower?	4.50	0
Have sexual relations?	5.25	0
Participate in moderate recreational activities like golf, bowling, dancing, and double tennis?	6.00	0
Participate in strenuous sports like swimming, single tennis, football, basketball or skiing?	7.50	0

(METs: metabolic equivalents)

TABLE 6: Reduced Duke Activity Status Index.

Activity	Weight
Degree of difficulty in the past 2 weeks for:	
• Walking indoor	1
• Walking a block or two	1
• Climbing a flight of stair	1
• Running a short distance	1
• Doing light housework	1.5
• Doing moderate housework	1.5
• Doing heavy housework	1.5
• Doing moderate to vigorous exercise	2.5

Note: A final score was calculated by the summary of giving each item a value of 3 = "done without difficulty", 2 = "done with difficulty", and 1 = "not done because of health reason". If any activity from 1 to 4 was not done because of health reason, it was skipped to activity 5.

class II), and 88% of the Duke classification (10% class III, 1% class II). For NYHA class III patients, 80% were SAS class III (5% class IV, 13% class II) and only 38% (42% class IV and 16% class II) of the Duke classification. Regarding NYHA class II patients, 74% were SAS class II (21% class III and 4% class I) and 26% of the Duke classification (39% class I, 29% class III and 3.6% class IV). Finally, among NYHA class I patients, 60% were SAS class I (34% class II, 5% class III) and 74% of the Duke classification (11% class II and 13% class III)".

UCLA (UNIVERSITY OF CALIFORNIA, LOS ANGELES) CONGENITAL HEART DISEASE FUNCTIONAL CLASS

This functional class[11] specifically deals with patient with congenital heart disease (**Box 1**).

WHO CLASSIFICATION OF FUNCTIONAL STATUS IN PULMONARY ARTERIAL HYPERTENSION

This A modified NYHA functional classification was adopted by World Health Organization (WHO) in 1998 for pulmonary arterial hypertension.[12] This NYHA/WHO classification includes syncope as a symptom in place of palpitation (**Box 2**). This functional class has a very important prognostic role. According to National Institutes of Health registry, the median survival for class I and II, class III, class IV are 6 years, 2.5 years, and 6 months, respectively.[12]

THE CANADIAN CARDIOVASCULAR SOCIETY SEVERITY OF ATRIAL FIBRILLATION SCALE

The CCS (Canadian Cardiovascular Society) SAF (Severity of Atrial Fibrillation) scale[13] is similar to the CCS angina functional class. The CCS-SAF score is calculated using three steps:
1. *Symptoms (S)*: To assess the symptoms.
2. *Association (A)*: To decide the association of symptoms with atrial fibrillation.
3. *Functionality (F)*: To assess the functional status and quality of life of the patient due to the association (**Boxes 3 and 4**).

BOX 1 | **UCLA (University of California, Los Angeles) congenital heart disease functional classes.**

- *Class I:* Asymptomatic
- *Class II:* Symptomatic, but does not interfere with normal activities
- *Class III:* Symptoms interfere with some but not most activities
- *Class IV:* Symptoms interfere with most if not all activities

---

BOX 2 | **Functional status in PAH—NYHA/WHO classification.**

- *Class I:* No limitation of usual physical activity
- *Class II:* No symptoms at rest; mild limitation of physical activity; normal physical activity causes increased dyspnea, fatigue, chest pain, or presyncope
- *Class III:* No symptoms at rest; marked limitation of physical activity; less than ordinary physical activity causes increased dyspnea, fatigue, chest pain or presyncope
- *Class IV:* Unable to perform any physical activity at rest; signs of right ventricular failure; dyspnea, fatigue, chest pain, or presyncope present at rest and symptoms are increased by any physical activity

(PAH: pulmonary arterial hypertension; NYHA: New York Heart Association; WHO: World Health Organization)

| BOX 3 | The Canadian Cardiovascular Society (CCS) Severity of Atrial Fibrillation (SAF). |

Step 1: Symptoms
Identify the presence of the following symptoms:
- Palpitation
- Dyspnea
- Dizziness, presyncope, or syncope
- Chest pain
- Weakness or fatigue

Step 2: Association
Is AF, when present, associated with the above-listed symptoms (A–E)?
For example: Ascertain if any of the above symptoms are present during atrial fibrillation (AF) and likely caused by AF (as opposed to some other cause)

Step 3: Functionality
Determine if the symptoms associated with AF (or the treatment of AF) affect the patient's functionality (subjective quality of life)

| BOX 4 | The Canadian Cardiovascular Society (CCS) Severity of Atrial Fibrillation (SAF) scale. |

Class 0:
Asymptomatic with respect to atrial fibrillation (AF)

Class I:
Symptoms attributable to AF have minimal effect on patient's general quality of life (QOL):
- Minimal and/or infrequent symptoms, or
- Single episode of AF without syncope or heart failure

Class II:
Symptoms attributable to AF have a minor effect on patient's general QOL:
- Mind awareness of symptoms in patients with persistent/permanent AF, or
- Rare episodes (e.g., less than a few per year) in patients with paroxysmal or intermittent AF

Class III:
Symptoms attributable of AF have a moderate effect on patient's general QOL:
- Moderate awareness of symptoms on most days in patients with persistent/permanent AF, or
- More common episodes (e.g., more than every few months) or more severe symptoms, or both, in patients with paroxysmal or intermittent AF

Class IV:
Symptoms attributable to AF have a severe effect on patient's general QOL:
- Very unpleasant symptoms in patient with persistent/paroxysmal AF and/or
- Frequent and highly symptomatic episodes in patients with paroxysmal or intermittent AF and/or
- Syncope thought to be due to AF and/or
- Congestive heart failure secondary to AF

EUROPEAN HEART RHYTHM ASSOCIATION FUNCTIONAL CLASSIFICATION OF ATRIAL FIBRILLATION

On 2014, European Heart Rhythm Association modified the functional classification of atrial fibrillation,[14] which was first proposed on 2007 (**Table 7**).

FUNCTIONAL CLASSIFICATION OF HEART FAILURE IN CARDIORENAL SYNDROME

More than 80% of patients with end-stage renal disease (ESRD) have concomitant cardiovascular disease.[15] Nearly all patients with ESRD presents with symptoms of heart failure, namely dyspnea and edema without renal replacement therapy, as severely diseased kidneys cannot excrete sodium and water. NYHA functional classification does not identify the variables of symptomology of the ESRD patients. In this context, a new functional classification was proposed.[15] The patients included are with ESRD before and after renal replacement therapy and it includes echocardiography, in addition to functional status (**Table 8**).

TABLE 7: Modified EHRA functional classification of AF.

mEHRA	Symptoms	Description
1	None	
2a	Mild	Normal daily activity not affected; symptoms not troublesome to patient
2b	Moderate	Normal daily activity not affected but patient troubled by symptoms
3	Severe	Normal daily activity affected
4	Disabling	Normal daily activity discontinued

(AF: atrial fibrillation; mEHRA: modified European Heart Rhythm Association)

TABLE 8: Functional classification of heart failure in ESRD.

Class	Presentation
1	Asymptomatic; echocardiographic evidence of heart disease
2R	Dyspnea on exertion that is relieved with RRT/UF to NYHA class I level
2NR	Dyspnea on exertion that cannot be relieved with RRT/UF to NYHA class I level
3R	Dyspnea on activity of daily life that is relieved with RRT/UF to NYHA class II level
3NR	Dyspnea on activity of daily life that cannot be relieved with RRT/UF to NYHA class II level
4R	Dyspnea on REST that is relieved with RRT/UF to NYHA class III level
4NR	Dyspnea on REST that cannot be relieved with RRT/UF to NYHA class III level

(ESRD: end-stage renal disease; NYHA: New York Heart Association; RRT: renal replacement therapy; UF: ultrafiltration)

SIX-MINUTE WALK TEST

The six-minute walk test[16] is a reliable, inexpensive, and simple objective test to assess functional capacity. It has wide application. In cardiology, indications of 6-minute walk test are:
- *Pretreatment and post-treatment comparison:*
  - Heart failure
  - Pulmonary hypertension
- *Functional status:*
  - Heart Failure
- *Prediction of prognosis:*
  - Heart failure
  - Pulmonary hypertension

Various test protocols, like 2-minute, 6-minute, and 12-minute walking tests have been used. The 6-minute walk test was first standardized by Lipkin and associates.[17]
- The test is carried out in a level enclosed corridor 20 m long.
- Each patient is instructed to cover as much ground as possible in 6 minutes.
- Patient is told to walk continuously, if possible but that they could slow down or stop, if necessary.
- The aim is that at the end of the test the patients believe that they could not have walked any further in the 6 minutes.
- The test may be repeated twice on the same day with at least 3–4 hours between tests.

This test may be less discriminating than the maximal or submaximal exercise test, but its simplicity and inexpensiveness are unique. It can be used as serial monitoring of patients with heart failure and pulmonary hypertension to assess the treatment.

Pretreatment and post-treatment result are interpreted on asking whether the patient has experienced a clinically significant improvement. The 6-minute walk distance is expressed as an absolute value. In chronic obstructive pulmonary disease, post-treatment walk distance >70 m is necessary to be 90% confident that the improvement is significant. In heart failure, 6-minute walk distance is more responsive to deterioration than to improvement. When single measurement is done to assess functional status, the walk distance in reference to matched healthy population is compared. In one study, median 6-minute walk distance was 580 m for healthy man and 500 m for healthy woman.[18] A low walk distance is nonspecific and nondiagnostic.

CONCLUSION

Functional classification has become a very important part of many cardiac disease. It not only helps to understand the severity of the disease, it also helps to decide specific therapeutic intervention. When to start medical management, when to implant device, and when to do surgical intervention, at every step functional classification is the decisive tool.

REFERENCES

1. The Criteria Committee of the New York Heart Association. Nomenclature and criteria for diagnosis of diseases of the heart and blood vessels. Boston: Little Brown; 1964.
2. The Criteria Committee of the New York Heart Association. Nomenclature and criteria for diagnosis of diseases of the heart and great vessels, 9th edition. Boston, Mass: Little, Brown & Co; 1994. p. 253.
3. Goldman L, Hashimoto B, Cook EF, et al. Comparative reproducibility and validity of systems for assessing cardiovascular functional class: advantages of a new specific activity scale. Circulation. 1981;64:1227-34.
4. Raphael C, Briscoe C, Davies J, et al. Limitations of the New York Heart Association functional classification system and self-reported walking distances in chronic heart failure. Heart. 2007;93:476.
5. Campeau L. Grading of angina pectoris. Circulation. 1976;54:522-3.
6. Hemingway H, Fitzpatrick NK, Gnani S, et al. Prospective validity of measuring angina severity with Canadian Cardiovascular Society class: The ACRE study. Can J Cardiol. 2004;20:305-9.
7. Kaul P, Naylor D, Armstrong PW, et al. Assessment of activity status and survival according to the Canadian Cardiovascular society angina classification. Can J Cardiol. 2009;25:e225-e231.
8. Hlatky MA, Boineau RE, Higginbotham MB, et al. A brief self-administered questionnaire to determine functional capacity (the Duke Activity Status Index). Am J Cardiol. 1989;64:651-4.
9. Alonso J, Permanyer-Miraldaf G, Cascantf P, et al. Measuring functional status of chronic coronary patients. Reliability, validity and responsiveness to clinical change of the reduced version of the Duke Activity Status Index (DASI). Eur Heart J. 1997;18:414.
10. Gibelin P, Poncelet P, Gallois H, et al. Evaluation of three functional classifications of cardiac insufficiency: a national multicenter study. National College of French Cardiologists. Ann Cardiol Angeiol. 1995;44(6):304.
11. Perloff JK, Child JS. Congenital heart disease in adults, 2nd edition. Philadelphia: WB Saunders; 1998:218.
12. McLaughlin VV, McGoon MD. Pulmonary arterial hypertension. Circulation. 2006;114(13):1417.
13. Dorian P, Cvitkovic SS, Kerr CR, et al. A novel, simple scale for assessing the symptom severity of atrial fibrillation at the bedside: The CCS SAF Scale. Can J Cardiol. 2006;22:383-6.
14. Wynn GJ, Todd DM, Webber M, et al. The European Heart Rhythm Association symptom classification for atrial fibrillation: validation and improvement through a simple modification. EP Europace. 2014;16:965-72.
15. Chawla LS, Herzog CA, Costanzo MR, et al. Proposal for a functional classification system of heart failure in patients with End-stage renal disease: Proceedings of the Acute Dialysis Quality initiative (ADQI) XI Workgroup. J Am Coll Cardiol. 2014;63:1246-52.
16. ATS statement: guidelines for the six-minute walk test. Am J Respir Crit Care Med. 2002;166:111-7.
17. Lipkin DP, Scriven AJ, Crake T. Six minute walking test for assessing exercise capacity in chronic heart failure. Br Med J. 1986;292:653.
18. Miyamoto S, Nagaya N, Satoh T, et al. Clinical correlates and prognostic significance of six-minute walk test in patients with primary pulmonary hypertension. Am J Respir Crit Care Med. 2000;161:487-92.

CHAPTER 3

A Triad: Cardinal Symptoms in Cardiovascular System

INTRODUCTION

Dyspnea, palpitation, and chest pain are the most important cardinal symptoms in cardiovascular system.

DYSPNEA

Definition

Dyspnea is a term used to characterize a subjective experience of breathing discomfort that consists of qualitatively distinct sensations that vary in intensity. American Thoracic Society defines dyspnea as "a subjective experience of breathing discomfort that consists of qualitatively distinct sensations that vary in intensity". The experience derives from interactions among multiple physiological, psychological, social, and environmental factors, and may induce secondary physiological and behavioural responses".[1] Braunwald defined dyspnea in simple word—an abnormally uncomfortable awareness of one's own breathing.[2]

Physiologic Components of Dyspnea

- Mechanoreceptors (respiratory muscles)
- Hypoxia (carotid and aortic bodies)
- Changes in PCO_2/pH (medullary center)
- Medullary center (afferent input and efferent output)
- Cortical function (sense of effort)

Basic Mechanism

Circuit

The circuit of dyspnea consists of receptors, sensory cortex, and motor cortex (**Fig. 1**). The mechanism of dyspnea lies in any incoordination of this complex circuit.

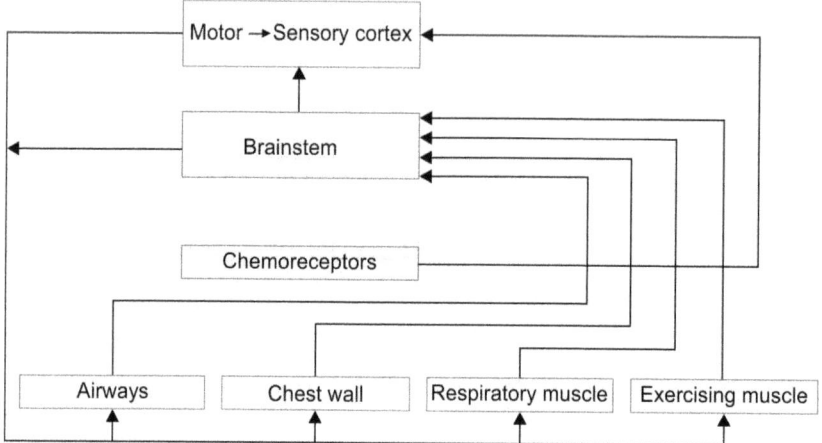

Fig. 1: Dyspnea circuit.

Receptor

Receptors include mechanoreceptors and chemoreceptors. Mechanoreceptors lie in upper airway and face, lungs, chest wall, and skeletal muscles including respiratory and exercising muscle. Receptors in upper airway and face, particularly in the distribution of trigeminal nerve modulate dyspnea.[2] A dyspneic patient gets relief, when he is exposed to fan or open window or cold air. Lungs consists of three type of mechanoreceptors:

1. Juxtacapillary receptors (J-receptor), supplied by C fibers, the unmyelinated nerve endings of vagus nerve, lie in alveoli and blood vessels. They are stimulated by interstitial congestion.
2. Stimulation of irritant receptors increase the sensation of dyspnea in the form of chest constriction and tightness. Dynamic airway compression causes deformation of these receptors which send afferent signal through vagus nerve to midbrain and sensory cortex.
3. Stimulation of pulmonary stretch receptors similarly send signal through vagus nerve only to reduce the sensation of dyspnea.

Receptors on chest wall muscles, including the respiratory muscles and diaphragm deform on chest wall movement send afferent signal.

Chemoreceptors play a lesser role in the mechanism of dyspnea. Hypoxia is not a major stimulus. Neither most of the hypoxic patients feel dyspneic, nor most of the dyspneic patients are hypoxic. Moreover, correction of hypoxia does not produce much improvement in symptoms. However, hypercapnia may cause dyspnea independent of any reflex increase in respiratory muscle activity. In experimental study,[3] patients on mechanical ventilation after induction of paralysis by neuromuscular-blocking drugs become dyspneic on rise of end-tidal carbon dioxide to 7–11 mm Hg. Hypercapnia and consequential change of pH stimulate central chemoreceptors and induce the feeling of dyspnea.

Length-tension Inappropriateness or Afferent Mismatch or Efferent-afferent Dissociation[4,5]

Dyspnea results when there is an imbalance between the perceived need to breathe and the perceived ability to breathe, resulting from mismatch between central respiratory motor activity and incoming afferent information from receptors in the airways, lungs, chest wall structures, and exercising muscle. This is a mismatch between the pressure (tension) generated by the respiratory muscle and the resulting tidal volume (change of length). The afferent feedback from peripheral sensory receptors may allow the brain to assess the effectiveness of the motor commands issued to the ventilatory muscles, i.e., the appropriateness of the response in terms of flow and volume for the command. When changes in respiratory pressure, airflow, or movement of the lungs and chest wall are not appropriate for the outgoing motor command, the intensity of dyspnea is heightened. Thus, any dissociation between the motor command and the mechanical response of the respiratory system may produce a sensation of respiratory discomfort, dyspnea.[6]

Dyspnea in Heart Failure

Lung Hypothesis

This is the time-old concept of explanation of exercise intolerance in heart failure, which leads to pulmonary venous hypertension and capillary congestion with interstitial edema. Lung becomes stiffer with reduced compliance. As mentioned earlier, the J-receptors are stimulated by this congestion leading to activation of Hering–Breuer reflex. This reflex does terminate the inspiratory effort before full inspiration is achieved, resulting in rapid and shallow breathing. On the other hand, increased tissue pressure leads to earlier closure of dependent airways with air trapping. These factors altogether behave as restrictive ventilatory defect. Work of breathing is increased to distend the stiff lungs. Tidal capacity is reduced, and respiratory rate is increased as compensation. Both engorged blood vessels and peribronchiolar cuffing may cause bronchoconstriction with increased airway resistance. There is also ventilation-perfusion mismatch, increased alveolar-arterial oxygen difference, and increased ratio of dead space to tidal volume.

Muscle Hypothesis[7]

According to this hypothesis, skeletal muscle, both respiratory and peripheral, plays the key role in the pathophysiology of exercise intolerance in heart failure. Heart failure leads to systemic inflammatory response along with an imbalance between anabolic and catabolic factor. There is muscle catabolism leading to respiratory muscle myopathy causing dyspnea, and peripheral myopathy causing fatigue.

Skeletal muscle abnormality induces ergoreflex, a muscle reflex stimulated by work done, through the ergoreceptors. Stimulation of the ergoreflex leads to greater ventilatory response to exercise than normal. This results in the sensation of dyspnea. At the same time, this reflex leads to greater sympathetic activation, another feature common during exercise in heart failure.

Heart failure also results in increased level of proinflammatory cytokines, interleukin-1, and interferon in skeletal muscles. Those cytokines increase the level of nitric oxide synthase. Intracellular nitric oxide level shoots up to a high level and inhibits mitochondrial oxidative phosphorylation. Exercise training reduces inflammation and inflammatory markers and increases mitochondrial volumes in skeletal muscle. Thus, muscle fatigue is reduced and exercise tolerance is improved in heart failure.

Assessment of Dyspnea
- Mode of onset
- Duration
- Progress
- Severity
- Functional status
- Special character
- Relieving factor
- Associated symptoms

Severity
Severity of symptom is scaled by the guideline of American Thoracic Society (**Table 1**).

Formal Measurement of Dyspnea
Dyspnea can be measured formally by provocative dyspnea scale and modified Borg scale.

Provocative Dyspnea Assessment Scale
Heart failure syndrome working group[8] described provocative dyspnea assessment (PDA) scale to measure dyspnea (**Box 1**).

After successfully completion of each stage of provocative dyspnea assessment scale, patient is asked 5 points of Likert scale: "worst possible shortness of breath, severely short of breath, moderately short of breath, mildly short of breath and not at all short of breath". Patient is continued to next stage. In this way, dyspnea severity scoring is done.

TABLE 1: Severity scale of dyspnea.

Grade	Degree	Characteristics
0	None	Only with strenuous activity
1	Slight	When hurrying on level ground or climbing a slight incline
2	Moderate	Needs to walk more slowly than others of the same age or has to stop for breath when walking at own pace on level ground
3	Severe	Stops for breath after 100 yards or after a few minutes
4	Very severe	Housebound or dyspnea when dressing or undressing

| BOX 1 | Provocative dyspnea assessment scale. |

- Sitting upright (>60°) with oxygen supplementation
- Sitting upright (>60°) without oxygen
- Supine (<20° head elevation) without oxygen
- Walking 50 m as fast as possible
- The six-minute walk test

TABLE 2: Modified Borg scale of dyspnea.

Scale	Severity
0	No breathlessness at all
0.5	Very very slight (just noticeable)
1	Very slight
2	Slight breathlessness
3	Moderate
4	Somewhat severe
5	Severe breathlessness
6	
7	Very severe breathlessness
8	
9	Very very severe (almost maximum)
10	Maximum

Modified Borg Scale

Modified Borg scale is a reliable assessment tool for dyspnea. Patients use to find that the language in this scale adequately expressed their dyspnea (**Table 2**).

Ventilatory capacity is measured prior to exercise, ventilation is measured during exercise, and these are related to the intensity of dyspnea rated using visual analog scale (VAS) which consists of a line, usually 100 mm in length, placed either horizontally or vertically upon a page, with anchors to indicate extremes of a sensation. The anchors on the scale have not been standardized, but "not breathless at all" to "extremely breathless" and "no shortness of breath" to "shortness of breath as bad as can be" are frequently used. Scoring is accomplished by measuring the distance from the bottom of the scale (or left side if oriented horizontally) to the level indicated by the subject. The reliability and validity of the VAS as a measure of dyspnea has been reported (**Fig. 2**).

Orthopnea

Orthopnea is defined as dyspnea during recumbency. In the horizontal position, there is redistribution of blood volume from the lower extremities and splanchnic beds to the lungs. Moreover, lung compliance and vital capacity are reduced

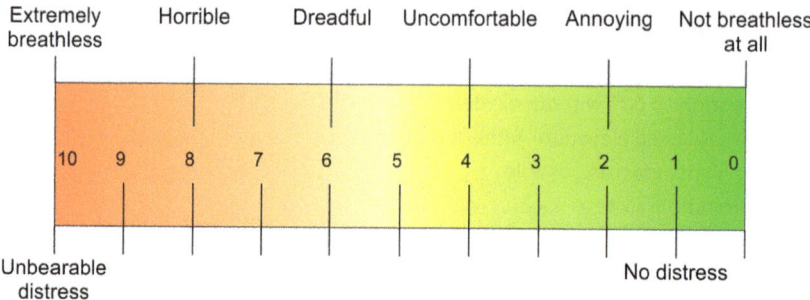

Fig. 2: Visual analog scale.

significantly, around 5% in normal population and 20% in obese patients on recumbent position.[9] In normal individuals, this has little effect, but in patients with heart failure, the dysfunctional left ventricle cannot pump the additional volume out. Besides, in heart failure, there may be reabsorption of edema fluid from previously dependent parts of the body. Venous return is increased by 250–500 cc of fluid.[10] In consequence, ventricular end-diastolic volume and pressure rise leading to more pulmonary congestion and orthopnea.

Orthopnea also occurs in massive ascites, pleural effusion, bilateral diaphragmatic paralysis, and morbid obesity.

Traditionally, orthopnea is classified as orthopnea of choice and orthopnea of necessity.[9] In orthopnea of choice, patient prefers to sit up, but they can lie down and remain comfortable. In orthopnea of necessity, patient takes upright position for self-preservation.

The correlation between orthopnea and raised pulmonary capillary wedge pressure (PCWP) is high with a sensitivity nearing 90%. In ESCAPE (Evaluation Study of Congestive Heart Failure and Pulmonary Artery Catheterization Effectiveness) study,[11] history of orthopnea requiring two or more pillows within 1 week predicted a PCWP of >30 mm Hg with an odd ratio of 3.6.

Dyspnea is said to be chronic, when it lasts >1 month.[12]

Paroxysmal Nocturnal Dyspnea

In a typical episode of paroxysmal nocturnal dyspnea (PND), patient is suddenly awakened 2–3 hours after going to sleep, gasping for air. He quickly sits up and puts his feet over the side of the bed, coughing, wheezing, and sweating or going to window for fresh air. He gets relief only after sitting for 10–15 minutes and usually sleeps the remainder of night. If the symptoms recur, it usually occurs 2–3 hours later.[13]

Pathophysiology

Pathophysiology is complex and different to that of orthopnea and acute pulmonary edema. PND is usually an early feature of heart failure, when patient usually is in NYHA I or II. There is no gross fluid overload. Thus, it takes 2–3 hours for fluid redistribution to lungs from periphery. Lymphatic system takes around 10–15 minutes to get redistributed interstitial fluid back into tissue. PND occurs only at night because of diurnal physiology. Sympathoadrenal dominance is replaced by vagal dominance at night. Failing left ventricle cannot pump out additional preload. However, it occurs during rapid eye movement phase of sleep, when there may be adrenergic surge. Respiratory center is also unresponsive during night-sleep. Nocturnal arrhythmia is another mechanism. During PND, there may be mild hypoxia and raised PCWP.

Cheyne-Stokes respiration, another cause of nocturnal dyspnea in heart failure, may simulate PND. The patient may awaken during the rapid, deep-breathing phase. However, in contrast to PND, it occurs immediate after patient going to sleep.[13] Acute pulmonary edema, another nocturnal dyspnea, is more dramatic than PND. Sputum may be profuse, frothy, watery or blood tinged. Heart rate and blood pressure may be very high. Hypoxia and central cyanosis may be significant. Lungs may be flooded with bubbling rales, wheezing, and rhonchi.

Most Common Diseases
These are mitral stenosis, other valvular heart diseases, ischemic heart disease, and dilated cardiomyopathy.

Noncardiac Causes
Noncardiac causes of nocturnal dyspnea are chronic pulmonary disease including nocturnal asthma and chronic obstructive pulmonary disease, pulmonary embolism, obstructive sleep apnea, anxiety, and hyperventilation. Nocturnal dyspnea associated with chronic pulmonary disease is preceded by paroxysm of cough before dyspnea and relieved by expectorating the secretion and not by sitting up. Anxious patient may awake from sleep, mostly after bad dream and shows similar features of PND. However, the episode may occur at anytime after going to sleep.

Trepopnea
Trepopnea may occur with asymmetric lung disease when the patient lies with the more affected lung down because of gravitational redistribution of blood flow. Left atrial myxoma, by obstructing mitral inflow in lateral decubitus, can cause trepopnea.

Platypnea-orthodeoxia Syndrome
Platypnea-orthodeoxia syndrome (POS) is characterized by dyspnea and objective evidence of hypoxemia in upright that resolves in supine posture. Patent foramen ovale (PFO) is present in around 25% of normal population. Combination of PFO (and other interatrial combinations), Chiari malformation, prominent Eustachian valve, and change in right atrial hemodynamic prepares the stage for POS. There must be two factors to cause POS: first is the anatomic factor including PFO, small or fenestrated atrial septal defect (ASD) and second is functional factors, including cardiac (pericardial effusion,

constrictive pericarditis), pulmonary (pneumectomy, emphysema, pulmonary AV malformation), abdominal (cirrhosis of liver or ileus) or vascular (aortic aneurysm, or elongation) producing deformity of atrial septum resulting in right-to-left shunt through PFO and small or fenestrated ASD in upright posture. Commoner conditions are after right pneumectomy, ascending aortic dilation, and arch surgery.[15]

How to explain right-to-left shunt across interatrial communication? Standing upright could stretch interatrial communication, allowing redirection of flow from inferior vena cava through stretched communication to left atrium. When present, Chiari malformation or Eustachian valve may play additional role in redirection. Normally, superior vena cava blood is directed to tricuspid valve, whereas inferior vena cava blood is directed to the upper part of interatrial septum, before turning downward toward tricuspid valve. The combination of these different flow pattern produces a clockwise vortex inside right atrium. The above-mentioned anatomical factors cause horizontal distortion of heart, right atrium, and interatrial septum, which change the hemodynamic of vortex. There is higher dynamic pressure in the outer layer of the vortex, resulting in differential pressure gradient across the interatrial septum. In consequence, there is right-to-left shunt across a more stretched interatrial communication on upright posture.[16]

Bendopnea

Bendopnea is dyspnea within 30 second of bending. In the first study on bendopnea,[17] Thibodeau et al. measured ventricular filling pressure on bending and found higher filling pressure of both ventricles in all patients on bending. Those with increased baseline filling pressure became more dyspneic on bending. They found that abdominal girth did not play any role in bendopnea. Rather, bending did increase intrathoracic pressure, which lead to increased filling pressure of both ventricles. All the patients with heart failure in their series, who had bendopnea, had orthopnea and increased jugular venous pressure. The triad, orthopnea, bendopnea, and increased jugular venous pressure may be the most specific and reasonably sensitive feature of chronic heart failure. Dyspnea, orthopnea, and PND have different statistical significance in heart failure (**Table 3**).

TABLE 3: Statistical significance of three symptoms of heart failure.[14]

Symptom	Sensitivity	Specificity	Positive predictive value	Negative predictive value
Dyspnea on effort	79%	84%	18.5%	99%
Orthopnea	25%	99%	64%	97%
PND	27%	99%	62%	96%

PALPITATION

Palpitation can be defined as uncomfortable awareness of one's own heartbeat. Patient describes the feeling as disagreeable sensation of palpitation, skipped or missed beat or a pounding sensation in chest. Though, occasionally it may indicate life-threatening arrhythmia, most often it is a benign symptom. Even if benign, palpitation is quiet a common symptom. Palpitation accounts for the 16% of the symptoms, for which patients visit their general physician.[18] Presenting symptom, second only to chest pain, to a cardiologist.

Pathophysiology

Pathophysiology of palpitation is poorly understood. The circuit involves sensory receptors (myocardial, pericardial, and peripheral mechanoreceptors and baroreceptors), afferent pathway (parasympathetic or sympathetic pathway), and brain centers (subcortical area and frontal lobe). Patient feels palpitation when cardiac contraction is too rapid or very slow and irregular. Patient may also feel palpitation, when vigorous contraction and anomalous movement of the heart occur in the chest.

Etiology

Most common causes of palpitation are arrhythmia and anxiety (**Table 4**).

Cardiac Cause

Cardiac cause of palpitation includes mostly arrhythmic and occasional nonarrhythmic. In one series,[18] arrhythmic causes of palpitation include atrial fibrillation (AF) (10%), supraventricular tachycardia (SVT) (9.5%), ventricular premature beat (VPB) (7.9%), atrial flutter (5.8%), premature atrial beats (3.2%), ventricular tachycardia (VT) (2.1%), mitral valve prolapse (MVP) (1.1%), sick sinus syndrome (1.1%), and pacemaker (1.1%). Nonarrhythmic causes of palpitation are aortic regurgitation, mitral regurgitation, mitral valve prolapse, hypertrophic cardiomyopathy, atrial myxoma, ASD, ventricular septal defect, etc.

Psychosomatic Cause

It is characterized by recurrent unexpected panic attack, more common in relatively younger women who somatize more frequently. However, one should

TABLE 4: **Etiological classification of palpitation.**[19]

Etiology	%
Cardiac (arrhythmic and structural)	43%
Psychosomatic	30.5%
Systemic causes and drugs	10%
Unknown	31%

not overdiagnose anxiety and should do a total evaluation, as arrhythmia can coexist with anxiety. Anxiety causes catecholamine surge and may induce ventricular tachycardia.

Systemic Cause
Fever, anemia, hypoglycemia, pheochromocytoma, and hyperthyroidism are some common noncardiac causes of palpitation.

Drugs
Beta agonist, theophylline, ephedrine, cocaine, alcohol, smoking, and caffeine cause palpitation.

Approach
Patient should be asked to describe the symptom in every detail. Its duration, onset and termination, slow or rapid, regular or irregular, activity and posture, associated giddiness, syncope, angina or dyspnea should be evaluated. Examiner himself can demonstrate or the patient may be asked to tap out the rhythm.

Clinical Types of Palpitation
European Heart Rhythm Association, in a position statement,[20] classified the clinical types of palpitation (**Box 2**).

Patient described extrasystolic palpitation as irregular skipped or missed beat or sinking of the heart. Onset and termination are sudden. Tachycardiac palpitation is described as regular or irregular accelerated beating wings in the chest with a sudden onset and termination and precipitated by physical effort. Anxiety-related palpitation is associated with anxiety and agitation, slightly accelerated, gradual onset and termination, and precipitated by stress and anxiety. Pulsation palpitation, mostly related to aortic regurgitation, or other structural heart disease with volume overload is described as pounding, regular, gradual onset and termination, nonrapid, and persistent.

Predictor of Cardiac Etiology
- Male sex
- Description of irregular heartbeat
- History of heart disease
- Duration of event >5 minutes

BOX 2	Clinical classification of palpitation.[20]
• Extrasystolic	• Anxiety-related
• Tachycardiac	• Pulsation

Clinical Evaluation

Symptoms

Feeling of flip-flopping in chest is suggestive of atrial or ventricular ectopic, whereas fluttering in chest is suggestive of atrial or ventricular tachyarrhythmia.

Rate and Rhythm

A rapid, irregular chaotic feeling, particularly in elderly is suggestive of atrial fibrillation. A fast-regular rhythm is suggestive of supraventricular or ventricular tachycardia. A pounding sensation in neck during tachycardia is suggestive that atrium is contracting against closed tricuspid valve and reflux of blood in superior vena cava. This may be regular in atrioventricular (AV) nodal reentrant tachycardia and known as frog sign (equivalent to cannon wave in JVP). In ventricular tachycardia, the frog sign is intermittent and indicative of atrioventricular dissociation, which produces intermittent simultaneous ventricular and atrial depolarization. Neck pounding produces a shirt-flipping sign. Visible neck pulsation only, as oppose to frog sign, is suggestive of accessory pathway-mediated AV re-entry tachycardia.

In presence of significant left ventricular dysfunction, rapid ventricular rate may not be sensed as palpitation due to poor ventricular contractility. In patients with dilated or ischemic cardiomyopathy, ventricular tachycardia produces palpitation only in 6-15% of patients, whereas 93-100% of patients present with palpitation in case of right ventricular dysplasia or idiopathic ventricular tachycardia.[20]

Onset and Termination

Very sudden onset and termination are suggestive of paroxysmal tachycardia, in contrast to sinus tachycardia, which occurs and terminate slowly. The caveats are supraventricular tachycardia and may become faster during exercise giving an impression of gradual onset and may have sinus tachycardia following termination giving impression of gradual cessation.

Circumstances

Palpitation and Syncope

Palpitation turns in an ominous symptom when palpitation is associated with dizziness, presyncope or syncope. Ventricular tachycardia is a strong probability. Supraventricular tachycardia can occasionally cause syncope, immediately after the onset. Rapid heart rate with low cardiac output and acute vasodilatation are the mechanism of syncope.

Palpitation and Dyspnea

Usually indicate arrhythmia associated with ventricular dysfunction, aortic stenosis, hypertrophic cardiomyopathy mitral stenosis, and ischemic heart disease.

Palpitation and Posture

Atrioventricular nodal reentrant tachycardia (AVNRT) may be initiated by standing posture from bending over and may be terminated after lying down. Patient with regurgitant lesion feels the pounding sensation more in lying or left lateral decubitus.

Palpitation and Catecholamine Excess

Exercised-induced disproportionate rapid palpitation may be due to catecholamine-induced idiopathic ventricular tachycardia, right ventricular outflow tract (RVOT) tachycardia, and AVNRT. Postexercise atrial fibrillation may occur due to increased vagal tone just after cessation of sympathetic tone. Mild exertion or emotional stress can cause palpitation in young female patient due to hypersensitivity of beta-adrenergic stimulation. It is called inappropriate sinus tachycardia.

Sleep

Palpitation during sleep is vagal-mediated atrial fibrillation or certain long-QT syndrome.

Polyuria

Any paroxysmal atrial arrhythmia, more commonly atrial fibrillation, induces polyuria due to over secretion of natriuretic peptide from atrial stretching. It is not very common (<5%) symptom.

CHEST PAIN

Chest pain is the most common symptom in regard to cardiovascular system. In USA, 7 million patients attend emergency department annually with chest pain. It is the important task for the clinician to establish whether the chest pain is cardiac or noncardiac. In an outpatient set up, <25% patient with chest pain will have cardiac cause and, in an emergency, set up, around 67% patient will have cardiac cause of chest pain (**Table 5**).

Cardiac Chest Pain

Stable Angina

One should determine three factors:
1. Substernal chest pain
2. Provoked by effort or emotional stress
3. Relieved by rest/nitroglycerine within minutes

When all the three characteristics are present, it is typical anginal chest pain. When two features are present, it is atypical angina. When only one feature is present, it is nonanginal chest pain. Pretest probability of obstructed coronary artery disease in 15,815 symptomatic patients, according to age, sex, and nature of symptom was studied in a pooled analysis (**Table 6**).[23]

TABLE 5: Common causes of chest pain.[21,22]

Diagnosis	Percentage of patient		Emergency (%)
	Primary care: USA (%)	Primary care: Europe (%)	
Musculoskeletal condition	36	29	7
Gastrointestinal	19	10	3
Serious cardiac cause (ACS, CHF, pulmonary embolism)	16	13	54
Stable CAD	10	8	13
Psychosomatic disease	8	17	9
Lung cause (pneumonia, pneumothorax, lung cancer)	5	20	12
Nonspecific chest pain	16	11	5

(ACS: acute coronary syndrome; CAD: coronary artery disease; CHF: congestive heart failure)

TABLE 6: Pretest probability of coronary artery disease according to type of angina.

	Typical angina		Atypical angina		Nonanginal chest pain	
Age	Male	Female	Male	Female	Male	Female
30–39	3%	5%	4%	3%	1%	1%
40–49	22%	10%	10%	6%	3%	2%
50–59	32%	13%	17%	6%	11%	3%
60–69	44%	16%	26%	11%	22%	6%
+70	52%	27%	34%	19%	24%	10%

TABLE 7: Predictivity of symptoms for acute ischemic pain.[24]

Predictive	Nonpredictive
Central, pressure-like, prolonged	Pressure-like pain
Radiation to one or both hands	Stabbing, pleuritic or positional
Similar type of pain during a prior presentation	Reproducible on palpation
Associated nausea and sweating	Response to nitrate

Acute Coronary Syndrome

In an acute chest pain presentation, 3% patient diagnosed as having noncardiac chest pain may suffer acute coronary syndrome (ACS) or death within 1 month. Hence, a clinical acumen added by optimum laboratory test can only help the emergency clinician to diagnose whether the chest pain is cardiac or noncardiac (**Table 7**).

TABLE 8: The HEART score for ACS at emergency department.

History	Highly suspicious	2
	Moderately suspicious	1
	Slightly suspicious	0
ECG	Significant ST-segment depression	2
	Nonspecific repolarization abnormality	1
	Normal	0
Age (years)	≥65	2
	45–65	1
	≤45	0
Risk factors	3 or more	2
	1–2	1
	No risk factor	0
Troponin	≥3 normal unit	2
	1–3	1
	Normal limit	0

(Low risk: 0–3 points; Non-low risk: ≥4 points)
(ACS: acute coronary syndrome; HEART: History, Electrocardiogram, Age, Risk factors, Troponin)

TABLE 9: Simplified EDACS score for ACS.

Age	18–39	0
	40–49	1
	50–59	2
	60–69	3
	70–79	4
	80–89	5
	90+	6
Known coronary artery disease or ≥3 cardiac risk factors		1
Male sex		1
Symptoms: Pain radiating to arm, shoulder, neck or jaw		1

Low risk 0–3 points; Non-low risk ≥ 4 points
(ACS: acute coronary syndrome; EDACS: Emergency Department Assessment of Chest pain Score)

There are several bedside scoring systems, which help to diagnose ACS with an added ECG or ischemic-injury biomarkers (**Tables 8** and **9**).

Pericardial Pain

Major part of pericardium is pain insensitive. Pain due to pericarditis is due to adjacent pleural involvement. Pain may radiate to neck, shoulder or back.

Radiation to trapezius ridge is specific symptom of acute pericardial pain. Most commonly, it is retrosternal, aggravated by coughing, deep breathing, and change in posture, all of which cause pleural movement. Sitting upright and leaning forward relieve pain.

Acute Aortic Syndrome

At the very beginning, pain reaches at peak, front, and back of the chest and is described as ripping, tearing, and severe sharp pain. Sudden-onset pain is very characteristic. Chest pain is more common in type A dissection in compare to type B dissection. There may be absence of pulse in one or both arms and patient may present with cerebrovascular accident or paraplegia or acute aortic regurgitation.

Pulmonary Embolism

Chest pain due to pulmonary embolism is due to dilatation of pulmonary artery or pulmonary infarction leading to pleural involvement. One can follow the Well model for clinical diagnosis (**Tables 10** and **11**).

Chest Wall Pain

History of osteoarthritis and rheumatoid arthritis and finding of local tenderness increase the likelihood of chest wall pain. Costochondral and costosternal syndrome are the common causes of chest wall pain. Tietze's syndrome, tenderness, swelling, and redness of costochondritis are infrequent findings. Chest wall pain distributed along a dermatome can be due to cervical root disease, intercostal muscle cramp, and herpes zoster.

TABLE 10: Well model for PE.

Clinical findings	Points
Clinical features of DVT	3
Heart rate >100 beats/min	1.5
Immobilization	1.5
Previous objectively diagnosed DVT or PE	1.5
Hemoptysis	1
Malignancy	1

Total point	Risk of PE	Probability of PE (%)
<2	Low	1–28
2–6	Moderate	28–40
>6	High	38–91

(DVT: deep vein thrombosis; PE: pulmonary embolism)

TABLE 11: Revised Geneva score for pulmonary embolism.

Clinical findings		Points
Age >65 years		1
Previous DVT or PE		3
Surgery under anesthesia or lower limb fracture in past month		2
Active malignant condition		2
Unilateral lower limb pain		3
Hemoptysis		2
Total point	Risk of PE	Probability of PE (%)
≤3	Low	7–9%
4–10	Intermediate	10–60%
≥11	High	>60%

(DVT: deep vein thrombosis; PE: pulmonary embolism)

Gastrointestinal Diseases

Esophageal pain due to acid reflux is a retrosternal burning pain, precipitated by some specific foods, more on lying down, early morning, and relieved by acid-reducing agent. Chest pain due to esophageal spasm is compressive in nature, may radiate down arms, and sometimes is relieved by antianginal medications. Pain due to peptic ulcer disease, gallbladder disease, and pancreatitis can radiate to lower chest wall.

Clinical Approach

A thorough history and clinical examination can diagnose most of the chest pain causes:
- Mode of onset, duration, and frequency
- Site of pain and radiation
- Character of pain
- Aggravating and relieving factors
- Associated symptoms.

CONCLUSION

William Heberden in 1768 described (*) cardiac chest pain as,- "Those who are afflicted with it are seized, while they are walking, and more particularly when they walk soon after eating, with a painful and most disagreeable sensation in the breast, which seems as if it would take their life away, if it were to increase or to continue: The moment they stand still, all this uneasiness vanishes.". After two and half centuries, when coronary imaging is at its peak, effort angina is a clinical diagnosis. Similarly, dyspnoea and palpitation help to initiate the diagnostic cascade in major cardiac diseases.

---

*A historical perspective towards a non-invasive treatment for patients with atherosclerosis. Slijkhuis W, Mali W, Appelman Y Neth Heart J. 2009;17:140-4.

REFERENCES

1. American Thoracic Society. Dyspnea. Mechanisms, assessment, and management: a consensus statement. American Thoracic Society. Am J Respir Crit Care Med. 1999;159: 321-40.
2. Schwartzstein RM, Lahive K, Pope A, Weinberger SE, Weiss JW. Cold facial stimulation reduces breathlessness induced in normal subjects. Am Rev Respir Dis. 1987;136:58-61.
3. Banzett RB, Lansing RW, Brown R, et al. 'Air hunger' from increased PCO_2 persists after complete neuromuscular block in humans. Respir Physiol. 1990;81:1-17.
4. Scano G, Ambrosino N. Pathophysiology of dyspnea. Lung. 2002;180:131-48.
5. Nishino T. Dyspnoea: Underlying mechanisms and treatment. Br J Anaesth. 2011;106(4): 463-74.
6. Manning HL, Schwartzstein RM. Pathophysiology of dyspnoea. N Engl J Med. 1995;333:1547.
7. Coats A JS, Clark AL, Piepoli M, et al. Symptoms and quality of heart failure: The muscle hypothesis. Heart. 1994;72;S36.
8. Pang PS, Cleland J GF, Teerlink JR, et al. A proposal to standardize dyspnoea measurement in clinical trials of acute heart failure syndromes: the need for a uniform approach. Eur Heart J. 2008;29:816-24.
9. Christie CD, Beams AJ. Orthopnea. Arch Int Med. 1920;25:306.
10. Gheorghiade M, Follath F, Ponikowski P, et al. Assessing and grading congestion in acute heart failure: a scientific statement from the Acute Heart Failure Committee of the Heart Failure Association of the European Society of Cardiology and endorsed by the European Society of Intensive Care Medicine. Eur J Heart Fail. 2010;12:423-33.
11. Drazner MH, Hellkamp AS, Leier CV, et al. Value of clinician assessment of hemodynamics in advanced heart failure: the ESCAPE trial. Circ Heart Fail. 2008;1:170-7.
12. Japp AG, Sumpson L, Pettit S, et al. Cardiovascular symptom. In: "The ESC Textbook of Cardiovascular Medicine". Oxford University Press; 2019. p. 11.
13. Spann JF. The recognition and management of heart failure. In JW Hurst (Ed). " The Heart". New York: McGraw-Hill Book Company; 1986.
14. Fonseca C, Morais H, Mota T, et al.; Epica investigators. The diagnosis of heart failure in primary care: value of symptoms and signs. Eur J Heart Fail. 2004;6:795-800.
15. Shah AH, Osten M, Leventhal A, et al. Percutaneous intervention to treat platypnea–orthodeoxia syndrome: the Toronto experience. J Am Coll Cardiol Intv. 2016;9:1928-38.
16. Cheng TO. Reversible orthodeoxia. Ann Intern Med. 1992;116:875.
17. Thibodeau JT, Turer AT, Gualano SK, et al. Characterization of a novel symptom of advanced heart failure: bendopnea. J Am Coll Cardiol HF. 2014;2:24-31.
18. Knudson MP. The natural history of palpitation in a family practice. J Fam Pract. 1987;24: 357-60.
19. Weber BE, Kapoor WN. Evaluation and outcomes of patients with palpitations. Am J Med. 1996;100:138.
20. Raviele A, Giada F, Bergfeldt L, et al. Management of patients with palpitations: a position paper from the European Heart Rhythm Association. Europace. 2011;13:920-34.
21. Klinkman MS, Stevens D, Gorenflw DW. Episodes of care for chest pain: a preliminary report from MIRNET. Michigan Research Network. J Fam Pract. 1994;38:345-52.
22. Buntinx F, Konckaret D, Bruyninckx R, et al. Chest pain in general practice or in the hospital emergency department: is it the same? Fam Pract. 2001;18:586-9.
23. Juarez-Orozco LE, Saraste A, Capodanno D, et al. Impact of a decreasing pre-test probability on the performance of diagnostic tests for coronary artery disease. Eur Heart J Cardiovasc Imaging. 2019;20(11):1198-207.
24. Japp AG, Sumpson L, Pettit S, et al. Cardiovascular symptom. In: "The ESC Textbook of Cardiovascular Medicine". Oxford University Press; 2019. p. 9.

CHAPTER 4

A Triad: Minor Symptoms in Cardiovascular System

INTRODUCTION

"Signs of fatigue soon manifested themselves more and more strongly, and slowly the men dropped out one by one, from sheer exhaustion. No murmur of complaint, however, would be heard."—said Fritz Kreisler. Murmur can easily be heard, when men with cardiac disease present with fatigue and other minor symptoms!

FATIGUE

Fatigue is defined as a subjective sensation of extreme and persistent exhaustion, tiredness, and lack of energy.[1] It is multidimensional and is influenced by physical and psychosocial factors.

How to Measure Fatigue?

Fatigue is measured by several subjective scale, most of which are used for fatigue assessment in cancer patients, or patients with chronic inflammatory disease or psychiatric disease. Fatigue Symptom Inventory (FSI), a 14-item self-report scale, measures fatigue intensity,[2] duration, and interference with activities of daily living over the past week. The scale score yields a score ranging from 0 to 10. Higher score reflects higher intensity of fatigue and more interference in daily activity. An intensity score ≥3 indicates clinically meaningful fatigue.

How Common is Fatigue as Symptom?

Fatigue is one of the most common symptoms reported to the physician and its prevalence in primary care ranges between 7% and 45%.[3] Both fatigue and dyspnea are manifestation of heart failure. Frequency of fatigue in heart failure is quite high, ranging from 69 to 88%.[4]

Mechanism of Fatigue in Heart Failure

Stroke index and cardiac index are decreased in healthy people with chronic fatigue syndrome, on rest and acute stress.[5]

Heart failure has two components—reduced forward flow and raised ventricular filling pressure. Fatigue is due to reduced forward flow and dyspnea is due to raised ventricular filling pressure. In heart failure muscle fatigue is expressed as fatigue. Muscle fatigue can arise due to alteration in the supply of oxygen to exercising muscle due to reduced forward flow or to a change of muscle itself in terms of total mass, structure, or metabolic and contractile function—the muscle hypothesis of heart failure.[6]

Feeling of fatigue, even at rest, indicates anxiety state, rather than low output, which is manifested as fatigue on exertion. Aggressive diuresis in heart failure leading to potassium depletion can cause significant fatigue.

EDEMA AND WEIGHT GAIN

Edema

In a normal subject, 60% of body mass consists of water, of which one-third is contained in extracellular space. Of this, 70% is distributed in interstitial space. Normally interstitial fluid confers a degree of turgor, which is not palpable. It takes several liters of fluid to accumulate in interstitial space, before it is palpable as edema.

Edema is defined as palpable swelling from fluid accumulation in body tissues produced by the expansion of interstitial fluid volume. Edema may be:
- Peripheral
- Edema in third space (pleural, pericardial, and ascitic)
- Pulmonary edema (fluid accumulation in pulmonary vascular interstitial or alveolar space)
- *Anasarca*: Fluid accumulation in all body tissue and cavities at the same time.

Grading of Edema

There are various methods to grade edema. Nearing 90 years back Harrison and Pilcher[6] suggested a simple grading of edema—"The term 'marked edema' has been used to describe those cases in which the entire lower extremity was involved. When the entire leg below the knee was swollen but the thighs were not, the cases were considered to have 'moderate' edema. Edema confined to the ankles and feet has been called 'slight' (**Table 1**)."

TABLE 1: Grading of edema.

	0	1+	2+	3+	4+
Visible	No	Yes	Yes	Yes	Yes
Pitting	No	Slight	>slight	>slight	Cannot reach tibia
Level	NA	NA	Below knee	Above knee	Above knee

TABLE 2: Grading of edema with physical characteristics.

Grade	Physical characteristics
1+	Slight pitting, no visible change in the shape of the extremity; depth of indentation 0–1/4" (<6 mm); disappears rapidly
2+	No marked change in the shape of the extremity; depth of indentation 1/4–1/2" (6–12 mm); disappears in 10–15 s
3+	Noticeably deep pitting, swollen extremity; depth of pitting 1/2–1" (1–2.5 cm); duration 1–2 min
4+	Very swollen, distorted extremity; depth of pitting >1" (>2.5 cm); duration 2–5 min

Another simple method[7] is to look for visibility of edema, pitting over the tibia, and whether edema rises above the knee.

Another way of grading is measuring the depth of pitting (**Table 2**).

Edema is a late sign of heart failure. It is usually preceded by dyspnea. At the same time, it is early to go with decongestant medications. Distribution of edema fluid is determined by local factor. In an ambulant patient, due to hydrostatic pressure, edema occurs in legs in daytime and diminishes at night. Fluid shifts from legs to sacral region in a patient, who is confined to bed. As tissue pressure around the eyes of children is low, fluid is accumulated in them as periorbital edema.

In MESA (Multi-Ethnic Study of Atherosclerosis), peripheral edema in isolation and heart failure was studied.[8] Peripheral edema was present in nearly one-third of community-dwelling patients without known cardiovascular disease. Peripheral edema was not associated with left or right ventricular systolic dysfunction. However, it was associated with other symptom of heart failure, abnormal NT-proBNP (N-terminal pro-brain natriuretic peptide) level, and incident hospitalized heart failure.

Weight Gain

There may be a weight gain of around 10 pounds before appearance of edema. Acute change in weight is a good marker of fluid balance, a gain indicating congestion and loss indicating response to decongestant medications. Increase in body weight is associated with hospitalization for heart failure and begins 1 week prior to admission. In fact, any sudden weight gains >2 kg in 3 days in heart failure patients should raise an alarm.[9] They should be instructed to contact health personal or to increase their diuretic doses. By simple weight monitoring, hospitalization can be prevented in many cases of chronic heart failure patients.

Congestion is not always associated with edema or weight gain. Pulmonary congestion may occur in MS or acute hypertensive heart failure, in euvolemic patient.

HEMOPTYSIS AND COUGH

Hemoptysis

Assessment

One should decide whether it is a brisk bleeding or slow bleeding. Brisk bleeding means coughing out large volume of liquid blood. Brisk bleeding usually indicates arterial bleeding associated with focal ulceration of the bronchus, which may occur in bronchiectasis, bronchogenic carcinoma or aortic aneurysm rupturing into tracheobronchial tree. Slow bleeding means coughing out of small quantities of dark or clotted blood. Slow bleeding indicates bleeding from low-pressure vessel or old bleeding. Common source is bronchial venous system, secondary to mitral stenosis. Blood, intimately mixed with pus, indicates deep-seated pulmonary infection. However, blood-streaked sputum may be due to cardiac cause. Source is the pulmonary capillaries, which yield to high intravascular pressure. This is the initial stage of pulmonary edema, interstitial pulmonary congestion. Frank pulmonary edema leads to pink frothy sputum.

Mitral Stenosis

Mitral stenosis is the most common cardiac cause of hemoptysis, which is an early feature of mitral stenosis. As classically described by Paul Wood, hemoptysis may be due to:
- Profuse bright red hemorrhage, due to rupture of bronchopulmonary varices, secondary to sudden rise of pulmonary venous pressure.
- Pink, frothy sputum associated with acute pulmonary edema.
- Blood-streaked sputum associated with paroxysmal dyspnea.
- Blood-streaked sputum associated with attacks of "winter-bronchitis." Mitral stenosis causes chronic passive pulmonary venous congestion, leading to chronic bronchial hyperemia. Hyperemia results in excessive bronchial mucous production, which presents as "winter-bronchitis."

Massive hemoptysis or pulmonary apoplexy was found in 18.3% cases and blood-stained sputum, or congestive hemoptysis in 16.5% cases.[10]

The systemic veins (bronchial veins) draining the mural vessels of extra-pulmonary bronchi and pulmonary arteries drain connects freely with pulmonary venous system. This network of veins is known as bronchopulmonary vein. The system which drains right side enters in azygos or superior vena cava and that drains left side enters in accessory azygos veins.

Bronchial veins located deep to bronchial mucosa of secondary and tertiary bronchi are the source of massive bleeding, because they rupture directly in the bronchial lumen. In presence of pulmonary venous hypertension in significant mitral stenosis, blood flow is channeled from the congested pulmonary veins via the bronchial veins into the low-pressure azygos-hemiazygos venous system. This high-pressure pulmonary venous flow makes the bronchial veins distended and varicosed, which yield relatively easily and bleed. The event is analogous to that leading from portal hypertension to hemorrhage from rupture of esophageal varices.[11,12]

Acute Mitral Regurgitation
Acute mitral regurgitation may result in a regurgitant jet directed toward the right upper pulmonary vein and this may result in right side pulmonary edema and alveolar hemorrhage, leading to hemoptysis.[13]

Eisenmenger Syndrome (Box 1)
Overall incidence of hemoptysis in Eisenmenger syndrome is 31%.[14] Incidence is uncommon before 20 years of age and, almost 100% over 40 years. More the complexity of the disease leading to Eisenmenger syndrome, more early the age of onset of hemoptysis. Hemoptysis does not affect overall prognosis in Eisenmenger syndrome. Neither the high pulmonary arterial pressure, nor the initial high pulmonary flow is responsible for hemoptysis. This is evidenced from the fact that incidence of hemoptysis in idiopathic hypertension is just 4% and in uncomplicated atrial septal defect (ASD) is around 3%. A combination of pulmonary arterial hypertension (PAH) and cyanosis is probably the causative factor. Hemoptysis in Eisenmenger syndrome may be due to various causes.[15]

One of the most important sources of hemoptysis is engorged bronchial arteries with abnormal collateral vessels formation. Pulmonary circulation is reduced at the level of the pulmonary arteriole due to vascular remodeling, hypoxemic vasoconstriction, and microthrombosis.[16] Due to reduced blood flow from pulmonary circulation, bronchial circulation grows up, either due to increased flow from aorta, or due to bronchial artery angiogenesis.[17] These bronchial vessels rupture due to elevated regional blood pressure and leak into the tracheobronchial tree, resulting in hemoptysis (**Box 2**).[18]

Cough: Assessment (Box 3)
Chronic cough is defined as cough persisting for >8 weeks. Chronic cough may arise from certain cardiac condition, whereas cough itself can lead to certain cardiac complication. A dry, nonproductive cough, more on recumbent posture, may be a manifestation of heart failure. A single bout of cough or chronic cough and syncope may be a presentation of ventricular premature beat. Pulmonary blood flow is augmented during ventricular premature beat and continuous wave Doppler echocardiography revealed a ventricular premature contraction (VPC)-induced transient increase in the calculated pulmonary artery blood flow, from 65 to 91 mL/s.[19] Distension of pulmonary artery may result in cough reflex.

BOX 1   **Hemoptysis in Eisenmenger syndrome.**

- Bronchitis
- Pulmonary thromboembolism
- Bleeding diathesis
- Rupture of bronchial arteries and collaterals
- Pulmonary artery or arteriole rupture

> **BOX 2** **Cardiac causes of hemoptysis.**
> - Mitral stenosis
> - Acute mitral regurgitation
> - Pulmonary infarction
> - Congenital cyanotic heart disease:
>   - Eisenmenger syndrome
>   - MAPCA
>   - Bleeding diathesis in cyanotic heart disease
>   - Pulmonary arteriovenous fistula with Osler-Weber-Rendu disease
> - Aortic aneurysm
> - Vasculitis in polyarteritis nodosa, systemic lupus erythematosus
>
> (MAPCA: major aortopulmonary collateral artery)

> **BOX 3** **Cardiac cause of cough.**
> - Heart failure
> - Ventricular or atrial premature beat
> - Drugs
> - Dilated pulmonary artery

Cardiac drugs causing chronic cough are angiotensin-converting enzyme (ACE) inhibitor, angiotensin receptor blocker (ARB), beta-blockers, and aspirin.

Cough due to pulmonary edema or paroxysmal nocturnal dyspnea is associated with frothy, pink, blood-tinged sputum. Cough due to chronic bronchitis is associated with white, mucoid sputum and cough due to pneumonia is associated with thick, yellow sputum.

CONCLUSION

Besides the major symptom like dyspnea, chest pain or palpitation, the minor symptom like fatigue, edema and cough should not be ignored, rather assessed critically, which might lead to detection of major cardiovascular disease.

REFERENCES

1. Aaronson LS, Teel CS, Cassmeyer V, et al. Defining and measuring fatigue. Image J Nurs Sch. 1999;31:45-50.
2. Hann DM, Denniston MM, Baker MM. Measurement of fatigue in cancer patients: Further validation of the fatigue symptom inventory. Qual Life Res. 2000;9:847-54.
3. Lewis G, Wessely S. The epidemiology of fatigue: more questions than answers. J Epid Com Health. 1992;46:92-7.
4. Nordgren L, Sorensen S. Symptoms experienced in the last six months of life in patients with end-stage heart failure. Eur J Cardiovasc Nurs. 2003;2:213-7.
5. Nelesen R, Dar Y, Joel E. The relation between fatigue and cardiac functioning. Arch Intern Med. 2008;168:943-9.

6. Harrison TR, Pilcher C. Studies in congestive heart failure-the effect of edema on oxygen utilization. J Clin Invest. 1930;8:259-90.
7. Coats AJS, Clark AL, Piepoli M, et al. Symptoms and quality of life in heart failure: the muscle hypothesis. Br Heart J. 1994;72(2 suppl.): S36-S39.
8. Yeboah J, Bertoni A, Qureshi W, et al. Pedal edema as an indicator of early heart failure in the community. Circ Heart Fail. 2016;9:e003415.
9. Chaudhry SI, Wang Y, Concato J, et al. Patterns of Weight Change Preceding Hospitalization for Heart Failure. Circulation. 2007;116:1549-54.
10. Wood P. An appreciation of mitral stenosis I-Clinical features. Br Med J. 1954;1:1051-63.
11. Nennhaus HP, Hunter JA. Massive hemorrhage from bronchial varices in mitral stenosis. Surgery. 1967;61:556-60.
12. Thompson AC, Stewart WC. Hemoptysis in mitral stenosis. JAMA. 1951;147(1):21-4.
13. Marak CP, Joy PS, Gupta P, et al. Diffuse alveolar hemorrhage due to acute mitral valve regurgitation. Case Rep Pulmonol. 2013;2013:179587.
14. Cantor WJ, Harrison DA, Moussadji JS, et al. Determinants of survival and length of survival in adults with Eisenmenger syndrome. Am J Cardiol. 1999;84:677-81.
15. Vongpatanasin W, Brickner ME, Hillis LD, et al. The Eisenmenger syndrome in adults. Ann Intern Med. 1998;128:745-55.
16. Deffenbach ME, Charan NB, Lakshminarayan S, et al. The bronchial circulation: small, but a vital attribute to the lung. Am Rev Respir Dis. 1987;135:463-81.
17. Liebow AA, Hales MR, Lindskog GE. Enlargement of the bronchial arteries, and their anastomosis with the pulmonary arteries in bronchiectasis. Am J Pathol. 1949;25:211-31.
18. Yoon W, Kim JK, Kim YH, et al. Bronchial and nonbronchial systemic artery embolization for life-threatening hemoptysis: a comprehensive review. Radiographics. 2002;22:1395-409.
19. Nimii A, Kihara Y, Sumita Y, et al. Cough reflex by premature ventricular contractions. Int Heart J. 2005;46:923-6.

CHAPTER 5

A Triad: Cardinal Symptoms in Left-to-Right Shunt

INTRODUCTION

Tachypnea/dyspnea, feeding difficulty and failure to thrive, the triad is the hallmark of congestive heart failure (CHF) in children. Important issue is—how does it occur in large left-to-right (L-R) shunt? As discussed, pulmonary structural changes rather than pulmonary congestion is responsible for the respiratory distress in L-R shunt in infancy. However, CHF does contribute in its' own ways.

MECHANISM

A large L-R shunt, particularly at post-tricuspid level, has the following effects:
- *Left ventricular volume overload*: Left ventricle gets dilated and hypertrophied, which lead to increased end-diastolic pressure. Eventually, ventricle may fail, which raises the left ventricular end-diastolic pressure (LVEDP) further.
- *Pulmonary overcirculation*: Excessive flow driven by systemic pressure through the pulmonary capillary bed increases the capillary pressure and alters the pressure relationship with the pulmonary interstitial space.

These two factors lead to interstitial edema, decreased lung compliance, and tachypnea or dyspnea. Occasionally, there may be frank pulmonary edema.

An infant with atrial septal defect (ASD) is less symptomatic. This is because of two factors. Firstly, increased left atrial pressure as a reflection of increased LVEDP is vented through the septal defect. Secondly, L-R shunt here is not driven by systemic pressure.

TACHYPNEA AND DYSPNEA

Tachypnea is a rapid, shallow breathing without apparent distress. In a quiet child, rate is usually above 60 breaths/min from birth to 6 weeks and above 40 breaths/min from 6 weeks to 2 years. It is a reflex-response mediated by J-receptors in the interstitial space, stimulated by interstitial edema. Even pulmonary venous pressure of only 8–10 mm Hg in the infant can lead to interstitial congestion, in contrast in the adult patient in whom a pressure of about 25–30 mm Hg is necessary to cause interstitial edema.

Breathing becomes more difficult along with tachypnea with further increase in pulmonary congestion. This difficult breathing, i.e., dyspnea, is manifested by grunting (forced expiration against a partially closed glottis), intercostal, subcostal and suprasternal retraction, and flaring of alae nasi.

FEEDING DIFFICULTY

The nursing mother can diagnose heart failure in her baby! Mother's description of the feeding pattern is very important. The tachypneic or dyspneic baby sweats and tires shortly during sucking. Feed is interrupted frequently. The exhausted kid falls asleep but to wake up again, being hungry and irritable. He may become lethargic. A normal infant can suck 4–8 oz in 20 minutes or less. The kid with CHF cannot finish it even after 40 minutes.

FAILURE TO THRIVE

Labored breathing increases the workload of the respiratory muscle. An infant with labored breathing costs around 30%, whereas normal breathing demands <5% of the total oxygen consumption. Besides, congenital heart disease is associated with reduced number of striated muscle and adipose tissue. A tachypneic infant takes less feed and often vomits out. There may be genetic cause of retarded growth. All the above factors lead to failure to thrive.

PULMONARY PROBLEMS IN LEFT-TO-RIGHT SHUNT

Children with large L-R shunt develop respiratory difficulties, which are better explained by pulmonary factors rather than CHF. Large pulmonary flow leads to dilated hypertensive pulmonary arteries, enlarged atrium and overall, dilated heart. Those structures compress the bronchi and lung parenchyma. Pulmonary problems, caused by this compression, are chronic and recurrent atelectasis, pneumonia, bronchiectasis and infantile lobar emphysema.

Left pulmonary artery arches over left main stem bronchus, courses posteriorly around the left upper lobe bronchus and descends to the lower lobe. Thus when dilated, it can compress the left main bronchus and the left upper lobe bronchus.

When dilated, right pulmonary artery can compress, most commonly the right middle lobe bronchus.

Dilated left atrium, lying just below the tracheal bifurcation can cause bronchial compression.

Complete obstruction of the bronchus results in atelectasis or pneumonia, whereas partial obstruction results in infantile lobar emphysema.

Those pulmonary complications due to L-R shunt commonly occurs between 2 and 9 months of age. In the first 2–3 months, smaller-sized pulmonary arteries and higher neonatal pulmonary vascular resistance (PVR) can limit the degree of L-R shunt. Over next few months, PVR comes down. It increases shunt and pulmonary vascular sizes. Infant becomes progressively symptomatic. Gradually the airways become larger in size and cartilaginous. They are now stiff enough to prevent the compressive effect of the cardiac structures. This is the most important cause of spontaneous improvement in respiratory symptoms. Decrease in defect's size, development of infundibular obstruction and pulmonary hypertension may also attenuate symptoms.

Infants are sometimes wheezy and their chest radiograph shows hyperinflated lungs. This lower airway obstruction correlates with degree of L-R shunt and pulmonary hypertension. Morphological studies showed smooth muscle hypertrophy of the bronchioles, which at the same time were compressed by hypertrophied arterioles. Thus, morphological changes of the airways are more important factors of the pulmonary symptoms, rather than pulmonary venous congestion or interstitial edema.

CONCLUSION

Frequent respiratory tract infection in a child does not denote that the child is having a large left-to-right shunt. Because, a child with low-flow situation may also suffer from the same. Feature of large left-to-right shunt is the feature of heart failure associated with respiratory tract infection, which is in most of the time, in the form of pneumonia necessiting hospital admission. A detail history from mother only can help to make a diagnosis of heart failure associated with respiratory tract infection.

FURTHER READING

1. Berlinger NT, Long C, Foker J, et al. Tracheobronchial compression in acyanotic congenital heart disease. Ann Otol Rhinol Laryngol. 1983;92:387.
2. Listar G, Pitt BR. Cardiopulmonary interaction in the infant with congenital cardiac disease. Clin Chest Med. 1983;4:219.
3. Motoyama EK. Peripheral airway obstruction in children with congenital heart disease and pulmonary hypertension (PAH). Am Rev Respir Dis. 1986;133:A10.
4. Stranger P, Lucas RV Jr, Edwards JE. Anatomic factors causing respiratory distress in acyanotic congenital heart disease. Pediatrics. 1969;97:195.

CHAPTER 6

A Triad: Cardinal Symptoms in Congenital Cyanotic Heart Disease

INTRODUCTION

All three presentations are dramatic! The baby starts his morning with spell. If he survives the spell and grows, child starts his or her walking on squatting posture. On further growth, the boy or the girl looks suffused and blue.

PAROXYSMAL HYPOXIC SPELL

Hypoxic spell is an ominous symptom, classically found in tetralogy of Fallot (TOF). But it may be a presenting symptom in other diseases of Fallot's physiology, as well as pulmonary atresia with ventricular septal defect (VSD). It may happen even in absence of cyanosis.

Age

Most common age of hypoxic spell is 4–12 months of age. Spell is uncommon in first month of infancy or beyond 2 years of age.

Typical Spell

Spell occurs usually in the morning, after a good sleep. It may be precipitated by a feed, crying, or bowel movement. The baby breathes quickly. Cyanosis as well as pallor deepens and hyperpnea increases. Occasionally, the baby may develop limpness, syncope, convulsion, stroke, and even death. Rudolph[1] explained the morning timing of spell as follows:
- Increased activity in the morning increases oxygen demand.
- Baby tries to stand on the crib, which reduces venous return.
- A reduction in circulating volume due to relative dehydration because of lack of fluid intake overnight.

Not all the spells lead to syncope. Many often, it is not described by parent as spell. Rather, it is described as colic, seizure disorder or a behavioral variation of an irritated spoiled infant. It is more common in presence of anemia and hypovolemia. Recurrent spell may affect intelligence quotient, learning, and other neurological development.

Mechanism

- Paul Wood,[2] long back in 1959, first proposed the mechanism of spell. He postulated the theory of increased resistance to right ventricular outflow, which increases right to left shunt, as the mechanism. This hypothesis is most acceptable. May be right ventricular infundibulum undergoes in spasm due to increased adrenergic activity precipitated by physical activity, crying, fever or infection. The number of β-adrenoreceptors in infundibular muscle has been found to be higher in children with TOF who have suffered hypoxic spells than in those who have not.[3] This theory is supported by the fact that spell can be effectively controlled by β-adrenoreceptor blocker. But it does not explain the mechanism of spell in pulmonary atresia with VSD.
- Guntheroth[4] suggested a hyperventilation theory. Spells are used to be precipitated by any stimulus producing hyperventilation, which leads to increased venous return. In view of fixed right ventricular obstruction, right to left shunt is increased. There is more hypoxemia and more hyperventilation, which increases the more work of the respiratory muscle and more oxygen consumption. However, increased venous return should increase pulmonary flow to some extent, which prevents deepening of cyanosis and hyperventilation appears during the spell rather than at its onset.
- Prolonged crying may not the mechanism but important additive factor in spell. During crying, prolonged expiration and Valsalva, both increases pulmonary vascular resistance. Breath holding produces inadequate ventilation. All these factors increase hypoxia and cyanosis.
- Kothari[5] presented a different theory for the spell, which may result from mechanoreceptor stimulation from right ventricle. Due to increased sympathoadrenal activity on crying, there is vigorous contraction of hypertrophied, small volume right ventricle, which can trigger a reflex, leading to hyperventilation and peripheral vasodilatation without bradycardia. This sets the stage for initiating the spell.
- Spell may be related to paroxysmal atrial tachycardia,[6] during which right ventricular volume is reduced due to shortened diastolic filling period. In consequence, narrowed right ventricular outflow in TOF is narrowed further. Effective result is increased right ventricular obstruction, increased right to left shunting, and eventually the spell.

Associated Finding

Tachycardia, a falling blood pressure, and disappearance of the ejection systolic murmur across the right ventricular outflow tract are the other physical findings.

SQUATTING

William Hunter noticed in 1784 that cyanotic patients obtained squatting posture to avoid fainting after exertion.[7] Taussig first observed that children with TOF assumed this posture for relief. Typically, a cyanotic child with right-to-left shunt may squat to rest after exertion like walking. Exertion causes dyspnea and fatigue in patients with TOF, because of increasing hypoxia, hypercarbia, and acidosis along with overreaction of blunted respiratory center and overdrive of the remodeled carotid chemoreceptor.

Diseases Associated with Squatting
- TOF is the classical example
- Tricuspid atresia[8]
- Transposition of great arteries[9]
- *Eisenmenger complex*: VSD with pulmonary hypertension.[10]

Mechanism
How squatting relieves symptoms is still illusive. In a simple way, squatting increases systemic arterial pressure. Right-to-left shunt is reduced and pulmonary flow in increased. However, the effect is more complex.

Effect of Squatting on Normal Hemodynamic
Squatting results in increase in cardiac output and central blood volume and in consequence, rise in systolic, diastolic, and pulse pressure immediately after squatting. This is followed by reflex bradycardia and reduction in forearm vascular resistance due to baroreceptor response to increased pulse pressure. What happens to peripheral vascular resistance? Many authors have suggested that the increase in blood pressure observed during squatting is caused by a rise in peripheral resistance which is attributed to muscular compression of vascular elements in the lower limbs.[11,12] Static leg muscle contraction during squatting may activate somatic pressor reflex, which contributes to the sustained rise in arterial blood pressure. Hanson et al.[13] measured peripheral resistance first time in their study on squatting and they suggested that increase in systemic pressure is contributed only by increase in cardiac output. Peripheral vascular resistance is rather reduced due to baroreceptor reflex.

Brotmacher Theory
Brotmacher studied the effect of squatting in TOF both in squatting in recumbent posture as well as squatting from standing posture.

Squatting in Recumbent Posture[14]
Tetralogy of Fallot babies used to become habitual squatter. Few of them assume squatting position, even when lying down in crib. Squatting makes them comfortable. During squatting, systemic blood flow increases. Momentarily, it may be due to increased preload, as venous blood is expressed from legs. The maintenance of the increased systemic flow cannot, however, be related to increases in venous return from the legs. This is because after a few beats, venous return from legs is reduced as a result of the kinking of vena cava and popliteal veins associated with squatting. The change from the resting state to the squatting

position leads to increase in cardiac output independent of venous return. With increased cardiac output, both, pulmonary flow as well as venoarterial shunt, are increased in the same tune, leading to increase in systemic flow. Due to kinking effect, leg flow is reduced dramatically. Thus, increased systemic flow is mostly distributed in upper-half of body. In lying down position, there is no increase in muscle tone or activity, except in the squatting legs. Thus, there is reduction in coefficient of oxygen utilization, less extraction of oxygen, and higher oxygen saturation in superior vena caval blood. Anoxia is significantly reduced in upper half of the body, where lie the vital centers of the body. Thus, patients feel comfortable on squatting equivalent even in lying down position.

Squatting during Recovery from Exertion[15]

During effort or exercise, lower limb saturation falls precipitously. Twenty movements of foot pedal against spring resistance may bring down iliac vein saturation to 31–51%. This desaturated blood reaches right side of the heart and is shunted to systemic circulation, resulting is further fall of saturation. On squatting after effort, femoral arteries and veins are angulated acutely in the groin between inguinal ligament and superior pubic rami. The popliteal veins are also angulated at popliteal fossa. Muscle of the legs and anterior abdominal wall are in tonic contraction. In consequence, venous return from legs is impeded, which prevents the fall in systemic saturation.

O'Donnell Theory[16]

On squatting, there is initial fall in saturation. As there is increase in venous return, desaturated blood may be shunted from right ventricle to aorta. This occurs immediately after squatting. However, immediate rise in peripheral resistance prevents further shunt and desaturation. Squatting increases central blood volume. At the same time, immediately after standing to squatting position, there is rise in systolic, diastolic, and pulse pressure. Usually about 4 beats after squatting, there is a bradycardia, due to baroreceptor response to rise of pulse pressure. Thus, right-to-left shunt is reduced, pulmonary flow is enhanced, and saturation is improved.

Squatting Equivalent

After exertion, patient chooses this posture effortlessly from intuition. There are some other postures, squatting equivalent namely knee-chest position, sitting with legs drawn underneath, standing with crossed-legs which can help the patient for relief.

HYPERVISCOSITY SYNDROME

Hypoxia leads to compensatory increase in red cell mass, known as polycythemia, to maintain the tissue oxygenation. It is better to name it as erythrocytosis, as it is a monoclonal response. With gradual rise of red blood cell (RBC) mass, it becomes a maladaptive situation, which includes increased viscosity,

TABLE 1: Grading hyperviscosity syndrome.[17]

Grade	Symptom	Pattern of limitation
0	Absent	Does not bother
1	Mild	Bothers without interfering with normal activities
2	Moderate	Interferes with some but not most activities
3	Severe	Interferes with most or all activities

BOX 1: Symptoms of hyperviscosity syndrome.

Erythrocytosis:
- Headache
- Faintness and dizziness
- Amaurosis fugax, blurred vision
- Myalgia, muscle weakness
- Depressed mentation
- Fatigue
- Chest and abdominal pain

Effect on bleeding parameters:
- Easy bruising
- Gingival bleeding
- Epistaxis
- Hemoptysis

Effect on urate metabolism:
- Arthralgia and arthritis

both pulmonary and systemic vascular resistance. Most importantly, increased viscosity leads to reduced tissue oxygenation and hyperviscosity syndrome. Symptoms can be graded as shown in **Table 1**.

Out of all these, symptoms due to erythrocytosis are related to hyperviscosity syndrome. An iron-depleted state produces more severe cerebrovascular hyperviscosity syndrome. As iron-depleted RBCs become more rigid in the microcirculation, tissue oxygenation becomes more affected. Fatigue is the most common symptom along with headache and giddiness (**Box 1**).

CONCLUSION

History gives even an anatomical diagnosis. Spell and squatting mean the underlying disease is TOF, unless and otherwise proved.

REFERENCES

1. Abraham Rudolph (Ed). Congenital disease of the heart clinical-physiological considerations, 3rd edition. San Francisco: Wiley-Blackwell; 2009. p. 350.
2. Wood P. Symposium on congenital heart disease; attacks of deeper cyanosis and loss of consciousness (syncope) in Fallot's Tetralogy. Br Heart J. 1958;20(2):282-6.
3. Sun LS, Du F, Quaegebeur JM. Right ventricular infundibular beta-adrenoceptor complex in tetralogy of Fallot patients. Pediatr Res. 1997;42:12-6.
4. Guntheroth WG, Morgan BC, Mullins GL. Physiologic studies of paroxysmal hyperpnea in cyanotic congenital heart disease. Circulation. 1965;31:70.
5. Kothari SS. Mechanism of cyanotic spells in tetralogy of Fallot--the missing link? Int J Cardiol. 1992;37(1):1-5.

6. King SB, Franch RH. Production of increased right-to-left shunting by rapid heart rates in patients with tetralogy of Fallot Circulation. 1971;44:265.
7. Hunter W. Three cases of malformation of heart. Medical observation and Inquiries' by a society of physician in London. 1784;6:291.
8. Keith JD, Rowe RD, Vlad P. Heart disease in infancy and childhood. New York: The Macmillan Company; 1958.
9. Campbell M, Suzman S. Transposition of aorta and pulmonary artery. Circulation. 1951;4:319.
10. Wood P. Disease of heart and circulation. Philadelphia: JB Lippincott company; 1956.
11. Sharpley-Shafer EP. Effects of squatting on the normal and failing circulation. BMJ. 1956;1:1072-4.
12. Bezucha GR, Lenser MC, Hanson PG, et al. Comparison of haemodynamic responses to static and dynamic exercise. J Appl Physiol. 1982;53:1584-93.
13. Hanson P, Slane PR, Rueckert PA, et al. Squatting revisited: comparison of hemodynamic response in normal individual and heart transplant recipients. Br Heart J. 1995;74:154-8.
14. Brotmacher L. Hemodynamic effect of squatting during repose. Br Heart J. 1957;19:559.
15. Brotmacher L. Hemodynamic effect of squatting during recovery from exertion. Br Heart J. 1957;19:567.
16. O'Donnell TV, McIlroy MB. The circulatory effect of squatting. Am Heart J. 1961;64:347-56.
17. Oechslin E. Hematological management of the cyanotic adult with congenital heart disease. Int J Cardiol. 2004;97 (Suppl 1):109-15.

CHAPTER 7

Syndrome and Measurements

INTRODUCTION

Antoine Bernard-Jean Marfan, a French paediatrician described a pattern of connective tissue disorder in a girl, named Gabrielle in 1896. Subsequently, the disease became known as a eponym after him, Marfan syndrome. Today, we know that Gabrielle was suffering from Conotruncal anomaly and not Marfan syndrome.

SYNDROME[1]

Marfan Syndrome (Figs. 1 and 2)

Marfan syndrome is a pleiotropic connective tissue disease.

Inheritance

Marfan syndrome is inherited as autosomal dominant trait, due to maturation in FBN1 gene encoding fibrillin 1, which is an extracellular matrix protein that

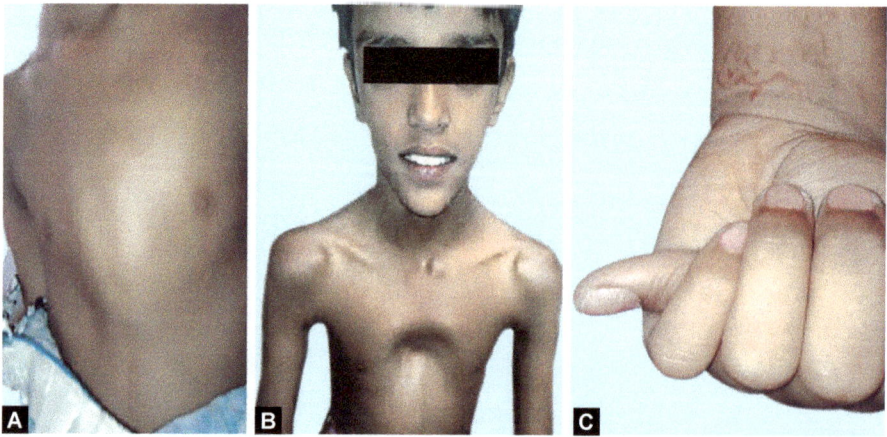

Figs. 1A to C: Marfan syndrome. (A) Pectus carinatum; (B) pectus excavatum; and (C) thumb sign.

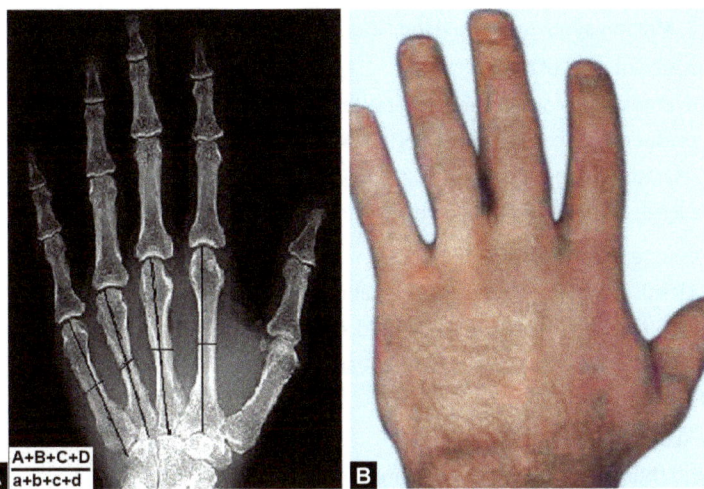

Figs. 2A and B: Marfan syndrome: Metacarpal index (values of between 8.4 and 9.4 have been used as cut-off for abnormal values) and arachnodactyly.

contributes to the final structure of myofibril. The FBN1 gene, which is made of 66 exons, is situated on the chromosome 15q21.1. Around 2,000 mutation has been described for FBN1 gene. In sporadic case, autosomal recessive transmission has been reported. Mutation in FBN1 gene can lead to other simulating diseases, like "myopia or mitral valve prolapse, mild aortic dilation, skeleton, and skin (MASS) syndrome" and "acromelic dysplasia, Weill–Marchesani syndrome, and stiff skin syndrome (SSS)."

Cardiac Defect

The major involvement is the thoracic and abdominal aorta in the form of aortic stiffness, aneurysm, and dissection due to accelerated vessel aging and maladaptive remodeling. By 60 years of age, 100% of patients of Marfan syndrome will develop aortic root dilatation of varying degree. Mitral valve elongation and myxomatous degeneration leading to mitral regurgitation occurs in 28–75% of patients. In children, mitral valve prolapse with severe mitral regurgitation can lead to heart failure. Aortic regurgitation is secondary to aortic dilatation or aortic dissection. Other abnormalities include atrial and VSDs and primary left ventricular dysfunction.

Phenotype

The presence of systemic feature (as mentioned in **Box 1**) with an increasing score classify following phenotype:
- *Score ≤4*: Nonspecific connective tissue disease
- *Score 5–6*: MASS syndrome
- *Score ≥7*: Potential Marfan syndrome
- *Score ≤4+MVP*: Mitral valve prolapse syndrome

BOX 1 — Marfan syndrome: Revised Ghent diagnostic criteria.[2]

In the absence of a FH of MFS:
- Aortic dilatation (Z-score ≥2) and ectopia lentis = MFS
- Aortic dilatation (Z-score ≥2) and FBN1* = MFS
- Aortic dilatation (Z-score ≥2) and Syst (≥7 points) = MFS[a]
- Ectopia lentis and FBN1 with known aortic dilatation = MFS

In the presence of a FH of MFS:
- Ectopia lentis and FH of MFS (as defined above) = MFS
- Syst (≥7 points) and FH of MFS (as defined above) = MFS
- Aortic dilatation (Z-score ≥2 above 20 years old, ≥3 below 20 years) + FH of MFS (as defined above) = MFS

Systemic score:
- Wrist and thumb sign –3 (Wrist or thumb sign –1)
- Pectus carinatum deformity –2 (pectus excavatum or chest asymmetry –1)
- Hindfoot deformity –2 (plain pes planus –1)
- Pneumothorax –2
- Dural ectasia –2
- Protrusio acetabuli –2
- Reduced US/LS and increased arm/height and no severe scoliosis –1
- Scoliosis or thoracolumbar kyphosis –1
- Reduced elbow extension –1
- Facial features (3/5) –1 (dolichocephaly, enophthalmos, downslanting palpebral fissures, malar hypoplasia, and retrognathia)
- Skin striae –1
- Myopia >3 diopters –1
- Mitral valve prolapse (all types) –1

Maximum total: 20 points; score ≥7 indicates systemic involvement.

Note: Aortic diameter at the sinuses of Valsalva above indicated Z-score or aortic root dissection.

*FBN1 (fibrillin 1) mutation defined according to the following criteria: (1) mutation previously shown to segregate in Marfan family; (2) de novo (with proven paternity and absence of disease in parents) mutation belonging to one of the five following categories: Nonsense mutation, in-frame and out-of-frame deletion/insertion, splice site mutation affecting canonical splice sequence or shown to alter splicing on mRNA/cDNA level, missense mutation affecting/creating cysteine residues, and missense mutation affecting conserved residues of the epidermal growth factor consensus sequence (D/N)X(D/N)(E/Q)Xm(D/N)Xn(Y/F), with m and n representing variable number of residues, D aspartic acid, N asparagine, E glutamic acid, Q glutamine, Y tyrosine, and F phenylalanine; (3) other missense mutations: Segregation in family if possible + absence in 400 ethnically matched control chromosomes; if no FH, absence in 400 ethnically matched control chromosomes; and (4) linkage of haplotype for n ≥6 meioses to the FBN1 locus.

[a]*Caveat*: Without discriminating features of Shprintzen–Goldberg syndrome, Loeys–Dietz syndrome, or vascular form of Ehlers–Danlos syndrome and after TGFBR1/2, collagen biochemistry, COL3A1 testing, if indicated.

(FH: family history; MFS: Marfan syndrome; Syst: systemic score; US/LS: upper segment/lower segment ratio; Z: Z-score)

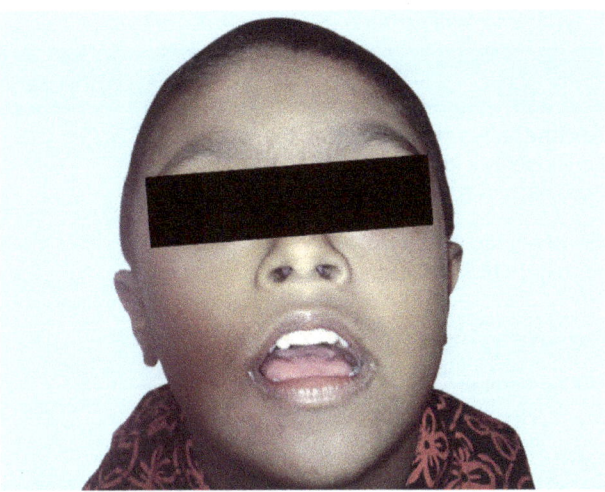

Fig. 3: Down syndrome.

Down Syndrome (Trisomy 21) (Fig. 3)

Inheritance

Ninety-five percent of infants with Down syndrome have full trisomy 21 due to nondisjunction. Around 2% infants have mosaic pattern with one trisomy 21 cell line and one normal cell line. Another 3% infants have translocation of the chromosome 21.

Cardiac Abnormalities

They are found in 40–50% cases. In order of frequencies, they are endocardial cushion defect, ventricular septal defect (VSD), and atrial septal defect (ASD). Uncommonly, tetralogy of Fallot (TOF) and transposition of the great arteries (TGA) may be found. Interestingly, cardiac involvements are more common in babies with trisomy 21 born to older mother than to younger mother. Babies are highly susceptible to develop pulmonary hypertension.

Phenotype

Phenotype includes hypotonia, flat facial profile, redundant skin around back of the neck, upward slant of the palpebral fissure, brushfield spots, small and rounded ears, closely spaced nipples, single (simian) palmar crease in 50% cases, clinodactyly (incurving of the fifth finger), single crease of the fifth finger, wide gap (sandal gap) between first and second toe.

Mental retardation is always present in Down syndrome with average IQ between 40 and 50. Life expectancy is reduced. At birth, it is about 16 years (**Tables 1** and **2**).

Turner Syndrome (Monosomy X) (Fig. 4)

It is not a very uncommon syndrome, occurring in 1 in 2,500 females.

TABLE 1: Down syndrome: Hall's criteria.

Signs	Frequency (percent of newborn affected)
Poor Moro reflex (the baby's muscles do not tighten when body support is suddenly withdrawn)	85
Hypotonia	80
Flat facial profile (the bridge of the nose tends to be low and the cheekbones high, which makes the face look flat and the nose look small)	90
Upward-slanting palpebral fissure	80
Morphologically simple, small round ears	60
Redundant loose neck skin	80
Single palmar crease	45
Hyperextensible large joints	80
Abnormal pelvis radiograph (X-ray of the pelvis shows that the pelvis is rather small and the bones less developed)	70
Hypoplasia fifth finger middle phalanx	60

TABLE 2: Down syndrome: Fried criteria.[3]

Signs	Frequency (percent of newborn affected)
Abundant neck skin	100
Mouth corners turned downward	80
General hypotonia	80
Flat face	96
Dysplastic ear	72
Epicanthic eye-fold	76
Gap between 1st and 2nd toes	60
Protruding tongue	64

Note: Each point scores 1. Score 0–2: Down syndrome disapproved, no further test; Score 3–5: Suspected Down syndrome, chromosomal analysis needed; Score 6–8: Clinically proven Down syndrome.

Inheritance

Patient with Turner syndrome can present with different karyotype, all of which lack X-chromosomal materials. About 40–50% of women with Turner syndrome present with the 45,X karyotype, 15–25% have mosaicism with 45,X/46,XX, and 20% of women have an isochromosome. In addition, ring X chromosomes are present in few women and 10–12% of women have differing amounts of Y chromosome material. *SHOX* gene, situated in the pseudoautosomal location of X-chromosome is responsible for the phenotype of Turner syndrome.

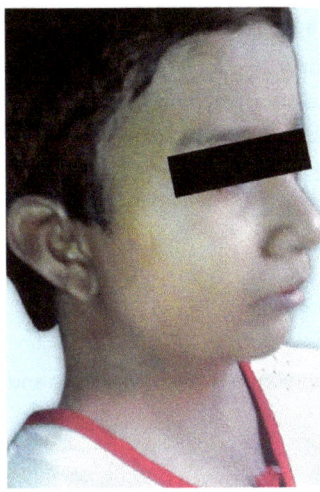

Fig. 4: Turner syndrome.

Cardiac Abnormalities

Most common congenital heart disease associated with Turner syndrome is bicuspid aortic valve, in 25% of cases, an influence of *TIMP1* and *TIMP2* genes. Coarctation of aorta is common and hypoplastic left heart syndrome is a part of other left-sided abnormalities. Abnormal pulmonary venous drainage, subaortic membrane, mitral valve dysplasia, and coronary artery anomalies are known association. Adult females are susceptible to aortic dissection, hypertension, and coronary artery disease. Aortic dissection is due to aortopathy in relation to bicuspid aortic valve, coarctation of aorta, and hypertension. Hypertension occurs in 50% of adult Turner syndrome. Estradiol deficiency, sympathetic-parasympathetic nervous system dysregulation, and coarctation of aorta—all may be responsible for hypertension. A blunted nocturnal dipping is the special feature of hypertension in Turner syndrome.

Phenotype

Short stature, primary amenorrhea, triangular face with down slanted palpebral fissures, epicanthal fold, ptosis, low set ears, short neck with marked webbing, broad chest with widely apart nipples, cubitus valgus with short fourth and fifth metacarpals, multiple nevi, and inguinal hernias are common features. Infertility with absence of secondary sexual characters is common due to hypergonadotropic hypogonadism with ovarian dysgenesis. Mental retardation is usually not present (**Box 2**).

Noonan Syndrome (Autosomal Dominant) (Fig. 5)

It is a rather common syndrome; its incidence is around 1 in 1,000 to 1 in 2,500 live births.

> **BOX 2** **Diagnostic criteria for Turner syndrome.**
>
> **Partial or complete X monosomy**
> - Phenotypic males regardless of karyotype
> - Women with 45,X cell lines but no clinical features, and
> - Women with small Xp deletions that do not include band Xp22.3 and Xp deletions distal to Xq24 (isolated premature ovarian failure). Karyotyping of at least 30 cells showing substantial proportion with absent or defective second sex chromosome
>
> **Short stature**
> - Height <2.5th percentile for age-matched girls.
>
> **Premature ovarian failure**
> - Absence of pubertal development or early menopause and increased level of gonadotropins
>
> **Congenital heart diseases**
> - Bicuspid aortic valve
> - Coarctation of aorta

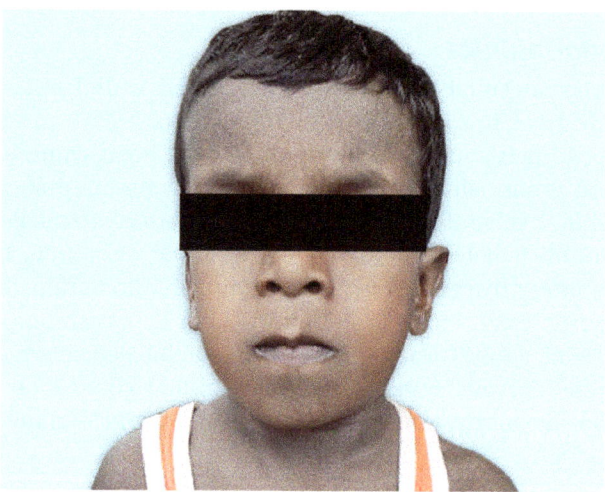

Fig. 5: Noonan syndrome.

Inheritance

Noonan syndrome may occur sporadically or shows autosomal dominant inheritance. In around 50% of patients with Noonan syndrome, a missense mutation is found in the *PTPN11* gene on chromosome 12. It is mostly inherited from mother, because fertility of males with this syndrome is decreased. Though recurrence rate is supposed to be 50%, actual figure is far less.

Cardiac Abnormalities

Incidence of cardiac abnormalities is in around 60–70% of cases. Most common is valvular pulmonary stenosis with dysplastic leaflets in 50–62% of cases. Hypertrophic obstructed cardiomyopathy occurs in 20% of cases. Other associations are ASD, VSD, and patent ductus arteriosus in 6-10%, 5%, and 3% of cases, respectively. Mitral valve prolapse and branch pulmonary artery stenosis are rare association.

Phenotype
Growth is retarded. Facial appearance changes with age. Large head, prominent eyes, depressed nasal root, short neck with webbing, curly or Woolly hairs, and pectus carinatum in upper part and pectus excavatum in lower part are common features. Male patients show cryptorchidism in 60% cases with infertility. Sexual development is delayed. Females are usually fertile. Mental retardation can be found in 35% cases (**Box 3**).

Differential Diagnosis
It includes Turner syndrome, Williams syndrome, fetal alcohol syndrome, and LEOPARD syndrome.

Holt–Oram Syndrome (Figs. 6A and B)
Holt–Oram syndrome belongs to heart-hand syndrome, a heterogenous group. The prevalence is estimated to be 0.95/100,000 births. In this syndrome, cardiac defect is associated with upper limb defect. There are three types of hand-heart syndrome.
1. *Type I*: Holt–Oram syndrome
2. *Type II*: Tabatznik's syndrome
3. *Type III*: Spanish type

Inheritance
The genetic background is the mutations in the *TBX5* transcription factor gene at human chromosome 12q2. This genetic mutation is specific to type I syndrome.

| BOX 3 | Diagnostic criteria for Noonan syndrome. |

Major characteristics
- Cardiac: Pulmonary valve stenosis (commonly dysplastic); Height: <3rd centile
- Chest wall: Pectus carinatum or excavatum
- Family history: First-degree relative with definite diagnosis
- Mental retardation, cryptorchidism, lymphatic dysplasia: All of the three present

Minor characteristics
- Cardiac: Other than pulmonary symptoms; Height: <10th centile; short stature
- Family: First-degree relative with suggestive diagnosis
- Mental retardation, cryptorchidism, lymphatic dysplasia: Any of the three present

Typical facial features with 1 major or 2 minor characteristics

Suggestive facial features with two major or three minor characteristics

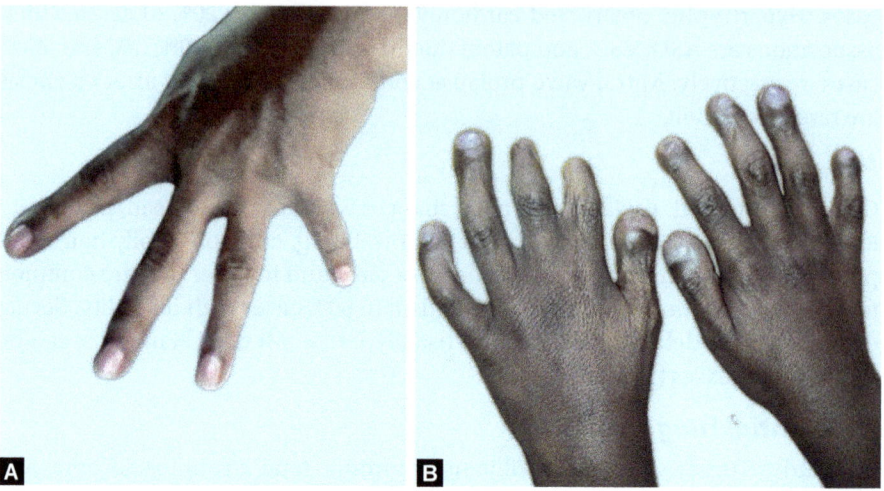

Figs. 6A and B: Holt–Oram syndrome: Smaller ring finger and thumb at same plane with other fingers.

The syndrome is transmitted as autosomal dominant inheritance with high penetrance. Females are affected more severely.

Cardiac Abnormalities
They are found in 75% cases. Most common is ASD, VSD, mitral valve prolapse, and other complex cardiac diseases. Conduction anomalies may be present in 40% of cases.

Phenotype
Skeletal abnormalities involving upper limb in its preaxial radial ray distribution, is always present. Preaxial radial ray distribution means the structures derived from the embryonic radial ray, typically the radial, carpal, and thenar bones. The abnormalities include aplasia, hypoplasia, and fusion of these structures. In consequence, there is triphalangeal or absent thumbs, foreshortened arms, and phocomelia. Left side is affected more, whereas lower limb involvement is rare.

Differential Diagnosis
It includes thalidomide embryopathy, Roberts syndrome, and Poland syndrome.

Williams Syndrome (Fig. 7)
Williams syndrome or Williams-Beuren syndrome, also known as "idiopathic infantile hypercalcemia" or "supravalvular aortic stenosis syndrome" is not an uncommon syndrome, with a prevalence of 1:7,500.

Inheritance
The genetic abnormality includes 1.5-1.8 Mb heterozygous microdeletion of elastin gene at chromosome 7q11.23.

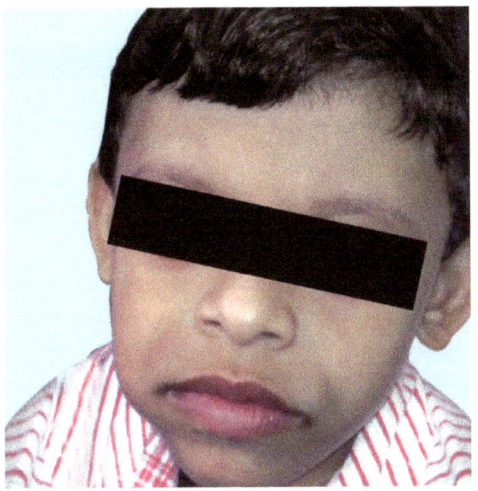

Fig. 7: Williams syndrome.

Cardiac Defects

Elastin arteriopathy is present in 75–80% of cases and can affect any artery. Most common is supravalvular stenosis, which may worsen within first 5 years of life. Middle aortic syndrome, diffuse narrowing of thoracic and abdominal aorta, is not very uncommon. Peripheral pulmonary artery stenosis is common in infancy and may improve spontaneously over years. ASD, VSD, and mitral valve prolapse are uncommon. Sudden cardiac death is not very infrequent. Coronary artery stenosis and QT prolongation may cause arrhythmic cardiac death. Hypertension is common and may be found in 45–50% of cases. Vascular stiffness and in few patients, renal artery stenosis are the contributory factors.

Hypercalcemia

Ionized calcium is high in 15–50% of cases and causes symptom of irritability, vomiting, and vomiting in first 2 years of life. Nephrocalcinosis is common. Impaired calcitonin metabolism can be the mechanism.

Phenotype

Typical face is described as elfin face characterized by periorbital fullness with crying, epicanthal fold with hypertelorism, depressed nasal bridge, stellate iris, and strabismus. Mouth is characterized by malar hypoplasia, wide mouth with prominent lower lip. Teeth are hypoplastic with gap and malocclusion. Neck is long with small head and hoarse voice. Pectus excavatum and inguinal hernia are commonly found. There is variable degree of mental retardation along with an outgoing personality (**Table 3**).

Velo-cardio-facial Syndrome

Velo-cardio-facial syndrome (VCFS) is one of the most common multiple anomaly syndromes. Its prevalence in population is roughly around 1:2,000. Other names

TABLE 3: Diagnostic criteria for Williams syndrome.

Characteristics	Points
Low birth weight	3
Feeding difficulty	3
Obstipation	3
Typical face	3
Supravalvular aortic stenosis	3
Mental deficiency	3
Overfriendliness	3
Strabismus	2
Developmental delay	2
Failure to thrive	1
Other congenital heart disease	1
Hypertension	1
Joint contracture	1
Hyperacusis	1
Hypoplastic nails	1
Total	31

Note: A feature scoring 20 points is strongly suggestive of William's syndrome. Total scoring below this value would indicate the need to carry out the fluorescent in situ hybridization (FISH) test, to confirm the elastin gene abnormality.

BOX 4   Conotruncal face.

- A long face with a prominent upper jaw
- Flattening of the cheeks
- An underdeveloped lower jaw
- Periorbital fullness with bluish color below the eyes
- Narrow upslanted palpebral fissure
- A prominent nose with large tip narrow and hypoplastic nares
- A long thin upper lip and a downslanting mouth
- Cleft palate or submucous cleft palate
- Small dysmorphic ears

---

are 22q11 deletion syndrome, conotruncal anomalies face syndrome, DiGeorge sequence, CATCH-22, etc. (**Box 4** and **Fig. 8**).

Inheritance

The syndrome shows autosomal dominant mode of inheritance, caused by a microdeletion from chromosome 22 at the q11.2 band, with a variable expression from near normal phenotype to life-impairing problems. The

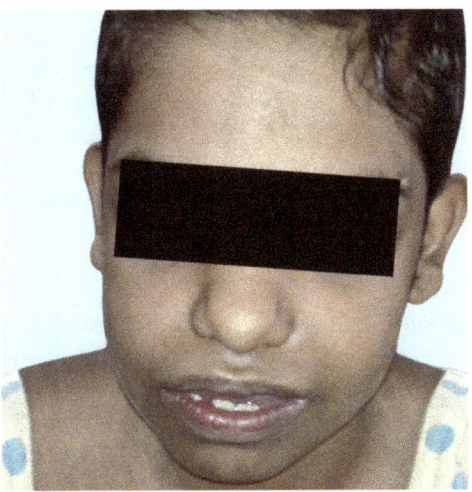

Fig. 8: Conotruncal facies.

diagnosis is therefore defined by the deletion of deoxyribonucleic acid (DNA) from chromosome 22 at the q11.2 band spanning the region that is regarded as the critical region. Fluorescent in situ hybridization (FISH) has a 100% accuracy for diagnosing VCFS. There is abnormal development of pharyngeal arch, leading to the defective development of conotruncal region of heart, thymus, and parathyroid gland.

Cardiac Defect

Congenital heart diseases are associated in VCFS in around 70% of cases. Most common is VSD. Others are conotruncal anomalies including aortic arch interruption type B, truncus arteriosus, TOF, VSD, and pulmonary atresia and subpulmonic VSD. Give the high prevalence of VCFS, a bay with conotruncal anomaly should be screened with FISH.[4]

Phenotype

There are about 180 phenotypes in VCFS. Cardiac anomaly, thymic hypoplasia, and hypocalcemia are the triad. Other common features are facial dysmorphism, cleft palate, vascular abnormalities, most commonly involving pharynx, ocular anomaly, cranial anomaly, renal anomaly, thyroid disorder, hypoparathyroidism, hypernasal speech, immune disorders, etc. VCFS has 25 times more probability to develop major psychosis including schizophrenia.

LEOPARD Syndrome

LEOPARD syndrome is a multiple congenital anomalies syndrome. In broad sense, the syndrome is overlapping Noonan syndrome with multiple lentigines. LEOPARD is an acronym (L: lentigines; E: ECG abnormalities; O: ocular abnormalities; P: pulmonary stenosis; A: abnormal genitalia; R: retardation of growth; D: deafness).

Inheritance

In about 85% of the cases, a heterozygous missense mutation is detected in exons 7, 12 or 13 of the *PTPN11* gene. Recently, missense mutations in the *RAF1* gene have been found in two out of six *PTPN11*-negative LEOPARD syndrome patients. The syndrome is an autosomal dominant condition, with full penetrance and variable expressivity. If one parent is affected, a 50% recurrence risk is appropriate.

Cardiac Defect

Electrocardiogram abnormalities are present in 75% of patients, including left axis deviation, P-wave abnormality, QT prolongation, conduction defect, and ventricular hypertrophy. Hypertrophic cardiomyopathy is the most common cardiac defect. In 40% of cases, it is obstructive. Sudden cardiac death is not uncommon. Pulmonary valvular stenosis with or without dysplasia is the second most common cardiac defect. Other abnormalities include mitral valve prolapse, mitral leaflet cleft, atrioventricular septal defect, multiple VSD, apical aneurysm, isolated LVH, and noncompaction of left ventricle.

Phenotype

Facial dysmorphism includes hypertelorism, flat nasal bridge, low-set dysmorphic ears, palpebral ptosis, deep nasolabial fold, and thick lips. Lentigines are characteristic flat, brown macular skin lesions involving face, neck, and upper part of the trunk. They appear at 4–5 years of age. In half of the patients, additional skin lesions are café-au-late spots. Other abnormalities include chest anomalies, cryptorchidism, delayed puberty, hypotonia, mild developmental delay, sensorineural deafness, and learning difficulties.

Poland Syndrome

Alfred Poland, a student-demonstrator in anatomy, first described this syndrome in 1841. Poland syndrome is also known as "pectoral-aplasia-dysdactylia syndrome" and "subclavian artery disruption sequence" (**Fig. 9**).

Inheritance

Poland syndrome is a nongenetic congenital disorder, with delayed mutation of an autosomal dominant gene leading to vertical transmission from parent to child or affected siblings with normal parents. Risk of recurrence in family is low. At the end of 6 weeks of gestation, upper limb bud lies adjacent to chest wall. Interruption of embryonic blood supply causes hypoplasia of ipsilateral subclavian artery. In consequence, there is hypoplasia of structures which are supplied by right subclavian artery and its branches.

Cardiac Defect

Isolated dextrocardia, in the form of dextroposition without inversion, is a strong association. In all cases of dextrocardia, chest wall abnormality is on left side. Dextrocardia may be a part of Poland syndrome, due to disturbance of vascular

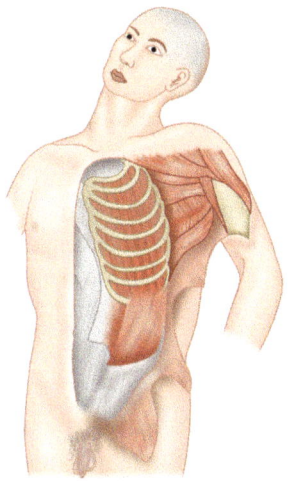

Fig. 9: Sketch of the autopsy done by Alfred Poland.
Source: Poland A. Deficiency of pectoral muscle. Guy's Hospital Report. 1841;6:191.

development. Though isolated dextrocardia is always associated with complex cardiac lesion, Poland syndrome is exceptional.

Phenotype

Most common chest wall deformity is absence of sternocostal head of pectoralis major muscle. Pectoris minor may also be affected. Breast involvement is in the form of mild hypoplasia to amastia. Hypoplasia of ribs involves 3rd to 5th. Hand abnormality is always on ipsilateral side of the affected chest. Abnormalities include cutaneous webbing, i.e., syndactyly and shortness of middle phalanges. Renal agenesis or duplication of urinary collection system may be associated and the combination is known as acro-pectoral-renal-field defect.

MEASUREMENTS[5]

Hypertelorism

True hypertelorism or wide spacing of eyes includes orbital and ocular hypertelorism. Large epicanthal fold leads to pseudohypertelorism, called telecanthus. Routine clinical measurements to identify the abnormality are (**Figs. 10A and B**):
- Interpupillary distance (IPD)
- Inner intercanthal distance (ICD)
- Outer intercanthal distance (OCD)

Radiological examination only, can measure:
- Inner interorbital distance (IID)
- Outer interorbital distance (OID)

By these measurements, one can identify:
Orbital hypertelorism: Increased OID or OCD
Ocular hypertelorism: Increased IPD
Both the above values vary with age and can be found in nomogram.

Telecanthus

It is defined as large distance between the two medial canthi (in normal adult, the width is up to 30 mm), in compare to interorbital distance. It can be expressed as Mustarde ratio (ICD/IPD) >0.55. Telecanthus is suspected when the lower lid puncta is lateral to the medial edge of iris in straight gaze.

Low Set Ears (Figs. 11 and 12)

An imaginary line is drawn from the outer canthus to the external occipital protuberance or the line joining inner and outer canthus and extending it. Normally, the superior attachment of the pinna is at or above this line. When it is below this line, it is a low set ear.

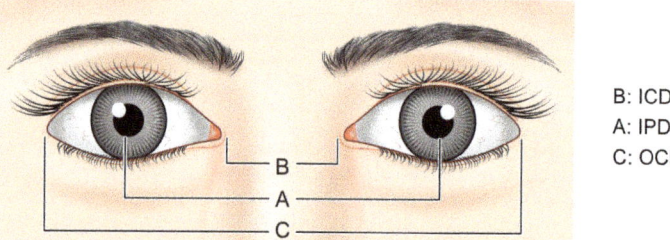

(ICD: inner intercanthal distance; OCD: outer intercanthal distance; IPD: interpupillary distance)

Figs. 10A and B: Hypertelorism. (A) Ocular hypertelorism and (B) telecanthus.

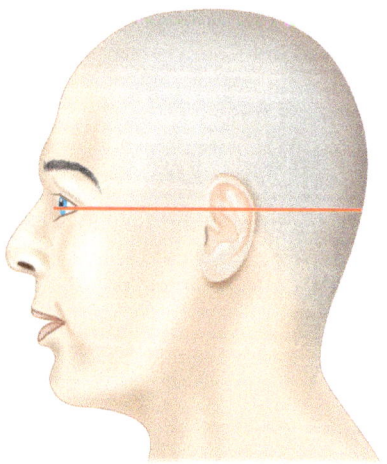

Fig. 11: Normal ear.

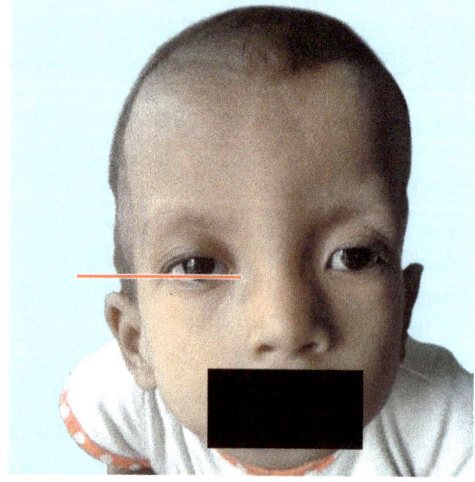

Fig. 12: Low set ear.

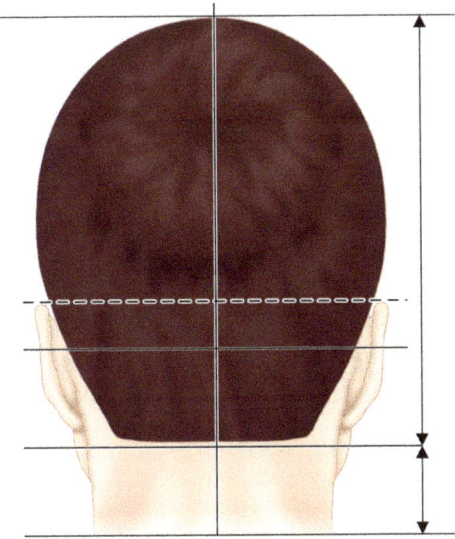

Fig. 13: Low hairline.

Low Hairline (Fig. 13)

There are two criteria:
1. Posterior hairline is below the level of 5th cervical spinous process.
2. Ratio of the distance between external occipital protuberance to the posterior hairline and distance between posterior hairlines to 7th cervical spinous process is >1/6 in men and >1/4 in women.

Short Neck

Neck length is measured as a linear distance between external occipital protuberance and the spinous process of C7 vertebra, with the patient standing upright and neck holding in neutral position. A criterion of short neck is the presence of Bird's index. This is the ratio between patient's standing height and neck length. Normal ratio is below 12.8. Short neck is said to be present when the ratio is >13.6.

Upper-to-lower Segment Ratio

It is the ratio of the length of the upper part of the body to the length of the lower part of body. Upper segment is measured from the middle part of pubic bone to the top of the head. Lower segment is measured from the middle part of the pubic bone to the sole of the foot. The ratio is >1 below 10 years and <1 above 10 years.

Span

It is the distance between the tips of the two middle fingers with the horizontally outstretched arms. In infancy and childhood, span is less than height. Beyond 10 years, span becomes higher than height. A normal span should be within 4 cm of the age-related median span.

High-arched Palate (Pseudo-cleft or Vaulted Palate)

High-arched palate is both high as well as narrowed. Measurement of palate is complex and ideally measured from X-ray skull. The palate height is measured by the shortest distance between midline of the junction of soft palate and hard palate to the reference plane, which passes either through the second primary molar/permanent first molar or through the canine tip.[6] At bedside, rough assessment is done. Palate is said to be high-arched, when the palatal height is greater than twice the height of the teeth. Palatal width is measured as the distance between right and left sided first maxillary molar teeth (**Figs. 14** and **15**).

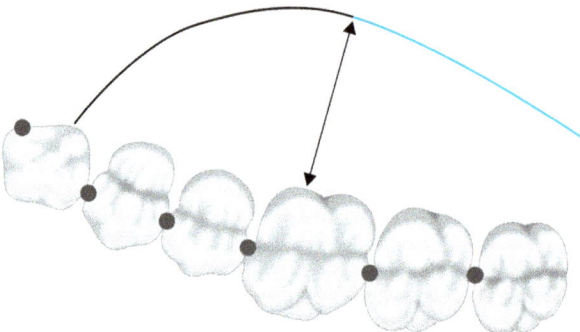

Fig. 14: Palate height: Shortest distance between a plane passing at the level of midline of the junction of soft and hard palate and another plane passing at the level of first maxillary molar teeth.

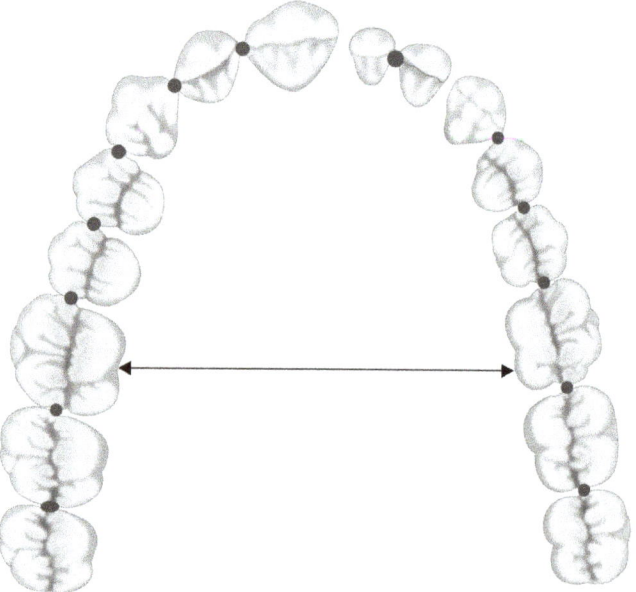

Fig. 15: Palate width: Distance between right and left first maxillary molar teeth.

CONCLUSION

Most of the syndromes have been described centuries back. We start knowing their genotypes only from few decades back. Decades to come when external measurement scale will be gradually replaced by genetic scale

REFERENCES

1. Grecha V, Gattb M. Syndromes and malformations associated with congenital heart disease in a population-based study. Int J Cardiol. 1999;68:151.
2. Loeys BL, Dietz HC, Braverman AC, et al, The revised Ghent nosology for the Marfan syndrome. J Med Zenet. 2012;47:476-85.
3. Fried K. A score based on eight signs in the diagnosis of Down syndrome in the newborn. J Ment Defic Res. 1980;24:181.
4. Shprintzen RJ. Velo-Cardio-Facial-Syndrome: 30 years of study. Dev Disabil Res Rev. 2008;14:3-10.
5. Hall JD, Allanson JE, Gripp KW, et al. Handbook of physical measurements, 2nd edition. New York: Oxford University Press; 2007.
6. Amirabadi GE, Golshah A, Derakshan S, et al. Palatal dimensions at different stages of dentition in 5 to 18-year-old Iranian children and adolescent with normal occlusion. BMC Oral Health. 2018;18:87.

CHAPTER 8

Clinical Instruments

INTRODUCTION

Stethoscope, the guardian of clinical instrument is having a crossroad moment. Many of the cardiologists are now in opinion that auscultation is superfluous. Before we announce stethoscope and other basic instrument's oblivion, we should re-explore its basic technology.

STETHOSCOPE

"Few modern stethoscopes show any significant acoustical improvement since the time of Laennec."[1]

In 1816, René Théophile Hyacinthe Laennec was called to a young lady "who presented the general symptoms of disease of the heart; the application of the hand to the chest, and percussion, afforded very little assistance, and immediate (meaning placement of his ear on the chest) auscultation was interdicted by the sex and embonpoint (a euphemism for breasts) of the patient."[2] In 1819, after trials with various materials of different density, Laennec started using a light wood cylinder as stethoscope. It took another 100 years to start the combined bell and diaphragm chest piece of the modern stethoscope.[3] Sound can be described by frequency or pitch and amplitude or loudness.

Frequency refers to vibrations per second and is measured in Hz. Its normal range is 20-20,000 Hz. The subjective perception of frequency is pitch. Amplitude is the degree of displacement of air molecules and is expressed as decibel. Loudness is the subjective perception of amplitude. Pitch is appreciated by inner hair cells of the cochlea. They have sensory innervation, while the outer hair cells have motor innervation. These outer hair calls have a feedback control over the inner hair cells to be more sensitive and selectively focused.

This has an important clinical application. This property helps a clinician to focus on particular frequency. During training class, the teacher should vocalize the sound to the student, rather than simply telling him to listen a sound of any pitch or amplitude. By hearing the vocalized sound, the student can tune and, thus focus the outer hair cells for a specific pitch during auscultation.[4]

Ideal Stethoscope

Littmann defined[5] ideal stethoscope as—*"Stethoscope should be able to deliver to the ear without important loss or distortion, all audible physiological phenomena."* The clinically significant sound mostly falls in the acoustic range between 60 Hz and 600 Hz, with the exception of some component of mitral diastolic murmur below 60 Hz and some pulmonary crept and rhonchi beyond 1,000 Hz. Stethoscope has three elements: The collector or accumulator of sound (diaphragm and bell), the connecting tube, and the binaural with spring and ear pieces. Littmann continued—*"Popular conceptions notwithstanding, no acoustic stethoscope amplifies or increases the original sounds. The very best ones transmit them to the examiner's ears with relatively few losses."*

Diaphragm

Stethoscope functions as acoustic filter. The diaphragm of the stethoscope normally is stretched and reduces the amplitude, specifically of lower frequency sound and unmasks the high frequency sound. Thus, it is the choice for high frequency sound. It should be of larger diameter and should be rigid, preferably made up of stainless steel. Diaphragm should be pressed firmly on chest to stretch skin for better transmission of high frequency sound.

Bell

Bell transmits all frequencies, but it amplifies the low frequency sound in the range of 30-150 Hz by 5-10 dB. Low frequency sound has higher amplitude; thus, bell is the choice for lower frequency sound. Firm pressure by the bell attenuates lower frequency. Further, pressing the bell stretches the skin, which acts as diaphragm and transmits the high frequency sound. Hence, it should be placed lightly on the skin. Moreover, a larger diameter bell collects greater intensity of sound. But large bell has two disadvantages. It may attenuate low frequency sound and it may not fit properly on chest wall. Hence, its diameter should be in between 1 and 1.5 inch and depth of ¼ inch.[5] Alternately, there may be provision of both large and small sized bells. Bell should have a detachable rubber ring, which allows light skin contact and prevents air leak at skin-bell interface.

Tubing

Tubing should be rigid and short to prevent transmission loss. However, it should not be too rigid to allow varying angulations of chest piece. Shorter the length, better is the transmission. Length around 12-14 inches and diameter around 1/8-3/16 inch are reasonable balance.[5] Double tubing transmits high frequency better[1] at the cost of high volume of air in two tubes, which have a hindrance on sound transmission.

Binaural

Binaural should be as short as possible and not >7 inches with an inner diameter closed to 1/8 inch. The earpieces should be as large as possible, nearing 5/8 inch in diameter.[5] Small earpieces invade external auditory canal and permit leakage of ambient sound.

ELECTRONIC (DIGITAL) STETHOSCOPE[6]

It can enhance the auscultatory skill, by electronic amplification of sounds, particularly the low frequency sound like S3, S4, and diastolic murmur of mitral stenosis, which are, otherwise, sometimes inaudible. This form of stethoscope is accomplished by its ability to record standard waveform, i.e., phonocardiographic display that can be transferred to a computer. One can visualize the sound when listening and it can be used as a simple form of phonocardiogram.

ULTRASOUND STETHOSCOPE

With the advent of ultraportable echocardiograph machine, including the laptop-based and handhold devices, issues have been raised, whether echocardiography should be used as ultrasound stethoscope, i.e., a part of bedside cardiology. Studies are coming up, comparing the efficacy of bedside clinics versus bedside echocardiography.

In one study,[7] 36 subjects had a complete cardiovascular examination by four board-certified cardiologists. They subsequently imaged each patient by portable echocardiogram (**Fig. 1**). The results of clinical examination and bedside echocardiography were compared using a complete echocardiographic study as the gold standard. Cardiac examination failed to detect 59% of the overall cardiovascular findings. Physician-performed echocardiography with

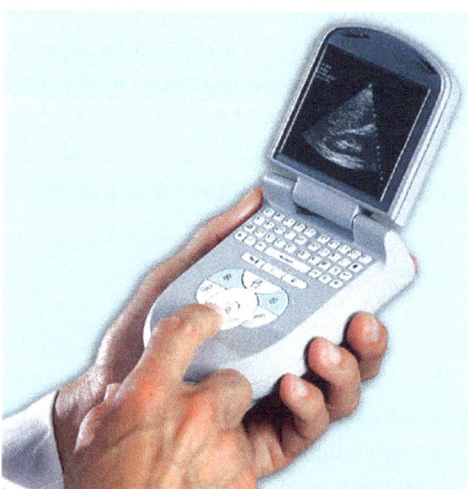

Fig. 1: Handheld echocardiogram.

the device missed 29% of the overall cardiovascular pathology. Only 3% of the findings, whether major or minor, were detected by clinical examination and missed by point-of-care echocardiography.

Clinical examination identified mitral and tricuspid regurgitation murmurs in 43% and 24% of subjects, respectively, aortic stenosis murmur in 88% cases, diastolic murmur of mitral stenosis and aortic regurgitation in 26% cases. Ventricular dysfunction, both systolic and diastolic, was missed by clinical examination in two-thirds of patient.

Even in high-grade aortic stenosis, mitral and tricuspid regurgitation, there can be high rate of missed diagnosis.[8,9] These data are consistent with previous studies demonstrating high rates of missed diagnosis for higher grades of systolic murmurs (14–50%).

Thus, this portable device, when used by clinician is superior to clinical examination alone, across all cardiovascular pathologies. As devices are ultra-portable, clinician can carry them easily during round or at their clinics. These devices are also relatively cheaper and can be owned by the physicians themselves, enabling immediate and accurate assessment.

Devices cannot replace clinical examination. They are complimentary to each other. Clinical examination can focus the echo assessment and echocardiogram can give immediate feedback to improve clinical skill.[7]

SPHYGMOMANOMETER

The sphygmomanometer[10] comprises a manometer and an inflation system. Inflation system consists of an inflatable bladder encased in a nondistensible cuff, an inflation bulb for manual inflation of the bladder in the cuff and connecting tubing.

Manometer

Manometers used are mercury, aneroid, automatic, and nonautomatic oscillometric manometer.

Mercury Manometer

Mercury manometer has been used over 100 years as a gold standard for blood pressure measurement. This is because of its simplicity, accuracy, and infrequent requirement of calibration. However, the mercury manometer has been discouraged worldwide for environment hazards, because of the risk of mercury spills. Maintenance of mercury manometer should be done at every 6 months.
- The mercury reservoir should be full to ensure the upper curve of the meniscus at the zero level.
- Any bouncing of the mercury, which should move freely in the column, indicates clogging of the air vent or dirt or air bubbles in the column.
- The condition of cuff, tubes, bulb, and fittings
- Scale visibility
- Contamination of the glass tube or mercury

- Cuff inflation and deflation control
- Security of mercury containment

Aneroid Manometer

Aneroid manometer translates pressure to mechanical force. Aneroid gauze consists of a metal bellow and watch-like movement connected to the compression cuff. Pressure variation causes the bellow to contract and expand, by which a gear is rotated. This rotational movement turns a pointer pivoted on bearings, across a calibrated dial.

Automated Nonauscultatory Electronic (Oscillometric) Manometer

Oscillometric automatic (electronic) manometer measures the oscillation of the artery. When the oscillation of pressure is recorded during slow deflation of sphygmomanometer cuff, the point of maximal oscillation corresponds to the mean intra-arterial pressure. The oscillations start before systolic pressure and continue below diastolic pressure. A preset algorithm determines systolic and diastolic pressure from the algorithm. As auscultatory skill is not necessary, it is the ideal device for home monitoring. As transducer need not be placed over brachial artery, position of cuff placement is not critical. On this device, observer errors like terminal digit preference, threshold avoidance and rapid deflation are eliminated. The devices are usually arm device. However, wrist and finger devices are also available. The limitation of this device is that in certain situations, which affect the oscillation nature of the arterial wall, like elderly, diabetes and pre-eclampsia, automated reading may not be accurate. In presence of atrial fibrillation, blood pressure measured by automated manometer was found higher in compared to auscultatory manometer in a large meta-analysis.[11] However, in a recent study, no difference of pressure was found in presence of atrial fibrillation between two devices.[12]

Auscultatory Electronic Manometer

Auscultatory electronic manometer uses pressure sensor and digital display. The cuff pressure is displayed as a simulated mercury column and digitally in LCD screen. During deflation of cuff, a button next to inflation cuff can be pressed on first and fifth Korotkoff sound, thus systolic and diastolic pressure digitally recorded. This eliminates terminal digit preference, common in other auscultatory manometer like mercury or aneroid ones. Thus, on this device, there is traditional auscultatory technique without relying on automated reading and without demerits of other auscultatory devices.

Which Device is Preferred?

When regular calibration is done, aneroid manometer closely matches mercury manometer in accuracy. The first study in the NHANES (National Health and Nutrition Examination Survey), found systolic BP to be minimally higher with the aneroid sphygmomanometer in children aged 8–17 years.[13] In SEARCH for Diabetes in Youth Study, no difference was found between the two methods in the mean systolic BP, while the diastolic BP was slightly lower with the aneroid monitor and a +1.8 correction factor was suggested.[14] In another study by Ma Y et al., no clinically significant difference was found between two devices.[15] In a large study[16] comprising >8,000 patients comparing oscillometric versus aneroid manometer, researchers used 604 sphygmomanometers (53% digital, 32% aneroid, 13% mercury, and 2% hybrid devices). They found that only 78% of the aneroid models were able to give accurate measures, while 88% digital devices were accurate, considering acceptable error of 3 mm Hg.

The 2018 ESC/ESH (European Society of Cardiology/European Society of Hypertension) guideline on hypertension recommends—*"Auscultatory or oscillometric semiautomatic or automatic sphygmomanometers are the preferred method for measuring BP in the doctor's office."* Similarly, 2017 ACC/AHA (American College of Cardiology/American Heart Association) hypertension guideline recommends—*"The clinical standard of auscultatory measures calibrated to a column of mercury has given way to oscillometric devices."*

Calibration

All sorts of manometer should be calibrated regularly: Mercury manometer at 3 years interval, aneroid manometer at 6 months interval, and automatic oscillometric manometer at 1-year interval (**Fig. 2**).[17] The pressure inlet of the desired manometer is connected to the reference manometer by Y-connector. With open valve, reference manometer should display zero and calibrating manometer's pressure is noted. Pressure is inflated to 200 mm Hg and then deflated slowly to 100 mm Hg. At this point, calibrating manometer's pressure is recorded. Then, the deflation is continuing to zero. Again, the calibrating manometer's pressure is noted. If the difference is >2 mm Hg, the manometer should be serviced.

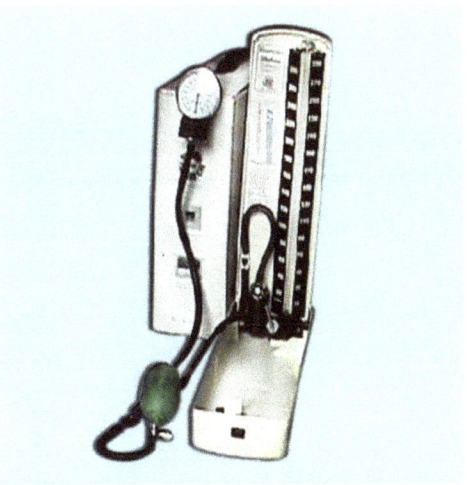

Fig. 2: Two aneroid manometers is getting calibrated, by connecting it through a Y-tube with mercury manometer.

Cuff and Bladder

Cuff is the inelastic cloth that encircles arm encloses the inflatable bladder (**Table 1**). Cuff is secured around arm, either by Velcro surface or by tapering end, which should be long enough, extending beyond of the bladder for 25 cm and then taper for a further 60 cm.[18] Bladder size inside the cuff is very important to avoid over- or undersizing. Too small and too narrow a cuff (undercuffing) overestimates blood pressure with a range of error 3.2–12 mm Hg (cuff-hypertension) and too long and too wide a cuff (overcuffing) underestimated blood pressure, with a range of error 10–30 mm Hg. Undercuffing is more common. Usually, the width of the cuff should be 20% more than the mid-arm diameter or 40% of the mid-arm circumference. Cuff size is used in reference to the inner inflatable bladder (**Fig. 3**). Length of the cuff should be adequate to encircle 80% of the limb in an

TABLE 1: Acceptable bladder dimensions (cm) for arms of different sizes.

Cuff	Bladder width (cm)	Bladder length (cm)	Arm circumference at midpoint (cm)
Newborn	3	6	<6
Infant	5	15	6–15
Child	8	21	16–21
Small adult	10	24	22–26
Adult	13	30	27–34
Large adult	16	38	35–44
Adult thigh	20	42	45–52

Note: When cuff size is not proper: 32−(1.05 × arm circumference in cm); if positive, to be added and if negative, to be subtracted from the recorded pressure.

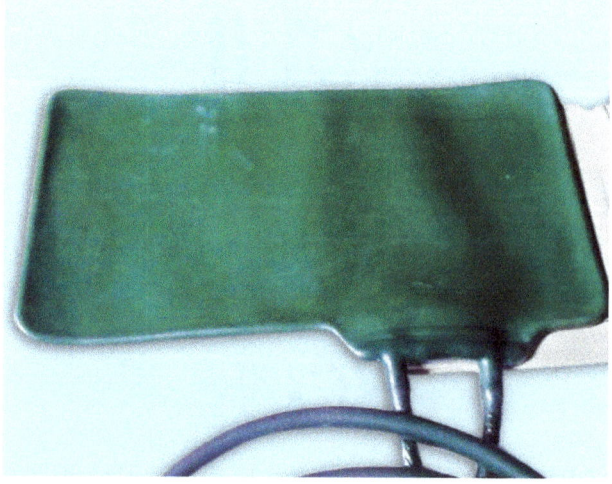

Fig. 3: The bladder.

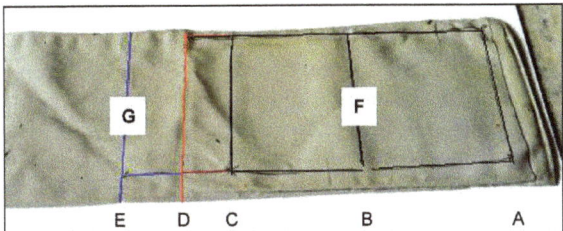

Fig. 4: The cuff. A to C: Bladder length; B: Central point of the bladder; A to D: Ideal arm circumference; C to E: Range of acceptable arm circumference; F: Bladder width; G: Cuff width.

adult and 100% in a child. An overlap does not cause much error. Width and length ratio should be around 1:2.

British Hypertension Society recommends[19] following cuff size:
- A standard cuff with a bladder measuring 12 × 26 cm for the majority of adult arms.
- A large cuff with a bladder measuring 12 × 40 cm for obese arm.
- A small cuff with a bladder measuring 12 × 18 cm for lean adult arms and children.

American Heart Association recommends[20] following cuff size:
- A small adult cuff with a bladder measuring 10 × 24 cm for arm circumference 22–26 cm.
- An adult cuff with a bladder measuring 13 × 30 cm for arm circumference 27–34 cm.
- A large adult cuff with a bladder measuring 16 × 38 cm for arm circumference 35–44 cm.
- An adult thigh cuff with a bladder measuring 20 × 42 cm for arm circumference 45–52 cm.

Cuff should be labeled with the dimensions of the enclosed bladder; a line should mark the center of the bladder, and two lines should indicate the range of arm circumference for which the bladder is suitable, i.e., encircling 80–100% of the circumference (**Fig. 4**).

CONCLUSION

Hearing the heart and measuring the blood pressure are still the bipod for a clinical cardiologist. We can keep the bipod surviving by improving our clinical skill and technology of the bipod.

REFERENCES

1. Ertel PY, Lawrence M, Brown RK, et al. Stethoscope acoustics: II. Transmission and Filtration Circulation. 1966;34:899.
2. Anonymous. Directions for use of the stethoscope. Lancet. 1826;ii:667.
3. Sprague HB. A new combined stethoscope chestpiece. JAMA. 1926;86:1909.

4. Welsby PD, Earis JE. Some high-pitched thoughts on chest examination. Postgrad Med J. 2001;77:617-20.
5. Littmann D. An approach to the ideal stethoscope. JAMA. 1961;178:504.
6. Hollins PJ. The stethoscope: Some facts and fallacies. Br J Hosp Med. 1971;5:509.
7. Spencer KT, Allen S, Anderson AS, et al. Physician-performed point-of-care echocardiography using a laptop platform compared with physical examination in the cardiovascular patient. J Am Coll Cardiol. 2001;37:2013.
8. Roldan CA, Shively BK, Crawford MH. Value of the cardiovascular physical examination for detecting valvular heart disease in asymptomatic subjects. Am J Cardiol. 1996;77:1327.
9. Rahko PS. Prevalence of regurgitant murmurs in patients with valvular regurgitation detected by Doppler echocardiography. Ann Intern Med. 1989;111:466.
10. Perloff D, Grim C, Flack J. Human blood pressure determination by sphygmomanometer. Circulation. 1993;88:2460.
11. Stergiou GS, Kollias A, Destounis A, et al. Automated blood pressure measurement in atrial fibrillation: a systematic review and meta-analysis. J Hypertens. 2012;30(11):2074-82.
12. Selmyte-Besuspare A, Barysiene J, Petrikonyte D, et al. Auscultatory versus oscillometric blood pressure measurement in patients with atrial fibrillation and arterial hypertension. BMC Cardiovascular Disorders. 2017;17:87.
13. Ostchega Y, Prineas RJ, Nwankwo T, et al. Assessing blood pressure accuracy of an aneroid sphygmomanometer in a national survey environment. Am J Hypertens. 2011;24(3):322-7.
14. Shah AS, Dolan LM, D'Agostino RB, Jr, et al. Comparison of Mercury and Aneroid Blood Pressure Measurements in Youth. Pediatrics. 2012;129(5): e1205-10 PMCID: PMC3340597.
15. Ma Y, Temporosa M, Fowler S, et al. Evaluating the Accuracy of an Aneroid Sphygmomanometer in a Clinical Trial Setting. Am J Hypertension. 2009;22:263-6.
16. A'Court C, Stevens R, Sanders S, et al. Type and accuracy of sphygmomanometers in primary care: a cross-sectional observational study. Br J Gen Pract. 2011;61(590):e598-603.
17. Turner MJ, Speechly C, Bignell N. Sphygmomanometer calibration when, how and how often? Aust Fam physician. 2007;36:834-7.
18. Beevers G, Lip GYH, O'Brien E. ABC of hypertension, 4th edition. London: BMJ Books; 2001.
19. O'Brien E, Petrie J, Littler WA, et al. Blood pressure measurement: recommendations of the British Hypertension Society, 3rd edition. London: BMJ Publishing Group; 1997.
20. Perloff D, Grim C, Flack J, et al. Human blood pressure determination by sphygmomanometry. Circulation. 1993;88:2460-70.

CHAPTER 9

A Triad: Cardinal Signs in Congenital Cyanotic Heart Disease

INTRODUCTION

De Senac in 1749, first described the pathogenesis of cyanosis. He thought that cyanosis was due to admixture of arterial and venous blood through a communication between two side of heart. He diagnosed it clinically and confirmed his clinical diagnosis by autopsy. We in modern era, diagnose cyanosis by oximeter, shunt lesion on echocardiogram and do confirm it on angiogram or cardiac MRI!

CYANOSIS

Cyanosis is defined as bluish discoloration of skin and mucous membrane. In 1761, Morgagni, father of medicine, first described cyanosis.[1] Cyanosis is due to presence of high level of deoxygenated blood flowing in superficial dermal capillaries and subpapillary venous plexus.

Ten Commandments

1. Clinical detection of cyanosis depends on dermal thickness, state of cutaneous capillaries, and cutaneous pigmentation (**Box 1**).
2. Cyanosis is best appreciated in places, where epidermis is thin and blood vessels are abundant. Thus, buccal mucosa, lips, ear lobules, cheeks, and nose are the best site to detect cyanosis.
3. Cyanosis is better appreciated under fluorescent light.[1]
4. Amount of reduced hemoglobin, which ultimately decides cyanosis, depends upon the total hemoglobin of the blood and amount of right-to-left shunt.

BOX 1   Congenital cyanotic heart disease without clinical cyanosis.
- Arterial saturation above 85%
- Anemia
- Small right-to-left shunt
- Dark skin

5. The arterial oxygen content is the sum of oxygen bonded to hemoglobin and dissolved in plasma, approximately 1.34 mL per 1 g of hemoglobin and 0.003 mL of oxygen per 100 mL of plasma.
6. Cyanosis is clinically visible only when 3–5 g or more deoxygenated hemoglobin per dL of blood is present in the capillaries of the dermal papillae and mucous membrane and in the subpapillary venous plexus of the dermis.
7. Cyanosis is clinically visible only when right-to-left shunt should contribute at least 40% of the systemic flow (40 mL of venous blood per 100 mL of aortic flow).
8. Central cyanosis implies arterial blood desaturation, which is caused by intracardiac or intrapulmonary right-to-left shunt.
9. Bluish discoloration of skin and mucous membrane is clinically detectable when the arterial oxygen saturation is below 85%. Corresponding oxygen tension will be around 42–54 mm Hg. However, detection of cyanosis depends on the amount of deoxyhemoglobin present in capillaries and not at arterial level.
10. Desaturation not enough to cause cyanosis, can cause reddish fingers and toes as an early sign.

Bluish Skin, No Cyanosis

- *Acrocyanosis*: Due to intermittent vasomotor changes in the skin, unusually prominent diffuse veins appear around lips, nose or eyes, simulating cyanosis.
- *Cutis marmorata*: It is a purple mottling of the skin, more commonly in children, on exposure of cold. Selective dermal constriction of the arterioles leads to the visibility of the dermal blue venules. Parents may complain of bluish discoloration of skin.
- *Methemoglobinemia*:[2] Hemoglobin contains iron in reduced or ferrous form. It combines with oxygen to form oxyhemoglobin. It can accept and release oxygen only in that reduced form. When hemoglobin is reduced, iron becomes in ferric form or methemoglobin (metHb). Circulation normally contains <1% metHb. When hemoglobin is pathologically oxidized in its ferric state, its oxygen-carrying capacity is reduced. Blood, containing metHb, looks dark reddish brown color. When its level is >1.5 g/dL, it imparts a blue color of the skin and mucous membrane. One should, in suspected case, measure arterial blood gas, which shows a saturation gap. There is cyanosis with normal SpO_2. Oxygen saturation measurement is often faulty in presence of metHb.
- *Hemoglobin M*: This hemoglobin is formed due to mild structural changes in the alpha and beta chains which keep it in an oxidized ferric state, thereby reducing oxygen carrying capacity and causing congenital cyanosis. Simple hemoglobin electrophoresis will detect hemoglobin M.
- Pseudocyanosis is bluish discoloration of skin due to drug effect, like amiodarone and metal effect like gold or silver. Pseudocyanosis does not respond to blanching effect by applying pressure, as peripheral cyanosis responds.

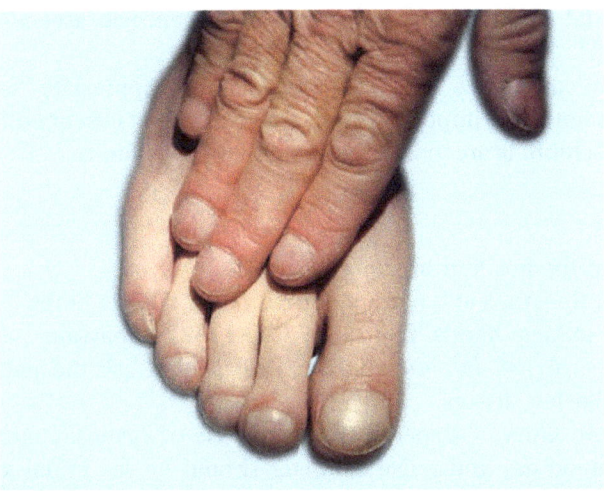

Fig. 1: Differential cyanosis.

Differential Cyanosis (Fig. 1)

Differential cyanosis is present, when right arm is pink and both lower limbs are blue. It occurs in patent ductus arteriosus (PDA) with pulmonary hypertension or PDA along with aortic arch interruption or coarctation of aorta with right-to-left shunt, and PDA with aortic arch interruption. Left arm saturation depends on whether PDA is presubclavian or postsubclavian. Differential cyanosis in a neonate indicates persistent pulmonary hypertension of the newborn and left heart abnormalities like interrupted aortic arch and critical coarctation.

Reverse Differential Cyanosis

Reverse differential cyanosis is present, when right arm saturation is lower than lower limbs. It is noted in neonatal age, in presence of transposition of the great arteries (TGA) with patent ductus and elevated pulmonary vascular resistance or in TGA, PDA and coarctation or interruption of aortic arch. In these conditions, oxygenated blood from the left ventricle passes into the pulmonary artery and through the PDA to the descending aorta, while systemic venous blood flows from the right ventricle into the ascending aorta and its branches. In TGA, however, intracardiac defects allow a high degree of mixing of the blood in the heart, and in the absence of obstruction to blood flow from the ascending to the descending aorta sufficient desaturated blood passes to the descending aorta to make the difference in cyanosis between the upper and the lower extremities slight and difficult or impossible to detect clinically.[2] Rarely, supracardiac total anomalous pulmonary venous connection can present with reverse differential cyanosis, in presence of PDA due to streaming of highly saturated superior vena cava blood into the right ventricle, out the main pulmonary artery, through a PDA, and to the descending aorta and lower limbs, with streaming of more desaturated blood from the inferior vena cava, directed by eustachian valve into the left atrium across the atrial septal defect/foramen ovale, left ventricle, ascending aorta, and upper limbs.[3,4]

Unless the difference is 10–20%, one cannot appreciate the differential cyanosis. It is not a very important clinical sign. Not very infrequently, upper limb cyanosis and clubbing are more prominent than lower limbs.

Approach
- To look in the lips and tongue.
- To look at fingertips and nails of both upper and lower limbs. Patient should be asked to keep hands by the site of feet for comparison.
- *Cyanosis expected, but unapparent*: One should ask the patient for light exercise like few sits-up.
- When hypoxemia is suspected for the cause of cyanosis, measurement of arterial blood gas and pulse oximeter should be the initial aid to clinical assessment.
- To differentiate between cardiac and pulmonary cause of cyanosis by hyperoxia test.

Arterial Blood Gas versus Pulse Oximeter versus Co-oximeter

Arterial blood gas shows the partial pressure of dissolved oxygen in blood and hemoglobin saturation. Pulse oximeter measures the absorption of light at two wavelengths which correspond to that of oxyhemoglobin and deoxyhemoglobin. Pulse oximeter cannot measure the wavelength corresponding to metHb. Co-oximeter can measure absorption of light at four different wavelengths corresponding to oxyhemoglobin, deoxyhemoglobin, carboxyhemoglobin, and metHb. Thus, it should be a better choice to determine methemoglobinemia.

Hyperoxia Test

This test is applicable mostly in neonate or infant presenting with cyanosis and immediate echocardiographic evaluation is not available. Arterial partial pressure of oxygen (PaO_2) is determined on room-air and after 100% oxygen for 10 minutes. Normal PaO_2 at room air is between 90 and 100 mm Hg. In a cyanotic infant, it may be between 10 and 80 mm Hg. When cyanosis is of cardiac in origin, PaO_2 will raise to maximum up to 150 mm Hg after oxygen inhalation. When cyanosis is of pulmonary in origin, PaO_2 will raise to between 400 and 500 mm Hg after oxygen inhalation. PaO_2 should be measured in all four limbs. It can be substituted by measuring simple saturation by using pulse oximeter (**Table 1**).

ANEMIA[5]

One should be vigilant to detect anemia, in presence of cyanosis. Clinical anemia is ominous in cyanotic heart disease. Relative anemia, even, can affect the

TABLE 1: Grading cyanotic burdens.

Grade	SpO$_2$ (%)	PCV (%)
Mild	>85	55–60
Moderate	75–85	60–65
Severe	65–75	65–70
Extreme	<65	>70

(SpO$_2$: oxygen saturation; PCV: packed-cell volume)

rheology significantly. It reduces oxygen-carrying capacity of blood and increases hypoxemia further. This in turn reduces systemic vascular resistance and increases right-to-left shunt. Relative anemia cannot be detected clinically in polycythemia patient.

A hemoglobin level at around 16 g/dL can be taken as relative anemia in a significantly cyanosed patient and one should examine other indices to detect iron deficiency.

These parameters include mean corpuscular volume (MCV), mean corpuscular hemoglobin (MCH), red cell distribution width (RDW), serum iron (SI), total iron binding capacity (TIBC), serum ferritin (SF), and serum transferrin (ST) levels. MCV, MCH, and RDW are simple and cost-effective parameters, rather than costly parameters like SI, TIBC, and SF. Iron deficiency is defined as a ferritin level <15 ng/mL or transferrin saturation <15%.

Red cell distribution width is a measure of deviation of the volumes of RBCs and not directly the diameter of RBCs. It is calculated with:

$$RDW = (\text{Standard deviation of MCV} \div \text{Mean MCV}) \times 100$$

Iron-deficiency anemia results in a varied size distribution of RBCs and shows an increased RWD. In simple word, increased RWD means red blood cells of unequal sizes, which is also termed as anisocytosis.

CLUBBING

"Clubbing is one of those phenomena with which we are all so familiar that we appear to know more about it than we really do."

Samuel West, 1897

Clubbing first described by Hippocrates in a patient of empyema in 460 BC[6] is a time-old sign. Digital clubbing is characterized by enlargement of the terminal segment of finger or toes due to proliferation of connective tissue between terminal phalanx and nail matrix. Clubbed fingers are also named as watch-glass nails, drumstick finger or Hippocratic nail. Hypoxemia leads to clubbing. Pulmonary hypoxemia is uncommon to cause clubbing. Hypoxemia secondary to cyanotic heart disease is more offending cause of clubbing.

Mechanism
- Hypoxemia and polycythemia lead to capillary engorgement, which results in thickening of tissue at the base of the nail.
- Normally megakaryocytes, after liberating from bone marrow, are trapped in pulmonary circulation and fragmented in platelets. In situation where megakaryocytes bypass the pulmonary circulation [when there is extrapulmonary shunting of blood in congenital cyanotic heart disease (CCHD) or carcinoma lungs] or there is aggregate of large number of platelets on left side of heart (infective endocarditis) or when there is platelets excess (inflammatory bowel disease) megakaryocytic factors are lodged in the capillaries of the terminal digits. They liberate vascular endothelial growth factors and platelet-derived growth factors. Those two factors induce vascular hyperplasia, edema, and fibroblast proliferation.[6,7]

What is Contained in Clubbed Fingers?
Digital angiography of clubbed finger shows increases in size and number of digital arteries and arteriovenous (AV) communications. MRI of the clubbed fingers shows the same features of hypervascularization.[8] There is increased number of fibroblasts, lymphocytes, and eosinophil.

How to Grade Clubbing?
Clubbing grows slowly. In the first stage, there is periungual erythema and spongy softening of nail beds. Gradually, the angle between nail bed and proximal nail fold increases due to increasing convexity of the nail. In the next stage, finger appears clubbed with increased depth of the terminal phalanx. Gradually the nail and periungual skin appear shiny with longitudinal ridge with a drumstick appearance. In the last stage, may develop hypertrophic osteoarthropathy. Grading does not have much clinical significance (**Box 2**).

How to Detect Clubbing?
- *Fluctuation test*: Either by palpation or by keeping the heads of two pins, one can demonstrate the fluctuation on the nail bed (**Fig. 2**).

BOX 2 | **Grading of clubbing.[9]**

- Proximal nail fold becomes glossy, shiny and soft
- Normal angle of the nail bed (around 160°), between proximal nail fold and nail plate, Lovibond angle becomes obliterated along with hypertrophy of the subungual tissue and fluctuation of nail bed
- Increased curvature of nail in both planes (accentuated convexity of nail) with a parrot beak appearance
- Swelling of the finger tissue at the end gives the fingers a drumstick appearance
- A shiny and glossy changes of the nail and adjacent skin with longitudinal striations
- In addition, there is painful bony involvement of the digits and may involve the wrist, elbow ankle, and knee-hypertrophic osteoarthropathy

- *Profile sign and profile angle*: To look from side at the terminal digit of the index finger and comparing it with a normal digit. Lovibond described profile sign and profile angle (Lovibond angle) in 1939.[9] Normally when viewed from the lateral aspect, an angle between nail and nail bed is around 160°. When the angle is >180°, that is suggestive of true clubbing (**Figs. 3A and B**).
- Lovibond angle has been modified as hyponychial angle, which is the angle between nail and nail fold.

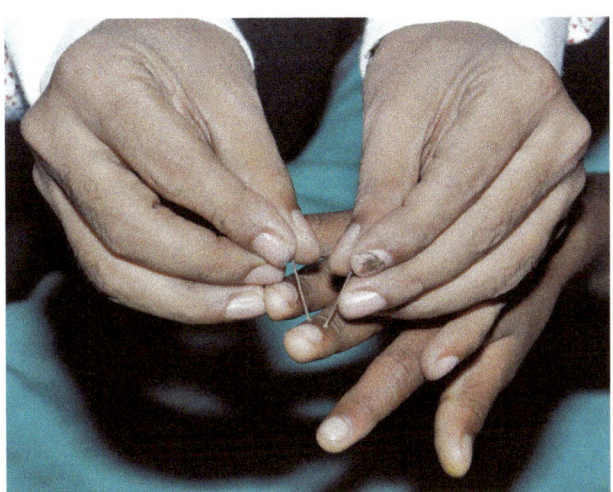

Fig. 2: Fluctuation test.

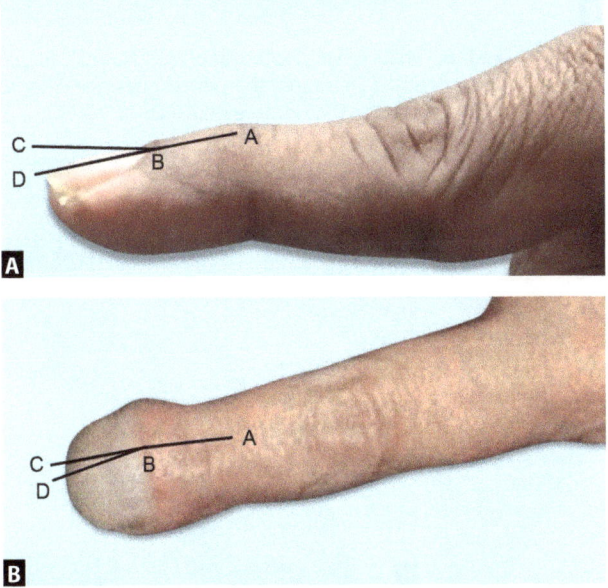

Figs. 3A and B: Lovibond angle and hyponychial angle. (A) ABC and ABD are the normal profile and hyponychial angle; (B) ABC and ABD are the increased profile and hyponychial angle in clubbed fingers.

- *Phalangeal depth ratio*: Rice and Rowland described this ratio.[10] Ratio of the depth of the index finger at the base of the nail and the depth of the terminal interphalangeal joint is measured. A ratio >1 is considered as feature of early clubbing. This sign is independent of age and sex (**Figs. 4A and B**). At bedside, this angle can be measured by using calipers.
- *Schamroth's sign*: When nails of two thumbs are placed face to face, there is a gap in between. In early clubbing, this gap is lost (**Figs. 5A and B**). Leo

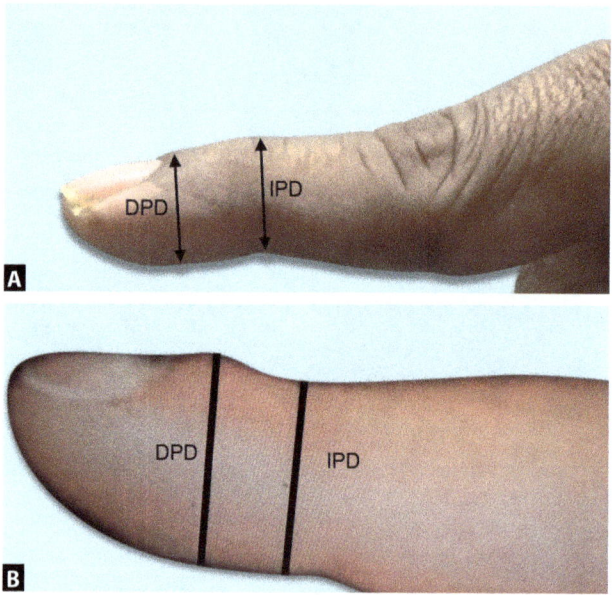

Figs. 4A and B: Phalangeal depth ratio. (A) Normal finger: interphalangeal depth (IPD) is more than distal phalangeal depth (DPD); (B) in clubbed finger, DPD is more than IPD.

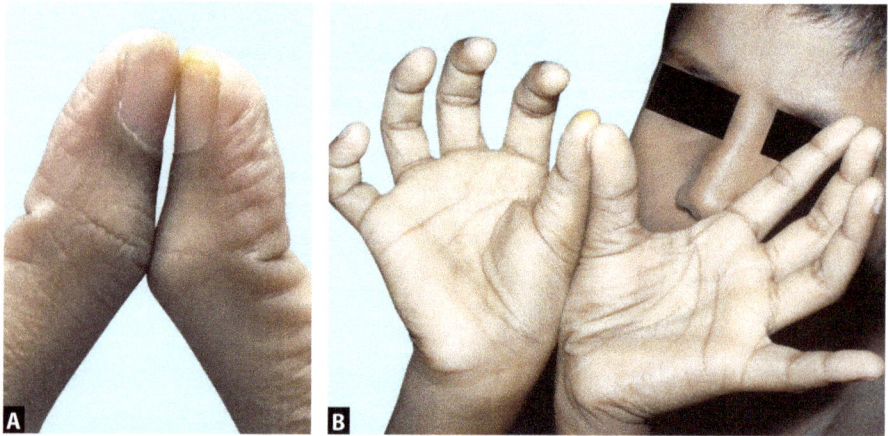

Figs. 5A and B: Schamroth's sign. (A) normally, there is a diamond-shaped space between thumb; (B) which is obliterated in clubbed finger.

Schamroth, the famous electrocardiologist, developed clubbing due to infective endocarditis. He observed this sign on himself.[11]

Cyanosis without Clubbing in CCHD

- CCHD in infant <3 months old.
- Clubbing may regress in presence of anemia in CCHD.
- In older children, cyanosis without clubbing indicates short duration of cyanosis and likely etiology is shunt reversal, due to developing high pulmonary vascular resistance.

Cardiac Cause: Clubbing without Cyanosis

- Saturation around 85–90% may not cause cyanosis but just reddening of fingers and toes along with clubbing.
- Infective endocarditis
- Cardiac myxoma

Unilateral Clubbing[12]

- Axillary artery aneurysm
- Brachial AV malformation
- AV fistula used for dialysis
- Palmar arch aneurysm
- Carcinoma right upper lobe bronchus
- Hemiplegia

Congenital Clubbing

This is found in congenital form of pulmonary osteoarthropathy-pachydermoperiostosis.

CONCLUSION

Cyanosis and clubbing, two most ancient signs in clinical medicine can never be replaced by any technology, even in far future.

REFERENCES

1. McGee SR. Evidence-Based Physical Diagnosis. Philadelphia: WB Saunders and Company; 2001.
2. Conkling PR. Brown B. Understanding methemoglobinemia. N C Med J. 1986;47(3):109.
3. Buckley MJ, Mason DT, Ross J, Jr., et al. Reversed differential cyanosis with equal desaturation of the upper limbs. Syndrome of complete transposition of the great vessels with complete interruption of the aortic arch. Am J Cardiol. 1965;15:111.
4. Yap SH, Anania N, Alborias ET, et al. Reversed differential cyanosis in the newborn: a clinical finding in the supracardiac total anomalous pulmonary venous connection. Pediatr Cardiol. 2009;30:359-62.
5. Onur CB, Sipahi T, Tavil B, et al. Diagnosing iron deficiency in cyanotic heart disease. Int J Ped. 2003;70:29.

6. Dickinson CJ, Martin JF. Megakaryocytes and platelet clumps as the cause of finger clubbing. Lancet. 1987;2:1434-5.
7. Martinez-Lavin M. Exploring the cause of the most ancient clinical sign of medicine: finger clubbing. Semin Arthritis Rheum. 2007;36:380-5.
8. Marrie TJ, Brown N. Clubbing of the digits. Am J Med. 2007;120:940-1.
9. Lovibond JL. Diagnosis of clubbed fingers. Lancet. 1938;1:363-4.
10. Myers KA, Farquhar DR. The rational clinical examination. Does this patient have clubbing? JAMA. 2001;286:341-7.
11. Cheng TO. A unique eponymous sign of finger clubbing (Schamroth sign) that is named not only after a physician who described it but also after the patient who happened to be the physician himself. Am J Cardiol. 2005;96:1614-5.
12. Sarkar M, Mahesh DM, Madhavabi I. Digital clubbing. Lung India. 2012;29:354-62.

CHAPTER 10

Jugular Venous Pulse

INTRODUCTION

Jugular venous pulse, both its waveforms as well as its pressure, denotes the hemodynamic of right atrium as well as the right ventricle. This is the bedside equivalent of the central venous pressure that is influenced by the volume of blood in the venous system, venous tone, right atrioventricular (AV) hemodynamic, and the intrathoracic pressure.

VEINS

Which vein: Internal jugular vein (IJV) is the preferred vein, rather than external jugular vein (EJV), for estimation of the venous pressure, because of the following reasons:
- IJV is the direct continuation of the superior vena cava.
- EJV joins superior vena cava indirectly through subclavian vein. It is compressible by fascial plane, smaller in caliber, and contains venous valves. When descents are visible on tis veins, EJV can be used to assess jugular venous waves. When descents are not visible and EJV is distended, it can be used for determination of mean pressure.
- Sometimes, the external jugular venous pressure (JVP) becomes high due to partial obstruction at the level of external jugular venous bulb due to thrombosis or obstruction by platysma muscle.
- Both the right and the left IJVs should be examined, as sometimes there may be disparity. In elderly, sometimes, the left JVP is higher than the right, because of the partial obstruction of the left innominate vein by the unfolded aorta.[1] This may also happen in persisting left superior vena cava draining in the coronary sinus.

What is actually seen: Jugular venous pulse is the oscillating top of the distended proximal portion of the IJV. The vein itself is not actually seen, but its pulsation is transmitted to the skin of the neck, which is appreciated as pulsation manometer.

Where to look for: The proximal internal jugular pulsation is best appreciated in the supraclavicular area in between the sternal and clavicular head of the sternomastoid muscle.

TABLE 1: Difference: Venous versus arterial pulsation.

Venous pulsation	Arterial pulsation
• Soft, diffuse undulant	• Sharp, external
• Lateral, superficial	• Medial, deeper
• Double undulations	• Single pulsation
• Definite upper level	• No such upper level
• Better visible than palpable	• Better palpable than visible
• Changes with maneuvers such as respiration, body position, etc.	• Does not change with maneuvers
• Can be obliterated by compressing at the root of neck	• Cannot be obliterated in this manner

How to identify venous pulsation: The characteristic of this pulsation is soft, diffuse. This is better seen than felt, having two crests and two troughs. Its upper level drops with inspiration and rises with expiration. Posture has the same effect due to the effect of the gravity, being higher in the horizontal position and lower in the vertical. And most importantly, a gentle compression by the finger or the stethoscope at the root of the neck obliterates the venous pulse (**Table 1**).

JUGULAR VENOUS PRESSURE

Basic Hemodynamics: 10 Commandments[2]

1. Jugular venous pressure is basically the mean of the positive and negative pulse waves.
2. Venous blood returning from systemic capillaries has a nonpulsatile flow.
3. Changes in the flow and pressure caused by the right atrial and right ventricular filling, give rise to pulsations in the central veins that are transmitted toward peripheral vein opposite to the direction of blood flow.
4. If the right atrial pressure is 10 cm of water, the jugular vein will be distended usually 10 cm above the center of the right atrium. The vein above this level is collapsed, because actual pressure within it is below the atmospheric pressure.
5. Tone of the venous system is decided both by the pressure of blood column and sympathetic tone. In consequence, the level of blood column may also be decided by sympathetic nerve for a given right atrial pressure.
6. At this top level, pulsation is very subtle. This is the fulcrum of the movement and the pressure is actually zero.
7. The pressure at any given point in the circulation is expressed in relation to a fixed reference point.
8. The fixed point or the base line of this manometric system is set at heart level. As a result, the reading actually becomes 10 cm of water, which represents the 10 cm height of water in the tube connecting the manometric base line to the needle in the vein.

9. Upper most crest of the pulsatile column is measured, which can be either *a* or *v* wave. Hemodynamically, it is not the mean pressure.
10. EJV is often nonpulsatile and venous pressure measured from it may simulate mean pressure.

Reference Point

- *Physiological zero point*: Physiological zero point is the site in the heart, where central venous pressure remains stable, irrespective of patient's body position. Right atrium is chosen as the zero point by most of the clinicians. A plane going through the intersection of the transverse plane through 4th intercostal space and a coronal plane midway between xiphoid and back is called phlebostatic axis. This axis passes through the posterior atrium. When zero mark of manometer is kept on phlebostatic axis, venous pressure does not change much in respective of body position, being supine, prone or in between.[3] As right atrium is not on the midline, others propose to make right ventricular inflow, just beyond the tricuspid valve, as the zero-point site.
- *External reference point—sternal angle*: As physiological zero point cannot be accessed, bony landmarks are taken. Sir Tomas Lewis first used sternal angle as reference point in 1930. Sternal angle is mostly followed, though there are several other suggestions. There is debate in the statement that normal jugular pulsation is up to 3 cm from sternal angle irrespective of body position, as observed by Lewis. This height has been described as 4 cm, 5 cm at 45° posture and 6 cm at 30° posture.[4] Debate starts when the statement is that normal venous pressure is 8 cm water, assuming the physiological zero point is 5 cm below the sternal angle. Such assumption may lead to underestimation of JVP.[5] Vertical distance between sternal angle and physiological zero-point changes along with change of body position. This distance was critically assessed in 160 patients by computed tomography (CT) of thorax.[6] The median value for the vertical distance was 5.4 cm in the supine position. However, when the CT images of the torso were rotated to 30°, 45°, and 60°, the median vertical distance was 8, 9.7, and 9.8 cm, respectively. It has been suggested that 10 cm should be added rather than 5 cm when torso is elevated >45°.[7]
- *External reference point—clavicle*: Simplest way to determine JVP is to use clavicle as reference point, which is 10 cm above the physiological zero point on sitting posture. A visible distended venous column above the clavicle in sitting posture indicates elevated JVP. This reference point was studied prospectively and clinical observation was correlated with cardiac catheterization.[8] The clinical observation showed the sensitivity and specificity of 65% and 85%, respectively. The limitation of this referral point is failure to detect low venous pressure. When suspected, patient should be examined in recumbent position.
- *External referral point—4th intercostal space*: Anterior end of 4th intercostal space lies at the same level of central point of right atrium or phebostatic axis

in sitting posture. When JVP is raised and venous column is visible at the base of the neck in sitting posture, the vertical distance between the anterior end of 4th intercostal space and upper venous column is the most approximate value of JVP.[9]

- *From clavicle to 4th intercostal space*: The upper end of the clavicle is 13–18 cm above right atrium and in erect posture similar to anterior end of 4th intercostal space. Thus, even when JVP is raised and >9 cm, the upper level of venous column may not be visible above the clavicle in sitting posture. In reclining posture, venous column is visible. However, in that posture the anterior end of 4th intercostal space will be higher in position than in sitting posture. In that case, the vertical distance between upper end of clavicle and 4th space will be reduced. To overcome this fallacy, the midpoint of the anteroposterior line from anterior end of 4th intercostal space and back is marked on lateral chest wall on sitting posture. Then in the reclined posture, the vertical distance between the marked point of lateral chest wall and upper venous column is measured.[10]

Body Position (Fig. 1)

The body angle in which the JVP is measured should be mentioned. JVP can be measured in any angle at which the upper level of the venous column can be seen. At 30–45° angle, upper level of the venous column remains at or just above the level of the clavicle, when the JVP is normal. For this reason, JVP is measured at this angle. If the upper level is found at around the level of the clavicle at this angle, JVP can be taken as normal without measuring it. When the JVP is very high, the upper level cannot be seen at 30–45° angle, because it goes up to earlobe. In that situation, body might have to be kept at 90° angle. If still not visible, patient should be asked to dangle the legs at bedside, to reduce the venous return. Even, patient may be asked to take standing posture. Similarly, when the JVP is low, the angle might have to be reduced to more horizontal position. If still not visible, abdomen may be compressed, or legs may be raised to enhance venous return.

Effect of Respiration

Inspiration causes decreased intrathoracic pressure with reduction of right atrial and jugular mean pressure, in spite of increased venous return. Increased venous return causes increased right atrial contraction and prominent *a* wave. Strong right atrial contraction is followed by rapid relaxation with a prominent *x* descent. Thus, inspiration can make an apparently unimpressive jugular venous pulse more visible. Moreover, inspiratory effect on jugular pulse is a special situation, where the mean pressure falls, but individual waves become prominent.

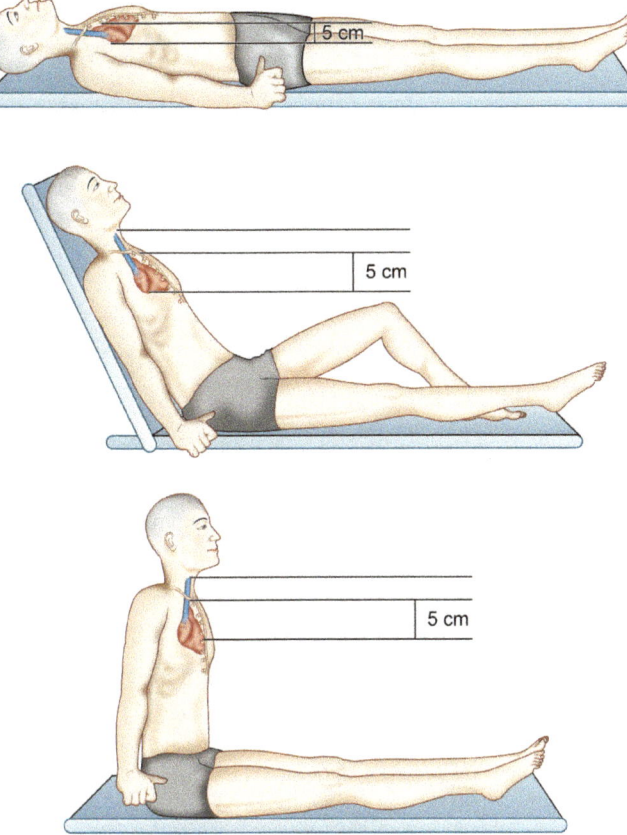

Fig. 1: Distance between center of right atrium and sternal angle is fixed (5 cm), irrespective of body position.

Method

Sternal angle as external reference point:
- Neck muscles should be relaxed.
- A light is shone tangentially from behind or in front of the neck overlying the IJV.
- By simultaneous palpation of the left carotid artery or auscultation helps to decide the time sequences of the pulse waves.
- Deep inspiration that increases venous return to the right heart may make jugular pulsations easier to see.
- When the patient is positioned, the angle should be subtended between the trunk and the bed. The trunk and the neck should be in the same line. Neck is slightly rotated toward left to make the sternomastoid muscle more prominent.
- A vertical line is drawn from sternal angle and another vertical line is drawn from the upper crest to the first vertical line (**Fig. 2**).

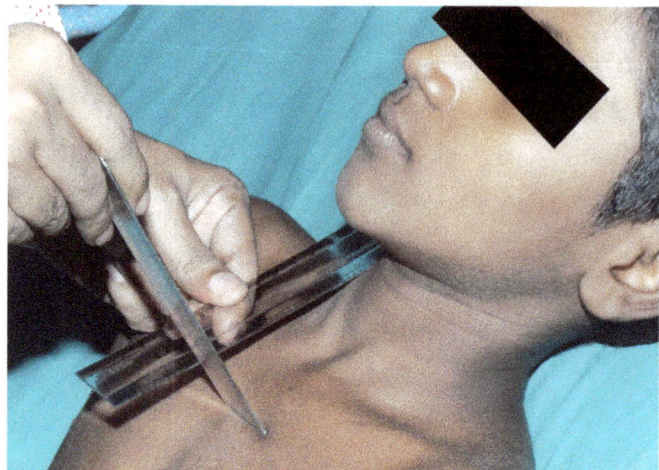

Fig. 2: How to measure jugular venous pressure: A scale is placed vertically from sternal angle. Then, the vertical distance from the top of the venous column to this scale is measured by another scale.

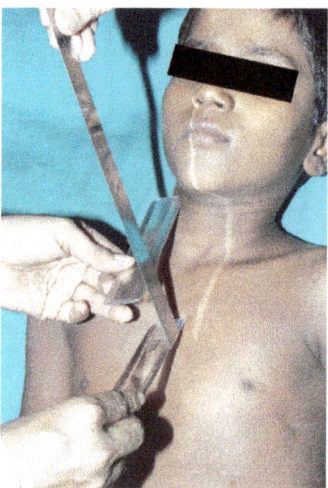

Fig. 3: How to measure jugular venous pressure: Alternately, two scales, horizontal to bed, are held from sternal angle and from top of the venous column, respectively. The vertical distance between these two scales is measured by another scale.

- Two horizontal lines in relation to floor are drawn, one from the sternal angle and the other from the upper level of the venous column. Vertical distance between these two lines is measured and 5 cm is added to it (**Fig. 3**). A simple approach to measure JVP is described in **Table 2**.

Normal Pressure and Units

Normally, this vertical distance is up to 3 cm. Hence, by adding the vertical distance of 5 cm from the center of the right atrium to the sternal angle, the normal

TABLE 2: Simple approach to measure jugular venous pressure (JVP).[11]

Patient inclined at 45°: Upper venous column	JVP
No visible pulsation at the level of clavicle	Normal or low <8 cm of water
Visible pulsation at clavicle level	10 cm of water
At midneck level	15 cm of water
At angle of jaw	20 cm of water

JVP becomes up to 8 cm of blood. This represents (disregarding the specific gravity of blood, which is 1.056) the central venous pressure of 8 cm of water. These figures roughly correlate the normal intracardiac mean right atrial pressure (up to 7–8 mm Hg; 1.3 cm column of water or blood is equal to 1 mm Hg).

Mean Jugular Venous Pressure

Paul Wood used the term "peak" JVP.[12] He described normal peak JVP range between +3 cm and about –5 cm with reference to sternal angle with the patient horizon. Peak of the *a* or *v* wave is not mean pressure, which is actually the mean of both positive and negative waves. Paul Wood also used the term "mean"' JVP. He described[12]—*"The normal jugular venous pulse oscillates gently around a mean level a little below zero with reference to the sternal angle".* Abrams[13] described in relation mean pressure—*"The height of the venous column at the peak of the a and v waves generally is taken as an indication of the venous pressure, although the actual mean jugular venous pressure will be slightly lower".* Applefeld[14] described the measurement of mean pressure—*"To determine the mean jugular venous pressure, the examiner should observe the nadir of the venous column on inspiration and then the crest of this column on expiration. Next, the midpoint of the excursion of the venous pulse during normal respiratory cycles is estimated visually…".* Vertical distance from this intersect point and sternal angle is the mean JVP. Common causes of elevated mean JVP is described in **Box 1**.

Hepatojugular Reflux (Abdominojugular Reflux)

Hepatojugular reflux was first described by Pasteur,[15] as a new sign of tricuspid regurgitation (TR). The concept was that compression must be on an enlarged liver only to induce the jugular reflux, hence the name hepatojugular reflux.

BOX 1 Elevated jugular venous pressure (JVP).
- Congestive heart failure
- Tricuspid stenosis or regurgitation
- An increased blood volume
- An increased intrathoracic or intra-abdominal pressure
- An increased pericardial pressure, such as pericardial tamponade or constrictive pericarditis
- Superior vena cava obstruction (nonpulsatile; sometimes, grossly increased intrapericardial pressure can lead to nonpulsatile elevated JVP)

Abdominal compression raises intra-abdominal pressure and sympathetic tone. Later may be due to patient's apprehension or compression-induced abdominal muscle contraction.[16]

In a normal person, jugular venous column either does not show any change or shows a transient rise. For two to three beats. Here, abdominal compression may transiently increase venous return to right heart chamber, or it has no effect, or it may reduce venous return. The last effect is due to raised intra-abdominal pressure, that obstructs femoral venous return.[17] Right ventricle with a normal end-diastolic pressure, accommodates this extra return without any change in venous pressure. If any rise in jugular venous, that is due to increased venous tone due to raised sympathetic tone.[18]

In congestive heart failure (CHF), there is significant amount of fluid pull in abdomen. Moreover, sympathetic tone is also increased. On abdominal compression, the pulled fluid is shifted to right heart. In CHF, extravenous return in right ventricle with high end-diastolic pressure is high and that extra return results in enhanced venous pressure, which is reflected in JVP. Moreover, venous tone is already high in CHF and the capacitance of thoracic great veins is already reduced due to venoconstriction. Increased sympathetic response on compression acts as an added factor. This enhanced venous tone is responsible for a rise of venous column >3 cm and persist for >15 seconds.[18] This is the basis for hepatojugular reflux in CHF.

Abdomen can be compressed at any place, but preferably, at right upper quadrant, by the palm of the warm hand firmly without hurting, for 15-60 seconds. The patient should be asked to breath normally during the compression. Sometimes, this might be the earliest sign of CHF.

Hepatojugular reflex may also be positive in constrictive pericarditis and tricuspid valve disease. Other conditions with high sympathetic tone without CHF, like thyrotoxicosis, anemia, etc., can produce this reflux.[18] In chronic obstructive pulmonary disease, a false positive result may occur due to high intrathoracic pressure due to change in breathing pattern in the dyspneic patient, which opposes the upward movement of diaphragm during abdominal compression.

NORMAL VENOUS PULSE

Hemodynamic

Normal jugular venous pulse consists of three positive waves and two negative waves (nadir of these negative waves is called troughs). First positive wave is the presystolic *a* wave produced by the right atrial contraction. First negative wave is the diastolic *x* descent produced by atrial relaxation. This trough reaches a plateau (*z* point) before the onset of right ventricular systole. Sometimes, the *x* descent is interrupted by a positive *c* wave, resulting from, bulging of the tricuspid valve into the right atrium during right ventricular isovolumetric systole and effect of the nearby carotid artery shuddering. After the *c* wave, the descent continues as a systolic *x* descent (someone ascribes it as *x'* wave), produced by the right ventricular systole (which pulls down its base that forms the floor of the atrium, resulting in fall of the pressure. Besides this, when the ventricle contracts, its volume shrinks that leads to fall in intrapericardial pressure which is transmitted to the right atrium). Subsequently, in the mid-systole, the right ventricular force of contraction is reduced that attenuates the descent of the base. As a result, the right atrial pressure starts building up due to increased venous return from the vena cava. This is reflected as late systolic positive *v* wave. When the right atrial pressure exceeds the right ventricular pressure, tricuspid valve opens and blood rapidly flows in the right ventricle, resulting in diastolic collapse or the *y* descent. The trough of the *y* descent is followed by its ascending limb, which is produced by the continued diastolic inflow of the blood in the right ventricle. When diastole is prolonged, this ascending limb of the *y* wave is followed by a brief small *h* wave, just prior to next *a* wave. Otherwise, there is a plateau phase.

Pressure wise *a, x, v, y* are 0, –4, 0, –3 mm Hg, respectively and the mean pressure is around zero in reference to sternal angle.[12] Hence, *a* and *v* waves are almost equal in amplitude, where as *x* descent shows the largest excursion.

At Bedside

At bedside, all jugular waves are not always appreciable unless there is slow heart rate or normal PR interval. In a normal jugular venous pulse, right atrial pressure waves, both *a* and *v*, have slow rise and small amplitude, hence normally not appreciable. On the other hand, descents are more appreciable, because:
- They have larger excursions.
- They are rapid movement, moving away from eye.
- Descents actually reflect flow acceleration.
- The reflected light from the skin varies on ascents and descents. During descents, less light is reflected from jugular and the overlying skin looks darker.[18]

Out of two descents, normally *x* wave is more appreciable in compare to *y* descent, as because it shows more excursion. *y* descent is visible in certain conditions with increased sympathetic tone (as explained later) such as in children, young adult, anemia, pregnancy, etc.

Thus, normal jugular venous pulse essentially is *x'* descent!

Time Sequences (Fig. 4)

In brief, *a* wave is diastolic (presystolic), whereas *c* and *v* waves are systolic in timing, though last part of *v* wave is actually in isovolumetric relaxation phase. Initial part of *x* and *y* descents are diastolic, whereas later part of *x* descent (*x'*) is systolic in timing.

Timing by pulse: *x'* descent corresponds with the radial pulse, whereas carotid pulse occurs before the *x'* descent.

Timing by heart sound: The *a* wave corresponds with S4 and approximately simultaneous with the S1, whereas nadir of the *x'* descent falls between S1 and S2 with its nadir occurs just before S2. The *v* wave peaks just after S2.

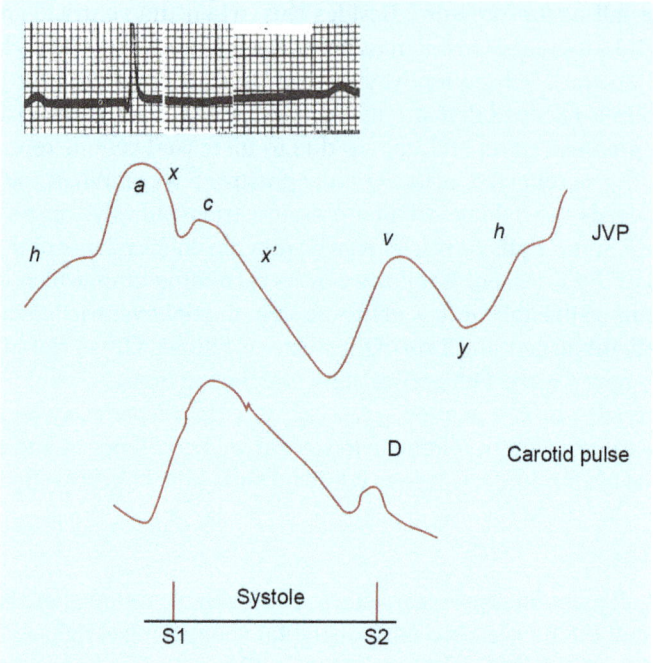

(JVP: jugular venous pressure)

Fig. 4: Time sequences: To identify the venous waves, timing with heart sound and carotid pulse.

ABNORMAL VENOUS PULSE

Pre-*a* Wave Pressure

This is in diastole, when slow filling phase occurs, and right atrial and right ventricular pressure become equal (**Fig. 5**). The tricuspid valve opens, and two chambers act as single chamber. All the pathological conditions affecting right ventricle and reducing its compliance and compressive physiology like constrictive pericarditis increase pre-*a* wave pressure. Pre-*a* wave pressure is the baseline for *a* and *v* waves. Its elevation will always elevate *a* and *v* waves.[19]

Prominent/Large and Giant *a* Waves (Figs. 6 and 7)

Sometimes, gradation is made between prominent/large (pressure corresponds to 3–6 mm Hg) and giant (6–15 mm Hg) *a* wave. These are presystolic, collapsing, and transmitted to liver and correspond to a right-sided S4. Change of posture does not affect, but inspiration increases its amplitude. These waves occur when right atrium contracts against an obstructed tricuspid valve or a noncompliant right ventricle (**Box 2**).

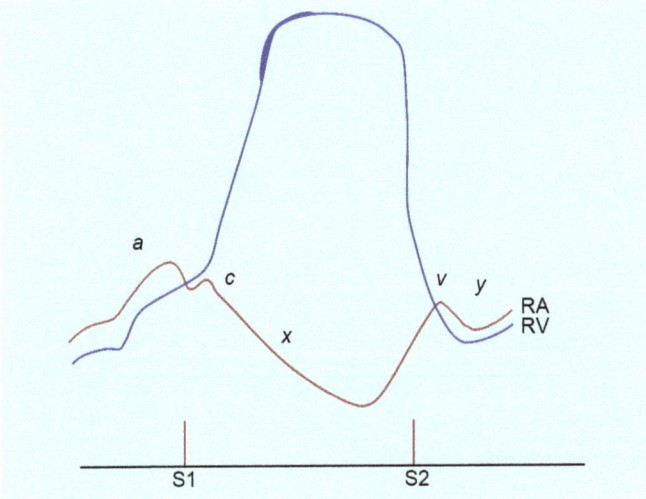

Fig. 5: Right atrial (RA) and right ventricular (RV) pressure curves.

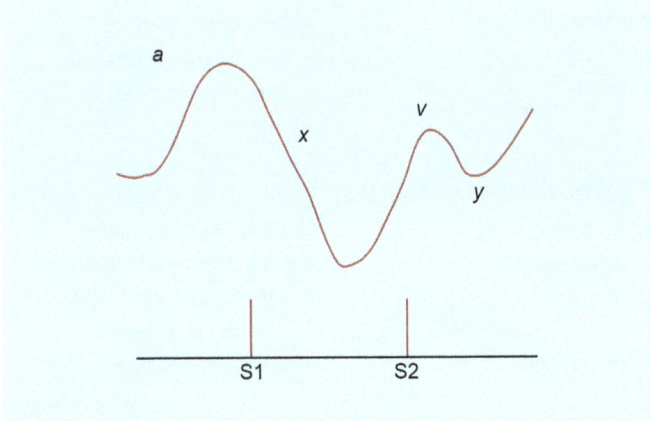

Fig. 6: Prominent *a* wave.

Cannon Wave

If the right atrium contracts against a closed tricuspid valve, the pressure is transmitted retrograde to form a very large *a* wave (roughly, >16 mm Hg), called cannon wave (**Box 3**).

Absent '*a*' Wave

In atrial fibrillation, *a* wave is absent (other features in atrial fibrillation are lesser excursion of *x* descent with a dominant *y* descent).

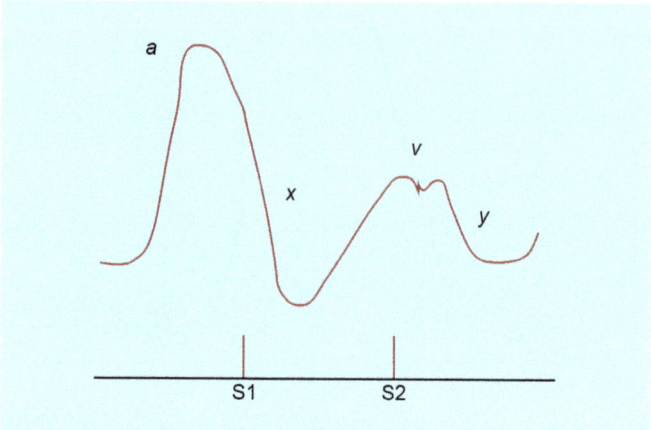

Fig. 7: Giant *a* wave.

BOX 2	Prominent '*a*' wave.
Right ventricular (RV) inflow obstruction: • Tricuspid stenosis • Tricuspid atresia	**RV outflow obstruction:** • Pulmonary stenosis • Pulmonary hypertension • Bernheim's syndrome

BOX 3	Causes of cannon wave.
Regular cannon waves: • Junctional tachycardia • Junctional rhythm • 2:1 atrioventricular block with a prolonged PR interval	**Irregular cannon waves:** • Complete heart block • Ventricular tachycardia • Ventricular ectopic • Ventricular pacing

Abnormal *x* Descent

The *x* descent occurs before the major systolic *x'* descent. In prolonged PR interval, *x* descent is delayed and even can occur at end-diastole and can be differentiated from diastolic descent by ECG only.

Abnormal *x'* Descent

A good *x'* descent indicates good right ventricular function, as its contraction contributes to movement of tricuspid valve and *x'* descent. Most important cause of blunted *x'* descent is right ventricular dysfunction. A small *x'* descent occurs in TR and atrial fibrillation. In TR, the descent even might be replaced by early systolic positive wave, produced by the regurgitant blood into the right atrium and reducing the usual systolic fall in venous pressure. Atrium fails to relax in atrial fibrillation, which causes diminished excursion of the descent. However, this wave is not obliterated, because of the other contributing factor for this wave, that is the descent of the base of the atrium by right ventricular systole. This wave is also obliterated in congenital absence of the pericardium. A prominent x' wave is sometimes found in constrictive pericarditis (**Box 4**).

Abnormal *v* Wave (Fig. 8)

How large the *v* wave should be in TR depends on its severity, whether low-pressure or high-pressure TR and the size of the right atrium. Even a moderate TR with a large accommodative right atrium produces only a prominent *v* wave. The *v* wave is followed by sharp *y* descent, from which *v* wave is identified, as descents dare always better appreciable. Higher the grade of the TR, larger is the systolic venous wave encroaching upon the *x* descent. Severe high-pressure TR produces a very large systolic wave that completely obliterates the *x* descent (ventricularization), looks like a venous Corrigan, and results in a pulsatile liver and sometimes even a pulsatile exophthalmoses. An elevated *v* wave has a longer duration and always increases mean JVP (**Box 5**).

Abnormal y Descent

Basic etiology is a large *v* wave and no restriction to early rapid filling phase of right ventricle. A rapid and sharp *y* descent is suggestive of TR, which is usually accompanied by a large *v* wave. A sharp *y* descent with a deep trough and a rapid

BOX 4	Reduced x' descent.

- Right ventricular systolic dysfunction
- Tricuspid regurgitation
- Atrial fibrillation

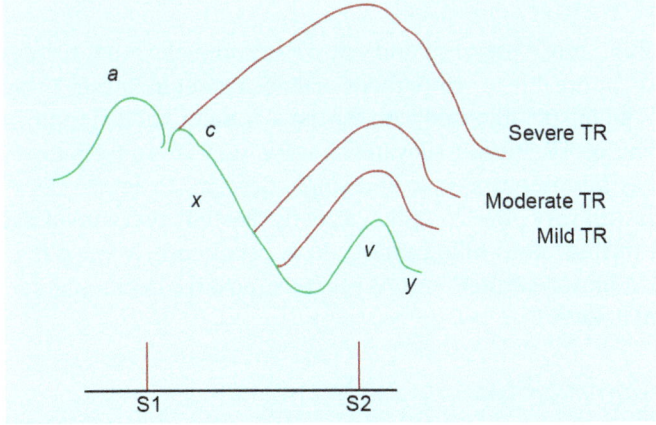

Fig. 8: Severe the tricuspid regurgitation (TR), larger will be the *v* wave. It will encroach upon *x* descent, that eventually will be obliterated in severe TR.

> **BOX 5** **Large v wave.**
> - Any condition raising pre-*a* wave pressure
> - Tricuspid regurgitation (due to regurgitant blood from right ventricle)
> - Atrial septal defect (due to shunted blood from left atrium; another explanation is the transmission of the left atrial pulse pressure through the defect in the venous pulse, thus equalizing the *a* and the *v* waves)
> - Anomalous pulmonary venous drainage in the right atrium
> - Congestive heart failure (due to high venous pressure or high right atrial and right ventricular pressure)
> - Constrictive pericarditis (due to decreased right atrial compliance)
> - Rapid circulation time, as in anemia, exercise, hyperthyroidism (due to rapid atrial filling)

> **BOX 6** **Prominent y descents.**
> - Increased sympathetic tone with rapid circulation time (children, anemia, thyrotoxicosis, pregnancy, etc.)
> - Constrictive pericarditis
> - Hypervolemia
> - Any condition, which increases right ventricular end-diastolic pressure, like pulmonary hypertension, right ventricular dysfunction, and cardiomyopathy

ascent is typical of constrictive pericarditis and severe right heart failure. In both conditions, venous pressure is high; however, the later condition is accompanied by the prominent systolic wave. A slow *y* descent is found in tricuspid stenosis and right atrial tumor, which prevent atrial emptying. Pericardial tamponade, due to high pericardial pressure, prevents ventricular filling and produces a slow *y* descent, in spite of elevated *v* wave (**Box 6**).

SPECIFIC SITUATIONS

Congestive Heart Failure

In heart failure, pre-*a* pressure and *v* wave become elevated. Increased venous tone in heart failure due to sympathetic activity further increases *v* wave pressure. *x'* descent is inconspicuous and with the development of TR, it is further reduced. Development of TR further elevates *v* wave and in consequence, *x'* is lost. Thus, there is prominent *v* wave and single descent. In severe right ventricular dysfunction with very poor compliance, early diastolic pressure of right ventricle is elevated during rapid filling phase. In consequence, *y* wave is lost. Jugular venous pulse shows elevated venous pressure, positive hepatojugular reflux, and a prominent *v* wave.

Jugular Venous Pulse in Arrhythmia

The *a* and *v* waves correspond with the P and QRS complex in the ECG and *a* wave falls on S1. Hence, in sinus rhythm, *a* wave is followed by *v* wave.

In first-degree AV block, *a* wave (P) will occur well before S1 (onset of ventricular systole/QRS complex), indicating a prolonged PR interval; with further prolongation, *a* wave merges with previous *v* wave (**Fig. 9**).

In second-degree type 1 AV block, *a-v* interval will gradually lengthen, ending with *a* wave not followed by *v* wave or S1. In type 2 block, if 2:1, there will be two *a* wave for each *v* wave; with a prolonged PR interval, alternate *a* wave will coincide the ventricular systole, resulting in regular cannon wave. In complete heart block, *a-v* interval will be variable, with more *a* waves than *v* wave and irregular cannon waves.

Irregular cannon waves are also found in ventricular ectopic or ventricular tachycardia, whereas this wave is regular in junctional rhythm (**Figs. 10 and 11**).

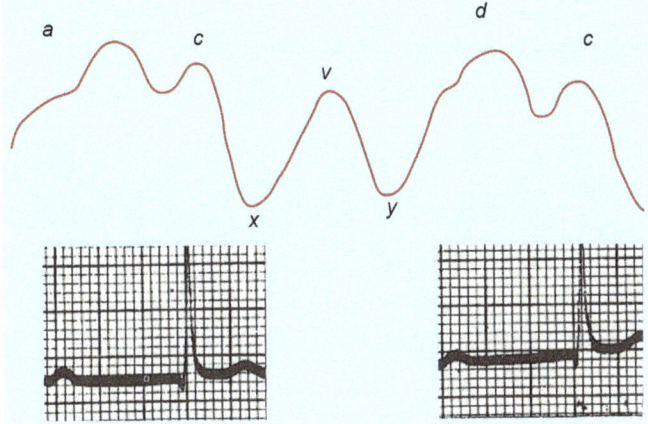

Fig. 9: First degree atrioventricular block: *a* wave (P) will occur well before S1 (onset of ventricular systole/QRS complex), indicating prolonged PR interval (normally, *a* wave corresponds with S1).

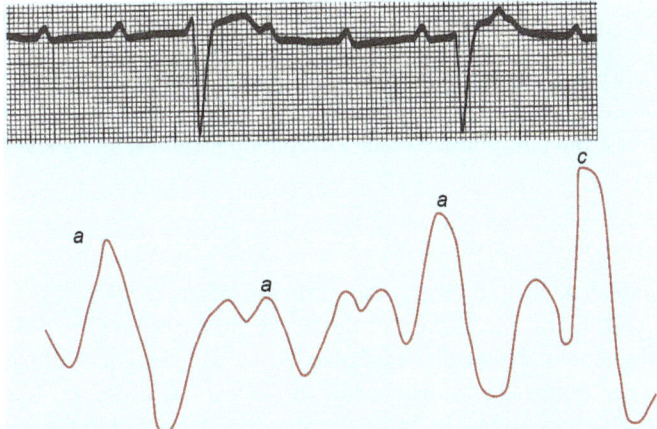

Fig. 10: Irregular cannon waves (c) in complete heart block. More *a* waves than *v* waves and intermittent cannon waves.

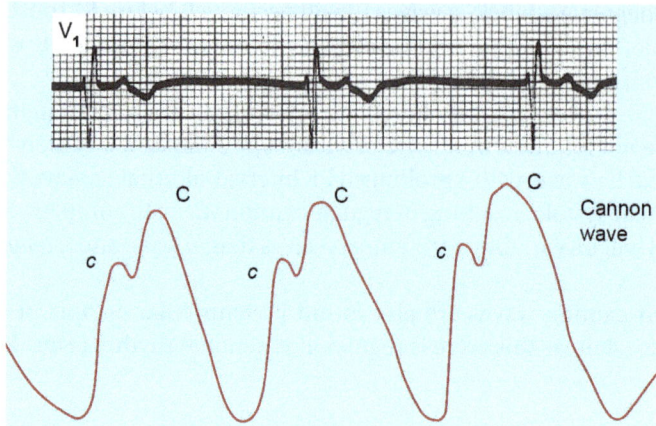

Fig. 11: Regular cannon waves in junctional rhythm.

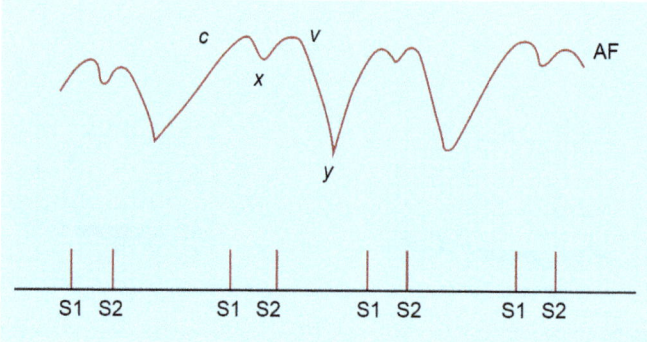

Fig. 12: Venous pulsation in atrial fibrillation (AF): Here, *a* wave is absent with diminished *x* descent, steeper *v* wave, and sharp *y* descent.

In atrial fibrillation, as mentioned earlier, *a* wave is absent. Due to absence of atrial booster, right ventricular contraction is poor, resulting in diminished *x* descent. Poor atrial compliance results in a steeper *v* wave and a sharp *y* descent (**Fig. 12**).

Jugular Venous Pulse in Pericardial Disease

Pericardial sac has a small reserve volume and when exceeded, the pericardial pressure operating on the surface of the heart increases rapidly; this pressure is transmitted inside of the cardiac chambers. So a component of the intracavitary filling pressure represents transmission of pericardial pressure. Besides these facts, respiratory changes in intrathoracic pressure are transmitted to the intracavitary pressure though pericardial space. When this space is obliterated, this transmission does not occur any more.

Cardiac tamponade: The above facts will explain the changes in JVP in pericardial diseases. Simple pericardial effusion, even if massive, does not produce any changes. But a tamponade, even with a small effusion, results in loss of *y* descent. Tamponade causes an elevated and equal intracavitary filling pressure and a fixed total heart volume. As a result, blood can enter the heart only when blood is leaving. *y* descent occurs in diastole, when tricuspid valve is opening (blood is not leaving the heart). Thus, no blood can enter the heart and *y* descent is inconspicuous. *x* descent occurs during ventricular ejection (blood is leaving the heart). Thus, venous inflow can increase normally, retaining the *x* descent.

Pericardial constriction causes markedly reduced filling of all the cardiac chambers resulting in equal elevation of filling pressure of all the cardiac chambers. As the end-systolic volume is small, there is rapid ventricular suction in early diastole; right atrial pressure is also elevated. These two factors cause rapid early diastolic filling and a prominent *y* descent. The normally prominent *x* descent is preserved. Thus, an elevated pressure with an M-shaped pulse constitutes the typical JVP in constrictive pericarditis (**Fig. 13**).

Inspiration causes decreased intrathoracic pressure with reduction of right atrial and jugular mean pressure, in spite of increased venous return. Increased venous return causes increased right atrial contraction and prominent *a* wave. Strong right atrial contraction is followed by rapid relaxation with a prominent *x* descent. Inspiratory fall of intrathoracic pressure is not transmitted to right heart chambers. As a result, right atrium does not expand on inspiration. Thus, mean JVP may remain same. Usual venous return makes the prominent *y* and *x* trough more prominent. Severe constriction makes right-sided chambers grossly noncompliant, so that they cannot accommodate the extra amount from venous return, resulting in inspiratory rise of mean venous pressure. This sign, JVP remaining same or rising on inspiration, is Kussmaul sign.

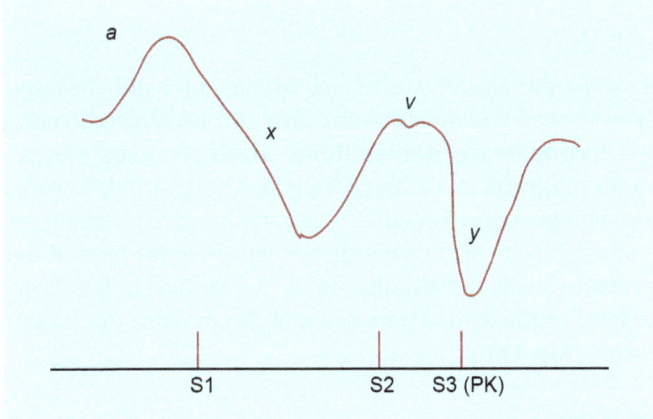

Fig. 13: Venous pulsation in constrictive pericarditis: There is prominent *y* descent corresponds with pericardial knock (PK). The normally prominent *x* descent is preserved. Thus, an elevated pressure with an M-shaped pulse constitutes jugular venous pressure.

Jugular Venous Pulse in Congenital Cyanotic Heart Disease

Jugular venous pulse is inconspicuous in the most common cyanotic groups—Fallot's physiology. In spite of the right ventricular outflow tract (RVOT) stenosis, *a* wave is not prominent because the right ventricle decompresses through ventricular septal defect (VSD). Only when the VSD becomes restrictive by the tricuspid leaflet or when there is associated hypertension or one with this disease reaches adulthood, prominent *a* wave is found. A prominent *a* wave is also found in tricuspid atresia, pulmonary stenosis with right to left shunt through stretched patent foramen ovale or pulmonary atresia with intact septum.

Jugular venous pulse in Ebstein's anomaly is characterized by prominent *c* wave. In fact, prominence of *c* wave correlates closely with the severity of displacement of the tricuspid valve and the size of the atrialized right ventricle.[20] Though TR may be severe, *v* wave is often inconspicuous, because large right atrium along with atrialized right ventricle accommodates low-pressure regurgitation volume without much elevation of venous pressure. Hence, prominent *v* and *a* waves are occasionally found.

OTHER VENOUS PULSES

Hepatic Pulse

Hepatic pulsations are in the same tune of jugular venous pulsations, transmitted through inferior vena cava to hepatic veins. Right palm should be placed in patient's right upper quadrant. Patient's breath should be held in mid-inspiration and palm edge should be in contact with hepatic edge. If pulsatile, its pulsation can be felt. In significant TR, hepatic pulsation can be felt.

Upper Arm Veins

Upper arm veins, particularly veins on dorsum of hand, become distended with increased central venous pressure. This can be utilized when anatomical abnormalities preclude assessment from jugular venous waves. Patient is positioned with the trunk at 30° angle from bed and hand is lowered below the sternal angle. Veins become distended. Then, arm is raised gradually and passively. With a normal venous pressure, veins get collapsed at the level of sternum. With increased pressure, veins remain distended. The vertical height from the sternal angle to the level of the arm, where veins of the dorsum get collapsed, is the venous pressure (**Fig. 14**).

CONCLUSION

Jugular venous pulse is one of the most impressive noninvasive bedside hemodynamic tool. Its role in modern cardiology is very much relevant.

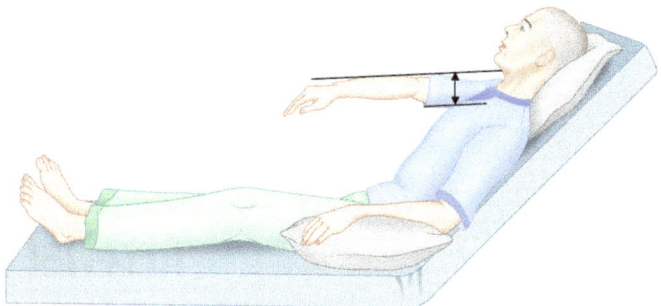

Fig. 14: How to measure venous pressure from upper arm: Arm raised to a height, when the veins on dorsum of hand collapses. A horizontal line is drawn from the hand and its vertical distance from the sternal angle is the jugular venous pressure.

REFERENCES

1. Sleight P. Unilateral elevation of the internal jugular pulse. Br Heart J. 1962;24:726-30.
2. Hurst JW, Schlant RC. Examination of the veins. In: The Heart, 4th edition. New York: McGraw-Hill Book Company; 1978. p. 193.
3. Winsar T, Burch GE. Phlebostatic level, reference levels for venous pressure and measurements in man. Proc Soc Exp Biol Med. 1945;58:165-9.
4. Swartz MH. Textbook of Physical Diagnosis: History and Examination, 5th edition. Edinburgh: Elsevier Inc; 2007. p. 418-21.
5. Chatterjee K, Otto CM, Yeon SB. Examination of the jugular venous pulse. UpToDate. 2009;17:2.
6. Seth R, Magner P, Matzinger F, et al. How far is the sternal angle from the mid-right atrium? J Gen Intern Med. 2002;17:852-6.
7. Devine PJ, Sullenberger LE, Bellin DA, et al. Jugular venous pulse: Window into the right heart. South Med J. 2007;100:1022.
8. Sinisalo J, Rapola J, Rossinen J, et al. Simplifying the estimation of jugular venous pressure Am J Cardiol. 2007;100:1779-81.
9. Bhattari MD. Prospects of jugular venous pulse assessment. J Nepal Med Assoc. 2010;49: 247-54.
10. LeBlond RF, DeGowin RL, Brown DD. DeGowin's Diagnostic Examination, 8th edition. Boston: Mc Graw Hill; 2004. pp. 365-8.
11. Miranda WR, Nishimura RA. The history, physical examination and cardiac auscultation. In: The Heart, 14th edition. New York: McGraw-Hill. 2017. p. 234.
12. Wood P. Diseases of the Heart and Circulation. Philadelphia: JB Lippincott; 1968.
13. Abrams J. The jugular venous pulse. In: Abrams J (Ed). Synopsis of Cardiac Physical Diagnosis, 2nd edition. Woburn: Butterworth-Heinemann; 2001.
14. Appelfeld MM. The jugular venous pressure and pulse contour. In: Walker HK, Hall WD, Hurst JW (Eds). Clinical Methods, 3rd edition. Boston: Butterworth; 1990.
15. Pasteur W. Note on a new physical sign of tricuspid regurgitation. Lancet. 1885;2:524.
16. Constant J, Lippschutz EJ. The one minute abdominal compression test or "the hepatojugular reflux," a useful bedside test. Am Heart J. 1964;67:701.
17. Constant J. Bedside Cardiology, 3rd edition. Boston: Little Brown; 1985.
18. Ranganathan N, Sivaciyan V, Saksena FB. The Art and Science of Cardiac Physical Examination. Humana Press, Springer; 2006. p. 84.
19. Ranganathan N, Sivaciyan V. Jugular venous flow velocity pattern, application to bedside recognition of jugular venous pulse contour and right heart hemodynamics. Am J Noninvas Cardiol. 1993;7:75-88.
20. Hosoi K, Fukuda N, Luchi A, et al. Characteristics of jugular venous pulse and its genesis in Ebstein's anomaly. J Cardiol. 1992;22:475-85.

CHAPTER 11

Arterial Pulse

"Quincke's sign is a waste of time.
de Musset was a master of rhyme
But, he was no doc;
His sign was ad hoc,
An aortic insufficiently mime".
—**Joseph D Sapira**

INTRODUCTION

"Abu Ali placed his hand on the patient's pulse, and mentioned the names of the different districts and continued until he reached the name of a quarter at the mention of which, as he uttered it, the patient's pulse gave a strange flutter. Then Abu Ali repeated the names of different streets of that district and different houses till he reached the name of a house at the mention of which the patient's pulse gave the same flutter. Finally, he uttered the name of different households of that house until he reached a name at the mention of which that strange flutter resumed. There upon he said: This man is in love with such-and-such a girl, in such-and-such a house, in such-and-such a street, in such-and-such a quarter: The girl's face is the patient's cure"!

Abu Ali Ibn Sina was a Persian physician of middle age, when pulse was used to diagnose every aspect in life!

(Quoted from: The Chahar Maqala of Nidhami-i-'Arudi-i-Samarqandi, S. Austin and Sons, Hertford, UK, 1899, Anecdote xxxv, translated into English by Edward Granville Browne).

ORIGIN OF PULSE

Prologue[1,2]

Arterial pulse wave begins with left ventricular ejection and aortic valve opening. Arterial pressure pulse enters the proximal aorta and travels distally as a velocity many times faster than blood flow. This wave is accompanied by a traveling wave distending the arterial wall. In the periphery, the arteries, being more branched and smaller, become stiffer, resulting in increased pulse wave velocity.

Aortic pressure rises rapidly in early systole. The rapid rising portion of the arterial pressure curve is termed anacrotic limb. After the peak, as ventricular ejection decreases and peripheral flow continues, pulse pressure has its descending limb.

During isovolumetric relaxation period, momentary reversal of flow occurs from aorta toward left ventricular before the aortic valve closure causing the incisura on the descending limb.

Incisura is followed by the secondary positive wave, due to elastic recoil of the aorta and aortic valve as well as reflected wave from the peripheral arterial system. Descending limb continues, as peripheral run off continues.

Proximal Aortic Pulse (Fig. 1)

There are two positive waves during systole: First shoulder is termed percussion wave and second one as tidal wave. Percussion wave is due to impulse generated by left ventricular ejection and the tidal wave is its echo from upper part of the body. Dicrotic wave following the incisura is due to reflection from lower part of the body.

Percussion wave is usually more prominent than tidal wave. However, in situations like aging, arteriosclerosis, and diabetes mellitus, tidal wave is equally or may be more prominent. At the same time, these factors make dicrotic wave less prominent.

Carotid Pulse

Carotid pulse has a smooth rapid ascending limb with a smooth dome. Dicrotic notch and waves are not very prominent. Descending wave is less rapid than ascending one. Percussion wave is usually more prominent than tidal wave.

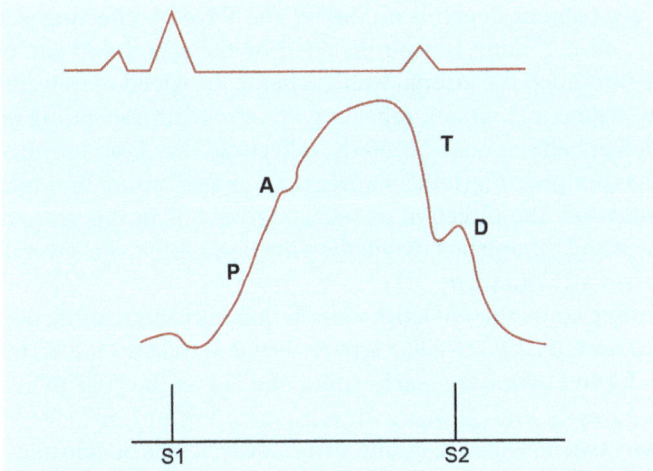

Fig. 1: Proximal aortic pulse: Initial part of the pulse in early systole is percussion wave (P), which is interrupted by anacrotic notch (A). Rest of the systolic wave is the tidal wave (T). The diastole starts with dicrotic notch or incisura, the nadir of which corresponds to A2, followed by the diastolic dicrotic wave (D).

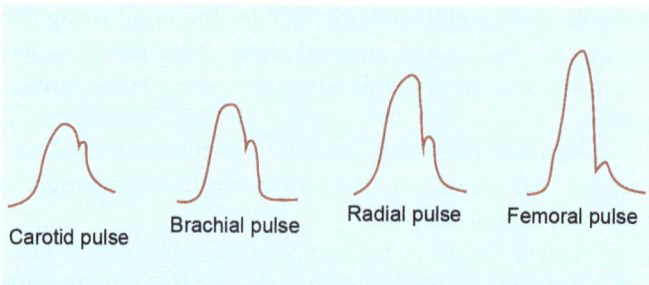

Fig. 2: Changes of pulse waves during peripheral transmission.

Changes during Peripheral Transmission (Fig. 2)

Ascending limb becomes steeper. Incisura is replaced by smoother dicrotic notch in a later part of the descending limb. There is high peak pressure and pulse pressure, whereas diastolic pressure and mean pressure are slightly lower. In a peripheral pulse, anacrotic notch, tidal wave, dicrotic notch, and dicrotic wave cannot be appreciated.

Reflecting Wave[3]

Incident pressure pulse is reflected back from the branching points of the periphery. This reflecting wave plays an important role in deciding the pulse wave contour. Normally, 80% of incident wave is reflected back. Aortic bifurcation is the major reflecting site. Rest of the reflection occurs from the arteriolar sites from both upper and lower body segment. Increased peripheral resistance increases reflection, whereas vasodilatation reduces it.

Pulse wave contour depends on timing and force of reflecting wave meeting the incident wave. Timing is again decided by the speed and site of reflecting wave. More thickened the arterial wall, higher is the speed of reflecting wave. As upper body segment is nearer, reflecting wave reaches ascending aorta earlier than from lower half segment. Similarly, reflecting wave from terminal arterioles reaches large peripheral arteries earlier than central aorta. The incident wave is enhanced, when the direction of reflecting wave is in the same direction of incident wave and diminished, when the direction is opposite. Overall, reflective wave facilitates incident wave.

In ascending aorta, the reflective wave augments central aortic pressure, both systolic and diastolic. In muscular arteries like femoral and radial, the reflective waves from further periphery reach earlier and fall on the peak of incident wave and enhance systolic and pulse pressure, more significantly in lower limbs. When the reflective wave reaches ascending aorta slowly, it falls on diastole and creates diastolic or dicrotic wave. When it reaches fast, it falls on systole and creates a second late systolic wave, the tidal wave.[4]

BOX 1	What one should look for?
• Rate, rhythm, and pulse deficit • Rate of rise/upstroke • Amplitude/volume • Special character/contour	• Condition of arterial wall • Synchrony • Scale

BOX 2	Pulsation and obstruction scale.
Pulsation scale: • *Grade 0*: Absent pulsation • *Grade 1*: Reduced pulsation • *Grade 2*: Comparably less than opposite side • *Grade 3*: Normal pulsation • *Grade 4*: Bounding pulsation	Obstruction scale (by auscultation of the artery): • *50% obstruction of artery*: Short systolic bruit • *80% obstruction of artery*: Continuous bruit • *>80% obstruction of artery*: No audible bruit

BASIC METHOD (BOXES 1 AND 2)

What one feels by the tactile receptors of the fingers is the movement of the arterial wall by the pressure wave. This movement is maximum in the proximal aorta in proportion to pulse pressure but minimum in the peripheral artery like radial artery.

Trisection: One should assess the upstroke, systolic peak, and the down stroke of the pulse by applying different degree of pressure.

With a few exceptions, in the carotid pulse, one should assess nature of the pulse, which is the direct reflection of the central aortic pulse. It can be timed by the S1, which occurs before the pulsation. Pulsus alternans is best appreciated in radial or femoral pulse, whereas pulsus bisferiens is best appreciated in carotid or brachial artery. Radial pulse is for the rate and the rhythm.

RATE AND RHYTHM

Bradyarrhythmia (Box 3)

A slow, regular pulse with regular cannon wave indicates slow junctional rhythm. A slow, regular pulse with variable amplitude, irregular cannon waves, and varying intensity of S1 indicate atrioventricular (AV) dissociation. Pulsus bigeminy may produce irregular slow pulse when weak ventricular contraction cannot open the aortic valve and not all the ectopic impulses are felt in the peripheral pulse. Auscultation will establish the sequence of short pause-weak beat versus long pause-strong beat sequence, characteristic of bigeminy.

BOX 3	Causes of bradyarrhythmia.
Regular: • Sinus bradycardia • Junctional rhythm • Complete heart block	**Irregular:** • Pulsus bigeminy

BOX 4	Causes of tachyarrhythmia.
Regular: • Sinus tachycardia • Paroxysmal supraventricular tachycardia • Atrial flutter • Ventricular tachycardia	**Irregular:** • Atrial fibrillation • Frequent ventricular premature beats • Chaotic atrial tachycardia/multifocal atrial tachycardia

Tachyarrhythmia (Box 4)

On carotid sinus massage, pulse rate will slow down gradually in sinus tachycardia and it will rise gradually on release. In atrial flutter, the change will be in a jerky pattern. In paroxysmal supraventricular tachycardia (PSVT), the tachycardia may be converted totally. In atrial fibrillation (AF), pulse is irregular in rhythm, amplitude, and pulse pressure with a pulse deficit (difference between heart and pulse rate) >10 beats/minute.

RATE OF RISE/UPSTROKE

Upstroke is the rate of rise of pulse from its onset to peak. Upstroke is best judged in carotid. Normal rate of rise in carotid is just a sharp and rapid tap against the palpating finger, this is because left ventricle ejects most of its volume in first third of systole. Slow rate of rise can be described as a push and indicates left ventricular outflow obstruction. Very rapid rise of pulse (brisk) is associated with high volume.

AMPLITUDE/VOLUME

Amplitude is the displacement of the arterial wall felt by palpating fingers. Displacement is decided by the tension in arterial wall created between diastole and systole. Tension increases as pressure and diameter increases. High stroke volume increases the arterial diameter and pulse amplitude. Pulse is called high-volume, which is loosely used in place of amplitude. Rise of pressure specifically pulse pressure increases amplitude. On the other hand, low stroke volume and low blood pressure cause reduced wall tension and poor displacement. This is low-volume pulse. It may be described as normal, low or high amplitude/volume pulse. Carotid is the usual place to assess amplitude.

Low Amplitude/Volume: Hypokinetic Pulse

Hypokinetic pulse is a small, weak pulse due to slow ejection of small stroke volume from left ventricle. It is associated with increased arterial resistance and narrow pulse pressure. Common causes are hypovolemia, left ventricular systolic dysfunction, and left ventricular inflow or outflow obstruction.

High Amplitude/Volume, Rapid Rise with Increased Pulse Pressure: Hyperkinetic Pulse

Hyperkinetic pulse is a large, bounding pulse due to rapid ejection of large volume of blood from left ventricle. It is associated with increased pulse pressure and decreased peripheral resistance. The pulse is better felt in brachial, radial, or femoral rather than carotid artery. Common causes are hyperdynamic circulation (exercise, fever, and anemia), conditions with increased stroke volume, and abnormal run off from arterial system.

Rapid Rise with Normal Pulse Pressure

It is found in mitral regurgitation and ventricular septal defect. Regurgitant volume and shunted volume increases left ventricular volume, which is rapidly ejected both in aorta and left atrium or right ventricle. This has two effects, brisk rise and not a very high stroke volume, resulting in a rapid rise of pulse with normal pulse pressure.

CHARACTER

Double-peaked/Double-beating Pulse (Fig. 3)

- Bisferiens pulse
- Dicrotic pulse
- Anacrotic pulse

At bedside, it is not always easy to distinguish between anacrotic, dicrotic, and bisferiens pulse. Anacrotic pulse—positive waves are on the ascending limb. Bisferiens—percussion and tidal waves are near the summit. Both peaks are in systole. Dicrotic pulse—percussion wave is near the summit and dicrotic wave is well down the descending limb. One peak is in systole and another is in diastole.

Bisferiens Pulse

In 1532, Galen first described pulsus bisferiens. Pulsus bisferiens consists of two positive waves during systole, with a mid-systolic dip. First wave is the rapid and forceful upstroke, the percussion wave. Second wave is the smaller and slow rising tidal wave reflected from the periphery. Usually best felt in carotid or brachial artery.

Clinical trial comparing central and peripheral arterial pressure pulses does not support the concept of a reflected component of the tidal wave and it is suggested that the anacrotic and bisferiens pulses do not consist of separate

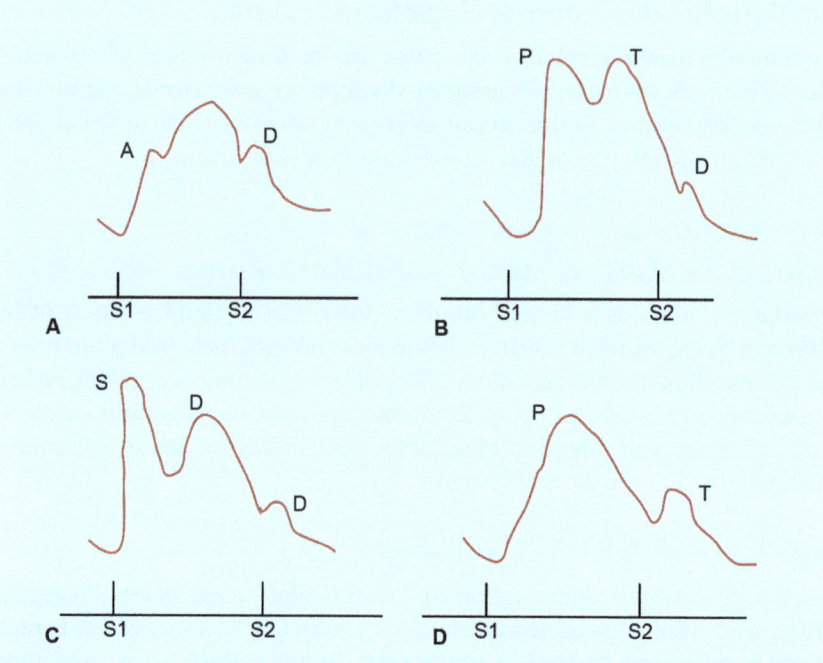

Figs. 3A to D: Double-peaked pulse. (A) Anacrotic pulse of severe aortic stenosis. It is of small amplitude, delayed peak with prominent anacrotic wave (A). Both waves are systolic; (B) pulsus bisferiens in aortic regurgitation. It is of high amplitude with rapid upstroke with percussion (P) and tidal (T) waves, both peaks in systole; (C) pulsus bisferiens in hypertrophic obstructive cardiomyopathy. It is of medium amplitude with rapid upstroke, the spike (S) with both waves is in systole. Second wave, the dome (D) is a sustained wave, like aortic stenosis and unlike of aortic regurgitation; (D) dicrotic pulse: It is of small amplitude gradual upstroke and down stroke with prominent dicrotic wave (D), which is diastolic in timing.

percussion and tidal waves, but are single wave deformed by the suction effect (Venturi effect) of a high-velocity bloodstream.[5] Thus, hemodynamics of pulsus bisferiens is Bernoulli effect. The rapid jet, at its peak, has a suction effect with decreased lateral force on the arterial wall. This causes midsystolic dip.

Common causes are significant aortic regurgitation with mild-to-moderate aortic stenosis, severe aortic regurgitation combined with mild aortic stenosis, any condition having large stroke volume with rapid upstroke from left ventricle, and hypertrophic obstructive cardiomyopathy (HOCM). The second wave is always larger than first wave in aortic regurgitation and stenosis situation, whereas in HOCM, first wave is prominent. Bisferiens nature is better appreciable in carotid. In the periphery, due to effect of reflective wave, the tidal wave becomes so prominent that it may mask the percussion wave.

Dicrotic Pulse

Dicrotic pulse has two peaks—one in systole and the other in diastole, latter is due to prominent diastolic wave. Physiologically, there is slow rate of rise and narrow pulse pressure, inconspicuous percussion and tidal waves, and low dicrotic notch and prominent dicrotic wave. It is best felt in carotid pulse. Dicrotic wave occurs after second heart sound.

There must be three physiological conditionings, when reflective wave may create prominent diastolic or dicrotic wave. They are low arterial pressure (slows down pulse wave), vasoconstriction (causes intensification of reflective wave), and shortened left ventricular ejection time (helps reflective wave to fall on incident wave after aortic valve closure).[3] These three conditionings are present in situations like severe left ventricular dysfunction associated with low stroke volume, cardiac tamponade, high systemic vascular resistance, young febrile patient, septic shock, and patient on intra-aortic balloon pump (diastolic augmentation).

Anacrotic Pulse/Pulsus Parvus et Tardus

Anacrotic pulse is a small amplitude pulse (Parvus) with delayed peak of the upstroke (Tardus) along with a shoulder on the upstroke, anacrotic notch. It is best felt in carotid artery, and can be felt in radial artery. When anacrotic notch is found immediately after the onset of upstroke, aortic stenosis is hemodynamically significant (gradient >70 mm Hg).

At bedside, delayed peak of the carotid pulse can be assessed by simultaneous auscultation and carotid artery palpation. Normally the carotid peak is closure to S1. In significant aortic stenosis, peak is delayed and gets closer to S2. Common causes are moderate or severe aortic stenosis and occasionally severe left ventricular systolic dysfunction. In elderly with aortic stenosis, due to noncompliant carotid artery, the pulse may not be typical.

Rapidly Rising, High Volume, Rapidly Collapsing Pulse (Fig. 4)

Water hammer, bounding, Corrigan, Cellar or Watson pulse should be described as rapidly rising, high amplitude/volume, collapsing pulse to denote the physiology better. In 1833, John Corrigan first described the pulse and in 1844, Thomas Watson used the term water hammer. High amplitude/volume is due to regurgitant volume increasing the stroke volume. Higher end-diastolic volume causes a forceful and rapid rate of rise of left ventricular pressure pulse, resulting in rapidly rising pulse.

Collapse occurs due to run off in two phases—in late systole and in diastole. Reflex vasodilatation and decreased peripheral resistance due to high stroke volume result in low diastolic pressure and peripheral run off. Central run off is due to back flow from high-pressure to low-pressure chamber (**Box 5**).

Mechanism

Water hammer is in reference to a toy in Victorian era, a sealed tube of vacuum partially filled with water. When the toy is raised and turned upside, the fluid falls rapidly with hammer-like slap on fingers.

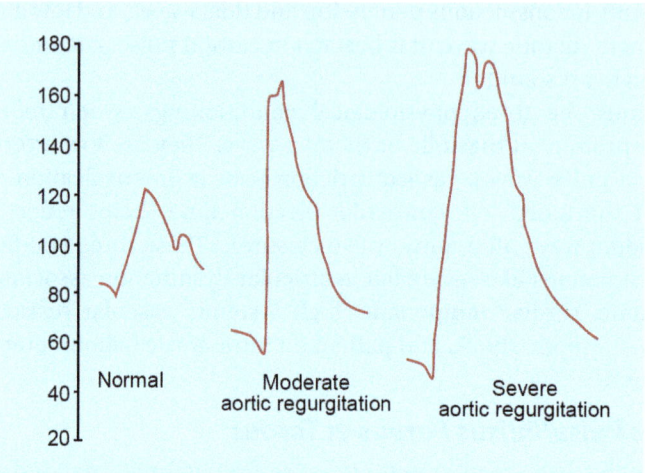

Fig. 4: Rapidly rising, high volume, rapidly collapsing pulse in aortic regurgitation. With increasing severity, pulse pressure widens.

BOX 5	Causes of rapidly rising, high volume, collapsing pulse.
Both central and peripheral run off:	**Peripheral run off:**
• Most common cause aortic regurgitation • Patent ductus arteriosus/ruptured sinus of Valsalva • Arteriovenous fistula • Truncus arteriosus	• Severe anemia, high fever, pregnancy, thyrotoxicosis

Raising the arm above the head causes rapid emptying of blood during diastole due to gravity. Fall in intra-arterial diastolic pressure with further widening of pulse pressure.[3] In consequence, pressure-volume curve is shifted with resultant increased arterial compliance.[6] Thus, amplitude of radial artery pulsation is increased. Raising the arm also brings the radial artery more in line with the outflow stream of the aorta. Pulsus bisferiens is best felt in the radial artery; patient's wrist is held in such a way, so that the pulps of the palm are rested on the radial artery and his arm is suddenly raised above his shoulder.

Unified Theory for Pulsus Bisferiens and Water Hammer Pulse

Long back, in 1876 Galabin demonstrated the graphical pattern of water hammer pulse, which he showed was characterized by sudden narrow peak in early systole followed by a sharp descent in midsystole, during ventricular ejection and the diastolic wave is relatively flat.[7] The study showed that the fall was in systole. This speaks against the diastolic theory of water hammer pulse. Very recently,

Chirinos et al.[8] proposed a unified theory for the radial water hammer and carotid bisferiens pulse. They used wave intensity analysis and demonstrated that—*"an abnormally pronounced forward-traveling mid-systolic suction wave, which immediately followed the initial forward-traveling compression wave from ventricular contraction, explained these pulse patterns. This suction wave likely resulted from blood inertia, arising from a ventricle ejecting a very large stroke volume into a vasodilated arterial tree."*

Pulsus Alternans (Mechanical Alternans)

Pulsus alternans is alternate strong and weak beat (small volume and slow, less powerful rate of rise). This is found in left ventricular systolic dysfunction, cardiac tamponade with pulsus paradoxus when respiratory rate is half of the heart rate, aortic stenosis, HOCM, sudden increase in preload, sudden increase in afterload, onset of tachyarrhythmia (**Box 6**).

Mechanism

Pulsus alternans is a normal phenomenon after a premature beat. Postextrasystolic beat is stronger due to postextrasystolic potentiation. This can be felt in two beats after extrasystole in normal subject. In presence of ventricular dysfunction, pulsus alternans is precipitated by extrasystolic beat. Here, the alternans is better appreciable and persist for a longer time. More severe the dysfunction, alternans becomes more appreciable and persist for longer time.

Mechanical Theory

Alternative change in contractility, preload, and afterload is the possible mechanism. Due to increased preload during pause, postextrasystolic beat is forceful. During pause, there is more peripheral run off and more fall in diastolic pressure along with fall in afterload, which also potentiates the contraction. A strong beat increases arterial pressure, afterload, and resistance to left ventricular ejection for the following beat. Depressed left ventricle is sensitive to afterload. Thus, the beat following the strong beat will be weaker beat.

Biochemical Theory[9]

Before released calcium from previous beat taken back by sarcoplasmic reticulum, the premature beat occurs. In consequence, postextrasystolic beat depolarization begins with a higher amount of total calcium. More the calcium, more is the actin–myosin interaction leading to forceful contraction of the

BOX 6	Causes of pulsus alternans.
• Left ventricular systolic dysfunction • Cardiac tamponade with pulsus paradoxus, when respiratory rate is half of the heart rate • Aortic stenosis	• Hypertrophic obstructive cardiomyopathy • Sudden increase in preload • Sudden increase in afterload • Onset of tachyarrhythmia

postextrasystolic beat. The uptake and release of calcium by sarcoplasmic reticulum may fluctuate every alternate beat and reaches a steady level after a few beats in normal situation. In presence of ventricular systolic dysfunction, steady state may be reached after a long duration.

How to Measure It?

It should be suspected when there is alternate strong and weak beat with a regular pulse. It can be confirmed by measuring blood pressure with the sphygmomanometer. Cuff pressure is released slowly till the phase I Korotkoff sound is appreciated, only during alternate strong beats. On further release, there is doubling of the sound, which now can be appreciated during both strong and weak beats. Patient should hold his breathing to obviate the effect of respiration on pulse volume. Lowering the filling pressure by standing or diuretics enhances the effect and the alternans can be appreciated better. By palpation only, difference in pulse pressure can be appreciated, when the beat-to-beat difference is >20 mm Hg. As here the difference is <10 mm Hg, blood pressure cuff is required.

Pulsus Paradoxus (Box 7)[10]

By definition, pulsus paradoxus is inspiratory fall of systolic pressure >10 mm Hg. In 1873, Adolf Kussmaul described the pulsus paradoxus as—*"pulse simultaneously slight and irregular, disappearing during inspiration and returning upon expiration."*

During inspiration, three events happen. First is a decrease in intrathoracic pressure. Second is increase in intra-abdominal pressure. And third is increase in lung volume. All these three factors interact with another factor, biventricular interdependence, and decide the mechanism of normal and exaggerated inspiratory fall of systolic pressure.

BOX 7 | **Pulsus paradoxus.**

- Classically in cardiac tamponade
- Uncommonly in constrictive pericarditis
- Severe acute bronchial asthma
- Chronic obstructive pulmonary disease
- Pulmonary embolism (right ventricular filling pressure is disproportionately higher than left ventricle; there is also sudden dilatation of right ventricular—all these compromise left ventricular volume further)
- Pregnancy, marked obesity
- Partial obstruction of superior vena cava

Pulsus paradoxus is absent, even in presence of tamponade
- Atrial septal defect (as there is reciprocal reduction in left to right shunt in inspiration—thus left ventricular volume is not much reduced in inspiration)
- Aortic regurgitation (regurgitant volume maintain the ventricular filling throughout the cardiac cycle)

Inspiratory fall in intrathoracic pressure lowers right atrial pressure, which is an intrathoracic chamber. Venous return is increased. Increase in preload increases right ventricular stroke volume. Pressure surrounding left ventricle, i.e., intrathoracic pressure is reduced on inspiration. However, pressure in extrathoracic arterial compartment remains same. Thus, left ventricle has to generate more force to eject blood in extrathoracic arterial compartment. This is a relative increase in left ventricular afterload on inspiration. Intra-abdominal pressure is increased on inspiration due to descent of diaphragm. Increased intra-abdominal pressure increases venous return and right ventricular preload. At the same time, it increases pressure of abdominal aorta and afterload to left ventricle. Inspiratory increases in lung volume compresses the intra-alveolar vessels and thus increases intra-alveolar vessel resistance, whereas increase in lung volume reduces extra-alveolar vessel resistance. Overall, in normal subjects, inspiration mildly increases pulmonary vascular resistance during tidal inspiration. Another important factor is biventricular interdependence, which may be in parallel or in series. Two ventricles are within a limited space of pericardium. Inspiratory increase in right ventricular volume and pressure makes the ventricular septum shifted toward left ventricle, reducing left ventricular filling. This is interdependence in parallel. The right ventricular stroke volume, which is maximum on inspiration, due to pulmonary transit time, reaches left ventricle during expiration and vice versa.

To summarize:
- During inspiration, intrathoracic pressure falls which is transmitted in the pericardial space.
- This causes increased venous return to right atrium and right ventricle.
- Increased intra-abdominal pressure also increases venous return.
- Increase in right ventricular volume causes interventricular shift of the septum and reduced volume of left ventricle with decreased stroke volume.
- During inspiration, there is increased lung volume with expansion of pulmonary vascular bed. This causes less venous return to left side.
- Due to pulmonary transit time, inspiratory stroke volume reaches left ventricle during expiration. Diminished intrathoracic pressure is also transmitted to the aorta.
- All these factors lead to inspiratory fall in aortic pressure. Normally, inspiratory fall of systolic pressure is <5 mm Hg and fall in left ventricular stroke volume is <10%. In consequence, inspiratory fall of systolic pressure is also small and <10 mm Hg.[11]

Cardiac Tamponade

In pulsus paradoxus, same things happen in an exaggerated form. As the effusion limits pericardial space, interventricular shift is more exaggerated, causing more compromised left ventricular volume and stroke volume. Left ventricular volume is further compromised by reduction of inflow due to diminished pulmonary vein—left atrial pressure gradient. Inspiratory fall in intrathoracic pressure is transmitted in the pulmonary veins, as they are extrapericardial structures. But this fall is not fully transmitted to left atrium or ventricle due to shielding effect by the pericardial fluid.

Why pulsus paradoxus more common in cardiac tamponade than constrictive pericarditis is difficult to define. May be inspiratory increase in right ventricle with compromise of left ventricular volume due to ventricular interdependency may be more aggressive in tamponade than constrictive pericarditis. The explanation has been offered that constricted pericardium can isolate the heart completely from the effect of respiration.

Acute Bronchial Asthma

Large decrease in intrathoracic pressure on inspiration and breathing at high lung volume are the features in acute bronchial asthma, which explain the occurrence of pulsus paradoxus. Inspiratory fall may be amounting to −30 to −20 mm Hg, which affect the fall of systolic pressure either directly by reducing aortic pressure and indirectly by reducing left ventricular stroke volume. During acute episode, functional residual capacity is markedly increased and as result, increased lung volume on inspiration increases right ventricular afterload significantly. Thus, increase in preload and afterload causes right ventricular distension and sets in the parallel ventricular interdependence mechanism with fall in left ventricular stroke volume on inspiration. There is an issue regarding preload in acute bronchial asthma. Right atrial pressure is not much high on expiration. When right atrial pressure falls short of atmospheric pressure, systemic veins entering right atrium may be collapsed and restrict venous return. Thus, right ventricular distension will be less and ventricular interdependence in series rather than parallel may be more important.

Acute Exacerbation of Chronic Obstructive Pulmonary Disease

Inspiratory fall of intrathoracic pressure and its effect are same as bronchial asthma. However, during expiration intrathoracic pressure is high due to lung hyperinflation and gas trapping. Venous return will be significantly less in compare to inspiration. As a result, right ventricular and in series left ventricular stroke volume show significant change between inspiration and expiration. Thus, there is swinging of intrathoracic pressure, in both phases of respiration, which is transmitted in intracardiac hemodynamics similar to tamponade. Here, pulse pressure, unlike in tamponade, is not reduced, as the fall in pressure affects both systolic and diastolic pressure.

How to Measure It?

Patient should be asked to take a moderate respiration. Cuff should be deflated slowly. Korotkoff sound first appears in expiration. On further deflation, Korotkoff sound can be heard in both phases of respiration. Blood pressure differences between these two observations are the amount of pulsus paradoxus. When the difference is >20 mm Hg, it can be appreciated on palpating the pulse. When pulse pressure is significantly reduced, pulsus paradoxus amounting to 6 mm Hg can be associated with significant tamponade. Alternate way to measure it is invasive

> **BOX 8** **Reverse pulsus paradoxus.**
> - Hypertrophic obstructive cardiomyopathy
> - Severe left heart failure on positive pressure breathing
> - Isorhythmic atrioventricular dissociation

measurement and pulse oximeter, in which respiratory waveform variation closely correlates to sphygmomanometric assessment of pulsus paradoxus.

Clinical Significance
Cardiac tamponade can be diagnosed by pulsus paradoxus in 98% of cases.[12] In acute bronchial asthma or chronic obstructive pulmonary disease, pulsus paradoxus and its grade are important point in severity scoring.

Reverse Pulsus Paradoxus (Box 8)
Reverse pulsus paradoxus is defined as inspiratory rise of arterial systolic and diastolic pressure, presumably related to inspiratory increase in left ventricular stroke volume. This pulse was first described by Massumi et al.[13] In HOCM, there is expiratory exaggeration of outflow obstruction and more powerful left ventricular contraction causing reduced stroke volume and fall in systemic arterial pressure. This reverse phenomenon cannot be explained by inspiratory-expiratory physiology. Left ventricle getting less pulmonary venous flow during inspiration, in which phase actually the left ventricular outflow gradient along with arterial pressure should have been exaggerated visa vis more pulmonary flow during expiration, in which phase left ventricular outflow gradient arterial pressure should have been reduced. During application of positive inspiratory pressure to airway, there is reduction of venous return and in turn reduction of right ventricular stroke volume. Severe heart failure produces pulmonary venous congestion. Inspiratory positive intra-alveolar pressure squeezes congested blood from pulmonary capillaries and venules to left ventricle and thus, increases left ventricular stroke volume along with arterial pressure. Isorhythmic AV dissociation is an arrhythmia, in which atria and ventricles are depolarized independently and almost simultaneously at same rate. Electrocardiographically, P wave falls on QRS wave. In consequence, atrial contribution to left ventricular output is absent, leading to fall in arterial pressure. This arrhythmia may be found in right ventricular pacing and after myocardial infarction. Increasing atrial rate places P wave before QRS, helps atrial kick added to ventricular stroke volume and increase in arterial pressure. Inspiration also increases sinus rate and place P wave before QRS complex, resulting in inspiratory increase in arterial pressure, i.e., reverse pulsus paradoxus.

CONDITION OF ARTERIAL WALL
Rigidity and elasticity of the arterial wall should be assessed; radial artery is best for this appreciation. Thickness and firmness of the arterial wall are felt by rolling

the radial artery against the bone. More the rigidity less will be the compressibility. A rigid artery usually indicates presence of systolic hypertension. As a definitive method, Osler's maneuver (described later) is done.

SYNCHRONY

Radio-radial synchrony is lost in:
- Subclavian artery obstructive disease (nonspecific, atherosclerotic or inflammatory).
- Coarctation of aorta (presubclavian).
- Dissection of aorta.
- Supravalvular stenosis.

Radiofemoral synchrony is lost in:
- Coarctation of aorta
- Aortic dissection
- Aortic arch syndrome
- Abdominal aortic disease such as giant cell arteritis.
- Leriche syndrome

PULSE IN SPECIAL SITUATION

Pulse in Hypertension

Pulse wave velocity is increased in hypertension. It causes quick return of the reflected waves from the lower half of the body to the central aorta in late systole in place of diastole. This wave merges with the reflected wave from the upper half of the body, resulting in prominent tidal wave, higher systolic pressure, and smaller diastolic wave.

Peripheral Sign in Aortic Regurgitation

Peripheral pulse and related signs in aortic regurgitation are related to huge stroke volume and increased ejection velocity, reduced peripheral resistance, wide pulse pressure, and reduced diastolic pressure. The last even is due to run off in left ventricle and dilated peripheral vasculature.
- Rapidly rising, high volume (pulsus magnus), rapidly collapsing (water hammer) pulse.
- Pulsus bisferiens
- Corrigan's sign is visible dancing carotid pulsation.
- Muller's sign is uvular pulsation.
- Minervini's sign is lingual pulsation, which can be appreciated by using tongue depressor.
- Landolfi's sign is alternate constriction and dilatation of pupil.
- Becker's sign is retinal artery pulsation.
- Mayne sign is fall of diastolic pressure >15 mm Hg, on arm elevation.
- Rosenbach's sign is hepatic pulsation.

- Gerhardt's sign is splenic pulsation.
- Dennison's sign is pulsatile cervix.
- Traube's sign is pistol shot sound over femoral artery.
- Palfrey's sign is pistol shot sound over radial artery, which he described in 1952.[14] He described it as auscultatory equivalence to water hammer pulse (**Fig. 5**). He graded aortic regurgitation severity according to the audibility of pistol shot sound from radial to brachial artery. He described—"Thus in all cases of aortic insuffiency, it is of interest to raise the arm vertically above the heart and to listen to the front of the wrist. If no arterial tone in heard it may be concluded that the insufficiency is not marked and may be slight. If the tone is heard over the elevated wrist but not lower it means a diastolic blood pressure of about 45 by mercurial manometer. This is evidence that the aortic regurgitation has caused a pronounced abnormality of the aortic circulation and, whether or not symptoms of failure of the left ventricle have developed, it is commonly reason for strict limitation of exercise. Next, with the arm still elevated, it is well to move the stethoscope gradually downward until at some the tone suddenly disappears. The lower the point, the less is the diastolic blood pressure; if the tone is present as low as the elbow it means a diastolic pressure of about 30 mm Hg".
- Quincke's sign (capillary pulsation) was described by Quincke in 1868. The pulse can be elicited on lips, face or hand compressing by a glass slide or compressing the nail bed (a flashlight against the finger pulp can enhance the effect). What one can appreciate is the capillary pulsation in the form of alternating blanching and reddening. Arterial pulse is transmitted through the dilated capillaries to the subpapillary venous plexus. This is not a specific sign of aortic regurgitation and may be present in any high-output state and even in a normal person. In aortic regurgitation with early heart failure, many of the peripheral signs may be retained, except this sign, which disappears early due to cutaneous vasoconstriction.

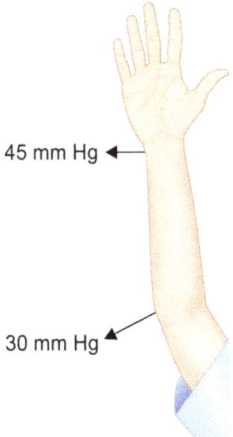

Fig. 5: Palfrey's sign: Auscultation for pistol shot sound at wrist and inching downward to elbow on a raised arm.

- de Musset's head bobbing sign is nodding of head, an eponym attributed to a patient Alfred de Musset, a French poet in 1900. Paul de Musset, the patient's brother described[15]—"One morning in the month of March (of 1842), during lunch, I observed that the head of my brother (Alfred) was showing a slight bobbing, which was involuntary, seemingly occurring with each heart beat...." This is an exaggerated ballistographic effect of large stroke volume and wide pulse pressure of severe aortic regurgitation. Ballistocardiograph was an old method, which was used to detect effect of ejection of blood on body movement.
- *Hill's sign*: Described in Chapter 12.
- Duroziez's murmur is also known as intermittent femoral double murmur of Duroziez. Paul Duroziez, a French physician described this sign in 1861.[16] The murmur has two components. Systolic component is due to excessive forward flow and diastolic component is due to backward flow toward aorta in diastole. There are two different ways to detect the murmur. One method described originally by Duroziez is to place the chest piece on the femoral artery and pressing the artery by finger 2 cm proximal to the chest piece 2 cm distal to the chest piece. Upstream pressure produces systolic murmur and downstream pressure produces the diastolic murmur. Another method is to place the stethoscope on femoral artery and pressing serially its proximal and distal end on femoral artery. Proximal pressing produces the systolic murmur and distal pressing produces the diastolic murmur. Duroziez's murmur is highly sensitive and specific for clinical detection of murmur.

Pulse in Hypertrophic Obstructive Cardiomyopathy

Hypertrophic obstructive cardiomyopathy is usually said to be associated with pulsus bisferiens. It is a rapidly rising pulse with normal pulse pressure. This brisk rise is the most characteristic. Forceful contraction of the grossly hypertrophied left ventricular is probably responsible for the brisk rise. 80% ejection takes place before the obstruction ensues. Rest of the ejection takes place slowly after the obstruction. Thus, there are two peaks of the pulsus bisferiens. First peak, percussion wave is larger than the second tidal wave.

Pulse in Coarctation of Aorta (Fig. 6)

From central aorta, pulse wave reaches at the peripheral pulses with progressive delay: Carotid 30 ms, brachial 60 ms, radial 80 ms, and femoral 75 ms. Thus, in a normal person, radial and femoral pulses occur almost simultaneously.

In coarctation, below the obstruction, pressure pulse rises and falls more slowly resulting in a delayed slow upstroke and smooth declining slope. This factor, rather than delayed transmission of pressure pulse from aorta to femoral artery, determines the radiofemoral delay. Thus, in comparison to the pulse proximal to coarctated segment, the slower rate of rise of the pulse wave, difference in the timing in the two peak, and narrow pulse pressure of pulse distal to coarctation cause the radiofemoral delay.

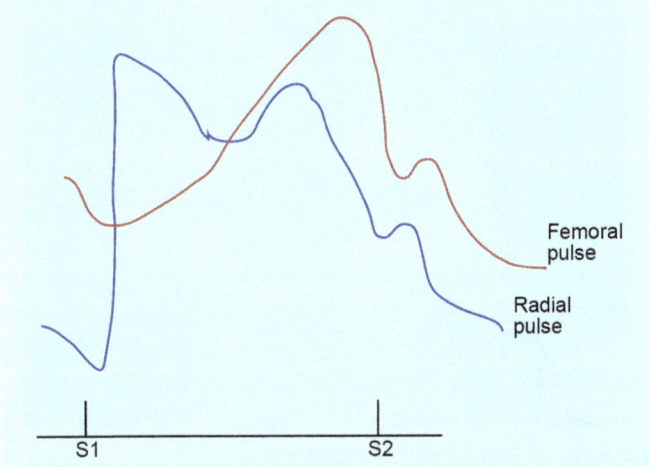

Fig. 6: Radiofemoral delay in coarctation of aorta: Delay is due to delayed peak of the femoral pulse.

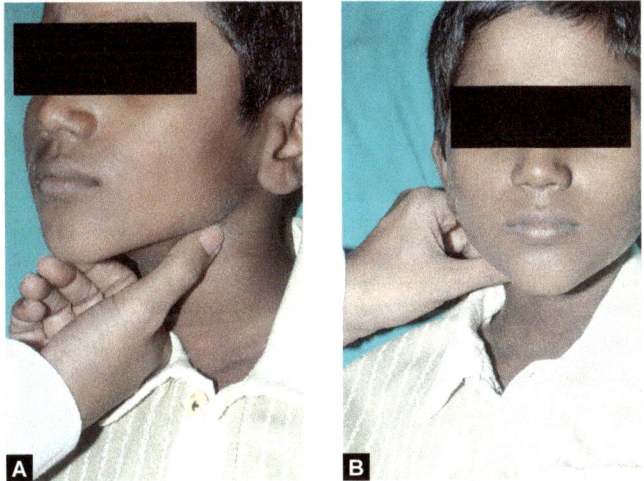

Figs. 7A and B: How to look for carotid arteries. (A) Left carotid artery: right thumb should be used. (B) Right carotid artery: left thumb should be used.

How to Look for?

Either radial or brachial pulse may be chosen. When radial artery is chosen, hand may be kept next to the patient's groin. Both should be palpated simultaneously. An absent right radial artery indicates origin of right subclavian artery from descending aorta below the coarctation. Absence of both the radial pulses with bounding carotids indicates origin of both subclavian arteries below the coarcted segment (**Figs. 7** to **10**).

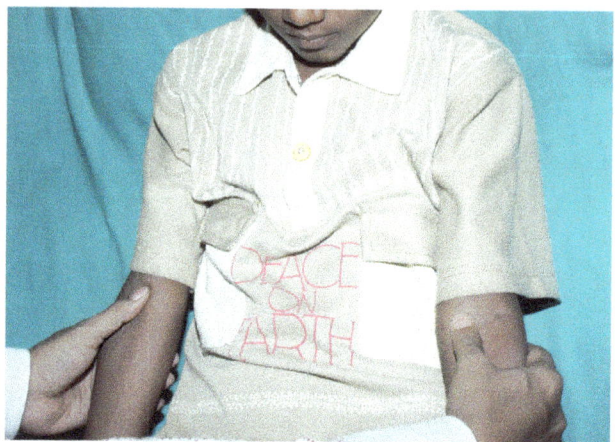

Fig. 8: Simultaneous palpation of both the brachial arteries.

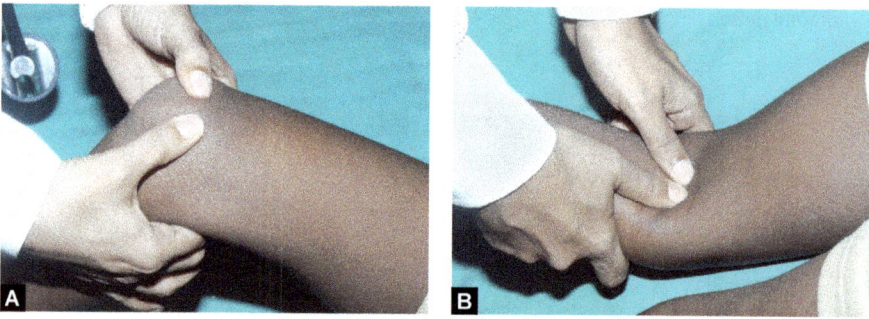

Figs. 9A and B: How to look for popliteal artery pulse. (A) Patient's knee is kept in semiflexed position. Examiner keeps the thumbs anteriorly and popliteal artery is palpated by the index fingers in the popliteal fossa; (B) patient in prone position. Knee in semiflexed position. Popliteal artery is palpated by both thumbs.

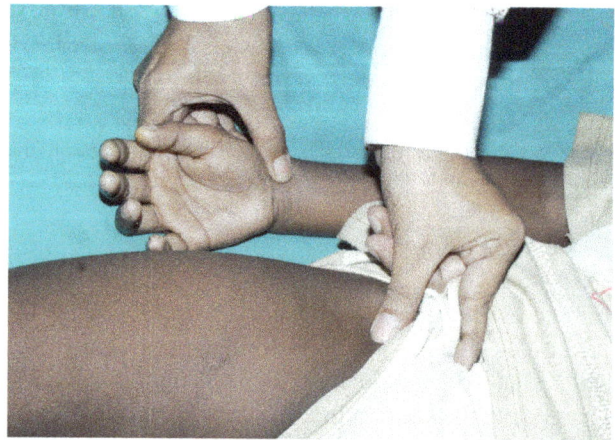

Fig. 10: Simultaneous palpation of radial and femoral arteries. Patient's hand is kept by the side of his thigh. This facilitates better appreciation of radiofemoral delay, if any.

Presence of aortic regurgitation, well-developed collaterals and obstruction <40–50% may obviate the radiofemoral delay.

ARTERIAL BRUIT

Bruits are audible noises due to turbulence in the arterial flow. They are usually systolic and results from partial obstruction of the arterial flow. Routine arterial auscultation should be done on carotid, subclavian, and femoral arteries. Bell of the stethoscope should be placed over the arteries. A diminished pulsation does not necessarily produce louder noises. Sometimes systolic murmur, specifically originating from aortic or mitral valve, may radiate to carotid artery. They can be differentiated from bruit by the site of best audibility. Carotid bruit is best audible on carotid artery, whereas radiating murmur is best audible at aortic area or apex.

Auscultation on thoracic aorta is done in coarctation of aorta. It is accomplished by auscultation by diaphragm of the stethoscope, over vertebral column, in between scapula. Patient should be in prone or supine position, with relaxed shoulder and chest.

Abdominal auscultation is done over both flanks to assess renal artery stenosis in a patient with hypertension. In iliofemoral obstructive disease, auscultation should be done over abdominal aortic bifurcation.

ABDOMINAL AORTA PALPATION

As abdominal aortic aneurysm (AAA) and its intervention is quiet a common procedure, palpation of abdominal aorta should be a part of clinical examination. About 10,000 annual death due to AAA occurs in United States. Palpation as a routine part of health examination in elderly population plays an important role in diagnosing one-third of new cases of AAA and may be more cost-effective for screening than ultrasound.[17] Usually a pulsatile mass is palpable at the level of umbilicus along with a bruit on auscultation. The sensitivity and specificity of palpability of AAA is 68% and 75%, respectively. Abdominal obesity, distension, and small aneurysm reduce the sensitivity of its detection by palpation. An abdominal girth >100 cm reduces the sensitivity significantly. When its pulsation is palpable over a wider area of abdomen, it is suggestive of aortic aneurysm. Another important sign is expansile nature of aneurysm. Two index fingers are placed on the abdominal aortic pulsation on 1 to 2 inches apart. A normal aortic pulsation lifts up the palpating fingers without separation, whereas expansile aneurysm lifts up the fingers with separation. Fink et al. concluded in their study[17] on palpability of AAA—"*Abdominal palpation to measure the width of the aortic pulsation thus remains the only physical finding of demonstrated value for AAA detection. It appears to be highly sensitive for diagnosis of AAA large enough to warrant elective intervention in patients who do not have a large girth, and it has good sensitivity even in patients with a large girth if the aorta is palpable. Patients with definite or suggestive findings for AAA on physical examination should have the diagnosis confirmed by an appropriate imaging study such as ultrasound.*"

CONCLUSION

"There are vessels from it to every limb. As to this, when any physician, any surgeon (lit. Sachmet-priest) or any exorcist applies the hand or his fingers to the head, to the back of the head, to the hands, to the place of the stomach, to the arms or to the feet, then he examines the heart, because all his limbs possess its vessels, that is: it (the heart) speaks out of the vessels of every limb".

Its true. Heart speaks out of the pule.

(Quoted from: Ebbell (B): The papyrus Ebers, Copenhagen: Levin & Munksgaard, 1937, pp 114-115)

REFERENCES

1. O'Rourke MF, Kelly R, Avolio A (Eds). The Arterial Pulse. Philadelphia: Lea & Febiger; 1992.
2. O'Rourke MF. The arterial pulse in health and disease. Am Heart J. 1971;82:687-702.
3. Ranganathan N, Sivaciyan V, Saksena FB. The Art and Science of Cardiac Physical Examination. Humana Press: Springer; 2006.
4. Murgo JP, Westerhof N, Giolma JP, et al. Aortic input impedance in normal man: relationship to pressure wave forms. Circulation. 1980;62:105-16.
5. Fleming PR. The mechanism of the pulsus bisferiens. Br Heart J. 1957;19:519.
6. Bonow RO. Chronic aortic regurgitation. In: Alpert JS, Dalen JE, Rahimtoola SH (Eds). Valvular Heart Disease. Philadelphia Lippincott Williams & Wilkins; 1999.
7. Galabin AL. On the causation of the water-hammer pulse, and its transformation in different arteries as illustrated by the graphic method. Med Chir Trans. 1876;59:361-88.
8. Chirinos JA, Akers SR, Virendeels JA, et al. A unified mechanism for the water hammer pulse and pulsus bisferiens in severe aortic regurgitation: Insights from wave intensity analysis. Artery Research. 2018;21:9-12.
9. Eisner DA, Diaz ME, Li Y, et al. Stability and instability of regulation of intracellular calcium. Exp Physiol. 2005;90:3-12.
10. Hamzaoui O, Monnet X, Teboul JL. Pulsus paradoxus. Eur Respir J. 2013;42:1696-705.
11. Ruskin J, Bache RJ, Rembert JC, et al. Pressure-flow studies in man: effect of respiration on left ventricular stroke volume. Circulation. 1973;48:79-85.
12. Guberman BA, Fowler NO, Engel PJ, et al. Cardiac tamponade in medical patients. Circulation. 1981;64:633-40.
13. Massumi RA, Mason DT, Vera Z, et al. Reversed pulsus paradoxus. N Engl J Med. 1973;289(24):1272-5.
14. Palfrey FW. Auscultation of the Corrigan or water hammer pulse. N Engl J Med. 1952;247:771-2.
15. Sapira JD. Quincke, de Musset, Duroziez, and Hill: some aortic regurgitations. South Med J. 1981;74:459-67.
16. Duroziez PL. Du souffle intermittent crural, comme signe de linsuffisance aortique. Arch Gen Med. 1861;17:417-23, 588-605.
17. Fink HA, Lederle FA, Roth CS, et al. The accuracy of physical examination to detect abdominal aortic aneurysm. Arch Intern Med. 2000;160(6):833-6.

CHAPTER 12

Blood Pressure

INTRODUCTION

Blood pressure was first measured by Stephen Hales in 1773. He was a British physiologist, who measured intra-arterial pressure of a white mare, whose carotid artery was opened and a brass pipe was introduced and connected to a glass tube. He measured the column of blood, eight feet tall above the level of horse's left ventricle. The horse was bled to death. But his concept is saving millions of human life.

DEFINITION

Blood pressure (BP) is defined as the lateral force per unit area of vascular wall. It is expressed as dynes/cm^2 or millimeter of mercury.

DETERMINANTS

Systolic pressure is determined by the volume and velocity of left ventricular ejection, distensibility, and end-diastolic volume of the arterial system and timing and amplitude of reflecting wave.

$$\text{Pressure} = \text{Cardiac output} \times \text{Peripheral resistance}$$

Diastolic pressure is determined by the peripheral resistance, arterial distensibility, viscosity, and the duration of cardiac cycle (duration of diastolic run-off).

DIFFERENT TERMINOLOGY

Pulse Pressure

Pulse pressure is the difference in systolic and diastolic pressure. It represents the pulse volume, which is determined by stroke volume and peripheral resistance. Average value is 40 mm Hg. Increased pulse pressure is found in fever, anemia, hyperthyroidism, aortic regurgitation, patent ductus arteriosus (PDA), arteriovenous fistula, sinus bradycardia, or complete heart block. Narrow pulse pressure is found in increased peripheral resistance (heart failure), decreased stroke volume (severe aortic stenosis), and decreased intravascular volume. A wide pulse pressure >80 mm Hg has a positive likelihood ratio of 10.9 for presence of moderate-to-severe aortic regurgitation.

Mean Pressure

Mean pressure determines the average pressure throughout the cardiac cycle. As diastole is prolonged than systole, mean pressure can be expressed as 60% of diastole and 40% of systole or:

Mean blood pressure = Diastolic pressure + 1/3rd of pulse pressure

Proportional Pulse Pressure

Proportional pulse pressure = Pulse pressure/Systolic pressure

More severe the left ventricular systolic function, lower will be the proportional pressure. Different methods to measure blood pressure are described in **Box 1**.

KOROTKOFF SOUND

This sound was described by a Russian physician NS Korotkoff in 1905. These are mostly low frequency sounds produced by the oscillation of the arterial walls. It has two major components: Initial transient (ki) and compression murmur (kc). BP measurement by Korotkoff sound shows a lower systolic and higher diastolic pressure in comparison to intra-arterial pressure (**Box 2**).

BOX 1 **Different methods to measure blood pressure.**

- Indirect method:
  - Sphygmomanometric method:
    - By palpation/auscultation
    - By flush method
  - Doppler method
  - Automated device
- Direct method

BOX 2 **Korotkoff sound is difficult to hear.**

- Poor blood flow
- Small pulse pressure
- Slow rate of rise (in aortic stenosis)

Korotkoff sound: How to augment it?

- Cuff to be inflated quickly
- To elevate the arm before inflation
- Patient should open and close his fist several times

- *Initial transient:* This initial sound occurs when the cuff pressure reaches arterial pressure and there is abrupt opening of the artery and its distension.
- *Compression murmur:* The compression murmur is due to the flow acceleration through the partially compressed artery.

Mechanism of Korotkoff Sound

The law of conservation of energy: The energy of a volume of fluid may be considered to be the sum of the energy expressed as lateral pressure, plus the kinetic energy of movement. As applied to the artery under the cuff, the following events take place. The artery is partially constricted by the cuff pressure. When blood is flowing through the stenotic portion, its velocity must increase which results in a reduction in lateral pressure energy at the constricted site. As a result, the lateral pressure at this point falls, the walls tend to move closer together, and the degree of constriction increases. The velocity of the stream through the constricted area increases further, the lateral pressure is reduced still more and the process of constriction becomes more marked. Gradually, vessel becomes almost entirely closed. At this point, velocity drops toward zero and all the energy of the column becomes available as lateral pressure. The walls of the constricted portion are then momentarily blown apart. Then the process of increased velocity with its progressive constriction begins again and the cycle is repeated. These fluttering of the walls are suggested as the mechanism of production of murmurs and palpable thrill. When the cuff pressure is above arterial pressure, a slight flow takes place but no flutter is produced. When cuff pressure has fallen to level at which no stenosis is produced, flutter is again absent since there is no site of high velocity flow.

Water hammer theory:[1] As the vessel opens from occluded state, the deceleration of the proximal high-velocity jet against the distal stationary jet produces the sound.

Korotkoff Sound: Five Phases

- *Phase I*: Clear tapping sound; it is initially soft and becomes louder when the cuff pressure equals to peak systolic pressure.
- *Phase II*: Further fall of cuff pressure results in a swishing sound or murmur.
- *Phase III*: Further augmentation of the murmur.
- *Phase IV*: Muffling of the sound; here the cuff pressure equals the diastolic pressure.
- *Phase V*: Complete disappearance of the sound; compression of the artery at this level of cuff pressure, does not produce any turbulence.

Diastolic Pressure[2]

American Heart Association (AHA) recommended in 1939 that phase IV should be adopted for diastolic pressure. They changed it to phase V in 1951 and then back to phase IV in 1967. In 1980, AHA again went back to phase V. Phase IV pressure may be 5–10 mm Hg than phase V pressure. Phase IV (muffling) is taken as diastolic pressure below 18 years, pregnancy and other hyperdynamic circulation, where the gap between muffling and disappearance is >10 mm Hg. In these situations, pressure in both the phases should be mentioned (like 150/70/40 mm Hg) and phase IV sound predicts diastolic pressure more accurately. The issue between phase IV and V is becoming less relevant, as automated blood pressure estimation is gradually replacing auscultatory blood pressure measurement.

AUSCULTATORY GAP

After the appearance, the Korotkoff sound may disappear. This gap is known as auscultatory gap, which may be up to 10–20 mm Hg. Inflation causes venous distension and increased tissue pressure distal to the cuff (forearm), thus reduction in antegrade arterial flow and disappearance of sound. This gap may lead to a falsely recorded lower systolic pressure. To note the systolic pressure at the point of disappearance of radial pulse may help to avoid the false reading. To avoid auscultatory gap, one should do the maneuver that augment Korotkoff sound. Essentially, "vibrations are present during the gap range, but these are subaudible; electronic amplification may bring these sounds to audible level."[3] The gap is more commonly found in elderly and hypertension with target organ damage with reduced flow to the peripheral artery. Systolic pressure, as measured by palpatory method, is 10 mm Hg lower than measured by auscultatory method.

SYNCHRONY: ARM VERSUS LEG PRESSURE

BP in Two Arms

When taken separately, 25% show a difference of around 10 mm Hg in systolic pressure between two arms. A simultaneous recording shows this difference only in 5% of patients. This difference is explained by the different angle of origin of innominate artery in right side and subclavian artery on left side of aorta. This different angle determines suction in two arms from aorta due to venturi effect of flow.[4] The arm with higher values should be taken for future blood pressure measurement. Pathological differences of >15 mm Hg is found in subclavian artery obstructive disease (atherosclerotic or inflammatory), presubclavian coarctation, dissection of aorta, and supravalvular aortic stenosis. A consistent difference of systolic pressure between two arms >15 mm Hg in elderly is associated with increased cardiovascular risk.[5]

Arm versus Leg Pressure

There is progressive rise of systolic pressure and fall of diastolic pressure from central aorta down to peripheral arteries when measured by cuff. Mean pressure is not much changed. As mentioned earlier, reflected wave is rapidly transmitted from the peripheral muscular arteries and amplifies the incident wave. This summated wave results in enhancement of systolic pressure. In a normal set up, peripheral amplification is higher in legs than arm, resulting in higher leg pressure even by 20 mm Hg. High upper limb pressure is found in coarctation or aortic dissection, aortic arch syndrome, abdominal aortic disease such as giant arteritis and Leriche syndrome. High leg pressure is found in significant aortic regurgitation.

HOW TO MEASURE LOWER LIMB PRESSURE (FIGS. 1 AND 2)

Leg Pressure

Patient should lie in prone position. Leg pressure is to be measured either by a large thigh cuff and auscultation at the popliteal artery or by the arm cuff on the calf and auscultation at the posterior tibial artery or dorsalis pedis.

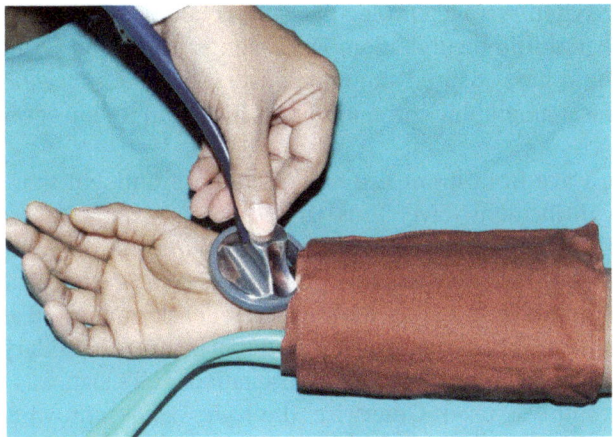

Fig. 1: How to look for forearm pressure?

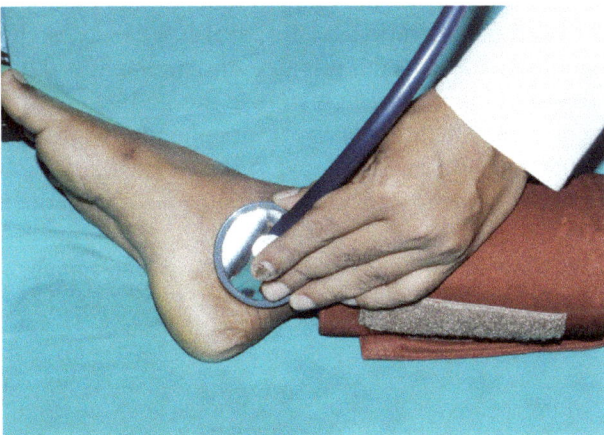

Fig. 2: How to look for leg pressure?

Blood Pressure in Thigh

As mentioned earlier, proper cuff size should be selected. Patient should lie on prone position. Otherwise, in supine position, knee should be flexed. Cuff is applied with the bladder over the posterior aspect of mid-thigh. Stethoscope is applied over the popliteal fossa. Systolic pressure measured in this way is 10–40 mm Hg higher than of arm pressure. Diastolic pressure is same in both upper and lower limbs. Intra-arterial pressure measurement shows only a minor difference, femoral systolic pressure a few mm higher, and diastolic pressure a few mm lower than the arm pressure.

BLOOD PRESSURE IN SPECIAL SITUATION

Aortic Regurgitation: Hill's Sign

Holtzmann actually first observed Hill's sign. He used to work with Sir Leonard Erskine Hill.[6] When systolic cuff-leg pressure is >20 mm Hg than systolic cuff-arm pressure in aortic regurgitation, Hill's sign is said to be positive. Both the pressures should be measured simultaneously or at quick succession. Frank et al. studied[7] the angiographic correlation of aortic regurgitation severity and Hill's sign (**Table 1**).

Reflecting wave from lower extremity is more prominent than upper limb, combining with incident wave. Thus, this standing wave is larger than that of upper limb. However, intra-arterial pressure measurement, even in severe aortic regurgitation, does not show this pressure difference and clinical validity of this sign has been questioned. In one study, Harmeet et al.[8] measured arm and thigh pressure using 12 and 19 cm cuff and intra-arterial pressure in axillary and femoral arteries in patients with severe aortic regurgitation. Hill's sign was positive only when 12 cm cuff was used. Otherwise, the sign was absent, when measuring pressure difference either by using 19 cm cuff or by intra-arterial pressure. In another study, Kutryk et al. studied cuff pressure and intra-arterial axillary and femoral arterial pressure and did not find any difference in intra-arterial pressure between axillary and femoral arteries.[9] This sign has been described as artifact of sphygmomanometric lower limb pressure measurement without any physiological basis. However, intra-arterial pressure in the studies are usually measured at femoral artery level, which is not that a peripheral artery and amplification effect of reflecting wave on incident wave may not be that prominent. On the other hand, leg blood pressure is measured at popliteal or posterior tibial arteries,

TABLE 1: Aortic regurgitation severity: Correlation between angiography and Hill's sign.

Angiographic grade	Hill's sign
I	<20 mm Hg
II	20–40 mm Hg
III	40–60 mm Hg
IV	>60 mm Hg

which are peripheral muscular arteries, in which reflecting wave shows maximal amplification effect. This may explain the fallacy between calf-leg pressure and intra-arterial femoral artery pressure.

Coarctation of Aorta

There is upper arm hypertension in coarctation of aorta and arm pressure is higher than leg pressure. In pre-subclavian coarctation, right arm pressure is higher than both left arm as well as lower limb. Hypertension in coarctation is due to mechanical factor, aortopathy with reduced smooth muscle cells, and increased collagen fibers accompanies coarctation leading to reduced arterial compliance and aortic distensibility, blunted carotid baroreceptor sensitivity resetting level of blood pressure response to a higher level, endothelial dysfunction, and poor renal blood supply with activation of renin-angiotensin-axis.

Pressure difference between upper and lower limb may be when narrowing of coarctated segment is <50%, associated significant aortic regurgitation, preductal coarctation (usually in neonates), and in presence of lot of collaterals.

Arrhythmia

Prevalence of atrial fibrillation and hypertension in elderly is 8% and 50%, respectively.[10] Thus, many of the elderly patients suffering from atrial fibrillation are hypertensive. Blood pressure measurement in presence of atrial fibrillation is uncertain because of beat-to-beat variability of filling time, contractility, and stroke volume. Because of all these factors, there is considerable beat-to-beat blood pressure fluctuation. Moreover, there is no generalized agreement in determining auscultatory endpoint. Either first appearance of Korotkoff sound or consistent presence of the sounds may be taken as level of systolic blood pressure (SBP).[11] Similar problem is also for diastolic pressure. When first appearance of sound and complete disappearance of all sound are taken as systolic and diastolic pressure respectively, the systolic pressure is overestimated and diastolic pressure is underestimated. Thus, whatever criteria is followed, blood pressure measurement in atrial fibrillation is always a rough estimate. To overcome the beat-to-beat variability, pressure must be estimated in several cycles (at least three cycles) on standard auscultatory blood pressure monitor and deflation rate should not be faster than 2 mm Hg per heartbeat.[11] As mentioned earlier, as oscillometric method for blood pressure estimation depends on a smooth profile of successive pressure waves, automated oscillometric method is usually not recommended for blood pressure estimation in presence of atrial fibrillation. However, in view of gradual replacement of auscultatory method by automated oscillometric method for its simplicity, the later method's validity in measuring pressure in presence of atrial fibrillation has been tried in several studies. A large meta-analysis[12] concluded—"These monitors appear to be accurate in measuring SBP but not diastolic blood pressure (DBP). Given that atrial fibrillation is common in the elderly, in whom systolic hypertension is more common and important than diastolic hypertension, automated monitors appear to be appropriate for self-home but not for office measurement." In presence of bradycardia, deflation rate should be slower than heart rate. Otherwise, too rapid deflation leads to overestimation of systolic and underestimation of diastolic pressure.

Children

Proper cuff size is very important and sizes including 4 × 13 cm, 8 × 18 cm and adult dimension 12 × 26 cm should be available for age range 0–18 years. Child must be in quiet condition because crying, eating or sucking can increase the pressure even up to 50 mm Hg. In children below 1 year, and in many younger than 5 years, Korotkoff sound may be too faint to appreciate. Here, other indirect methods such as flush methods, Doppler or oscillometry method can be used. In Flush method, cuff is wrapped in patient's forearm, which is elevated. Hand distal to cuff is wrapped firmly by elastic bandage or is massaged till it gets blanched. Cuff is then inflated well above the expected systolic pressure with the arm elevated and blanched. Then it is placed in the horizontal position and cuff is deflated gradually till the blanched hand gets flushed. The pressure measured at this point is the mean pressure. In Doppler method, transducer is placed over the artery of interest. Oscillation of the arterial wall is transmitted as audible sound signal at the peak systolic arterial pressure. Oscillation and the sound signal disappear at the end diastolic pressure.

Elderly People

Elderly shows considerable blood pressure variation with changing diurnal pattern. Ambulatory blood pressure monitoring (ABPM) can detect theses variation better than office blood pressure measurement. Isolated systolic hypertension is common in elderly people. SBP in them, measured by conventional method shows 20 mm Hg more than day time ABPM measurement and that can lead to overestimation and excessive treatment. Postural hypotension is common in elderly and should be checked regularly. Postprandial hypotension is not very uncommon in this age group and may be symptomatic. This should be detected by ABPM more convincingly. Autonomic failure develops on aging. This is manifested as period of hypotension interspersed with hypertension. As elderly are more susceptible to adverse effect of antihypertensive medicines, ABPM can detect this variability and help to decide the timing of antihypertensive medicine.

Pseudohypertension is common in elderly people. When sphygmomanometric pressure is far higher than the intra-arterial pressure, it is called pseudohypertension. This is common in elderly, because due to thickened calcified, noncompressible artery. This can be recognized by Osler maneuver, where radial pulses are still palpable, with an occlusive pressure (more than systolic) over the more proximal brachial artery.

Vascular stiffness is another characteristic feature of elderly population. Bedside features of vascular stiffness are Osler's sign and wide pulse pressure, in absence of any diastolic runoff. However, these are parameters of peripheral stiffness. It is undecided, how much they correlate with central aortic stiffness, which is an important factor in relation to optimum control of blood pressure. Stiffer the aorta, quicker will be the reflection wave merging with the forward wave in the more proximal segment of aorta. Thus, central aortic pressure becomes higher than the peripheral arteries. As a result, BP measured in the peripheral artery underestimates the central aortic pressure. Augmentation index is the index of how much the percent increase of systolic pressure due to early return of reflection wave during late systole. It is measured by peripheral tonometry and converted into central stiffness indices.

Exercise

On dynamic exercise, systolic pressure rises and diastolic pressure remains same or moderately lower. Debate continues, when one should call high blood pressure on exercise. Exercise-induced exaggeration of blood pressure response is associated with more chance of future development of hypertension, left ventricular hypertrophy (LVH), and increased cardiovascular mortality. Measurement of blood pressure during exercise is cumbersome. Systolic pressure can be measured comfortably by conventional sphygmomanometer or automated monitor, but diastolic pressure measurement shows either overestimation or underestimation. As most of the prognostic studies on exercise-induced hypertension are on systolic pressure, only systolic pressure estimation can be done during exercise. Age-independent upper limit of 180 mm Hg systolic for exercise blood pressure at 100 W standardized bicycle test may be taken as upper normal limit.[13]

CHECKPOINTS DURING BP MEASUREMENT

- *Bell versus diaphragm*: As Korotkoff sound are of low frequency, it is a general recommendation that bell should be placed over artery rather the diaphragm. However, there is not much difference between bell and diaphragm in picking up Korotkoff sound. As diaphragm covers a greater area and is easier to hold on artery than the bell piece, diaphragm is used for routine clinical measurement of blood pressure.[14]
- BP should be measured in sitting position with arm at heart level, roughly at 4th intercostal space.
- Gravity has its effect on BP. At the xiphoid level, BP is 5 mm Hg higher and at sternal level, it is 5 mm Hg lower.
- Patient should sit comfortably with supported arm, unsupported back, and uncrossed legs.
- In lying-down position, hand should be raised by a pillow to keep it at mid-chest level.
- After coming to the clinic, patient should have rested for 5–10 minutes.
- No smoking or ingestion of coffee.
- Subject should not talk during measurement.

- It is measured usually in working hand; if measured in both arms, higher pressure one should be taken as pressure of that individual.
- Cuff should be wrapped snugly around the arm, 1 inch above the antecubital crease.
- Bladder should be placed on the inner side of the arm.
- Initial assessment is done by palpatory method (systolic pressure is few mm less than auscultatory method).
- Another measurement should be done at least 30-second after the first measurement and average of the two should be taken.

HYPERTENSION

Grade of Hypertension
Hypertension is graded differently by different cardiac society (**Tables 2** and **3**).

True Normotension and Sustained Hypertension
True normotension is when both office and out-of-office (ABPM and home monitoring) BP are normal. Sustained hypertension is when both office and out-of-office BP are high (**Table 4**).

TABLE 2: The 2018 ESC/EHA guideline.

Category	Systolic BP (mm Hg)		Diastolic BP (mm Hg)
Optimal	<120	and	<80
Normal	120–129	and/or	80–84
High normal	130–139	and/or	85–89
Grade 1 hypertension	140–159	and/or	90–99
Grade 2 hypertension	160–179	and/or	>100–109
Grade 3 hypertension	≥180	and/or	≥110
Isolated systolic hypertension	≥140	and	<90

(BP: blood pressure; ESC: European Society of Cardiology; ESH: European Society of Hypertension)

TABLE 3: The 2017 ACC/AHA guideline.

	Systolic BP (mm Hg)	Diastolic BP (mm Hg)
Normal	<120	<80
Elevated	120–129	<80
Stage I	130–139	80–89
Stage II	≥140	≥80
Isolated systolic hypertension	≥140	<90

(ACC: American College of Cardiology; AHA: American Heart Association; BP: blood pressure)

TABLE 4: Definition of hypertension according to office, ABPM, and home monitoring.

Category	Systolic BP (mm Hg)		Diastolic BP (mm Hg)
Office	≥140	and	≥90
ABPM			
Day time (or awake) mean	≥135	and/or	≥85
Night-time (or asleep mean)	≥120	and/or	≥70
24-hour mean	≥130	and/or	≥80
Home BP mean	≥135		≥85

(ABPM: ambulatory blood pressure monitoring; BP: blood pressure)

White Coat Hypertension

White coat hypertension is defined as BP measured at office being higher than BP measured by home BP or ABPM or both. At least three clinic BP >140/90 mm Hg and two home BP <135/85 mm Hg without target organ damage is defined as white coat hypertension. Its prevalence is 30–40% of people with elevated office BP. White coat hypertension is more common in elderly, female, and nonsmoker. Risk of cardiovascular complication is lower with white coat hypertensive than with sustained hypertensive. However, patients with white coat hypertension are susceptible to increased adrenergic activity, cardiovascular complication, development of diabetes mellitus, and sustained hypertension in the long run.[15]

Masked Hypertension (Reverse White Coat)

Masked hypertension is defined as normal office BP and higher out-of-office BP, i.e., home BP or ABPM. It is more common in younger population and in those who show high-normal office BP. Identifying masked hypertensives is clinically important, because they are susceptible to develop all complication of sustained hypertension, including enhanced cardiovascular mortality, sustained hypertension, LVH, and diabetes mellitus.

Masked Uncontrolled Hypertension

Masked uncontrolled hypertension (MUCH) is defined as controlled office BP on hypertension management, but high out-of-office BP, i.e., uncontrolled on measurement by ABPM or home BP measurement. MUCH is not uncommon and may be found in 30% of treated hypertensive patients.[16] BP remains uncontrolled more at night-time than daytime, as detected by ABPM. MUCH is common in patients with diabetes mellitus and chronic kidney disease (CKD).

Isolated Systolic Hypertension in Young

Some young individual may show isolated systolic hypertension on office BP, but a normal intra-arterial central aortic pressure. Excessive peripheral augmentation of systolic pressure is the mechanism. It is common in smoker and its longstanding cardiovascular risk is similar to that of patients with high-normal BP.[17]

Orthostatic Hypotension[18]

Orthostatic hypotension (OH), a feature of autonomic failure, is quiet a common entity. OH consists of three variants: Classical OH, delayed OH, and initial OH. Classical OH is defined as fall of systolic and or diastolic pressure >20 and 10 mm Hg, respectively within 3 minutes on standing or head-up tilt-table testing. Delayed OH is defined as postural fall of BP after 3 minutes of standing or upright tilt. Initial OH is a transient fall of pressure defined as fall of systolic pressure >40 mm Hg and diastolic pressure >20 mm Hg within 15 second of standing. Giddiness or vertigo, presyncope and syncope, fatigue, blurring of vision, cognitive impairment, and "coat-hanger headache" or neck and shoulder pain are the presenting symptoms. Precipitating factors are warm environment, which causes vasodilatation and prolonged standing. Standing from a prolonged sitting, which pulls around 500–1,000 mL blood to lower extremity can lead to significant giddiness and even syncope. Symptom is also common in early morning hours, during going to bathroom. This is more common in patients with supine hypertension. Normal diurnal fluid shift and nocturnal diuresis cause hypotension in early morning. This factor may add in precipitating postural hypotension.

Postprandial Hypotension

Patient with autonomic dysfunction may develop hypotension after taking meal, known as postprandial hypotension. It is defined as fall of systolic BP >20 mm Hg or systolic BP becoming <90 mm Hg with a preprandial BP >100 mm Hg within 2 hours of meal.[18] Symptoms are similar to OH. However, patient may be symptomatic at sitting posture. Preventive measures are small meals, low-carbohydrate meal, taking less hot stuff, and avoiding alcohol with meals.

Supine Hypertension–Orthostatic Hypotension

Supine hypertension–orthostatic hypotension (SH–OH) is a form of autonomic dysfunction, where patient is hypertensive on supine posture and develops OH on standing. Supine hypertension is defined as SBP at least 150 mm Hg and diastolic pressure at least 90 mm Hg, when supine.[19] Supine hypertension develops due to abnormal baroreceptor setting, increased volume overload, reduced natriuresis, and residual sympathetic output in the setting of hypersensitive postsynaptic adrenergic receptors.

CONCLUSION

Measuring blood pressure is a simple method. Blood pressure instruments are also simple. Those simple things can prevent consequence of very complex cardiovascular disease, hypertension.

REFERENCES

1. Erlanger J. Studies in blood pressure estimation by indirect method. Part II. The mechanisms of the compression sounds of Korotkoff. Am J Physiol. 1916;40:82-125.
2. Levine SR. "True" diastolic blood pressure. N Engl Med J. 1981;304:362-3.
3. Roadbard S, Margolis J. The auscultatory gap in arteriosclerotic heart disease. Circulation. 1957;15:850-4.
4. Ranganathan N, Sivaciyan V, Saksena FB. The art and science of cardiac physical examination. Humana press: Springer; 2006. p. 53.
5. Clark CE, Taylor RS, Shore AC, et al. Association. of a difference in systolic blood pressure between arms with vascular. disease and mortality: a systematic review and meta-analysis. Lancet. 2012;379:905–914.
6. Hill L. The measurement of systolic blood pressure in man. Heart. 1909;1:73-82.
7. Frank MJ, Casanegra P, Levinson GE. Evaluation of aortic insufficiency: clinical, radiologic and hemodynamic criteria of severity. Circulation. 1963;28:723.
8. Harmeet KK, Andrews GR, Ramamoorthy S. A study to evaluate the clinical values of Hill's sign in the assessment of aortic regurgitation. Nurs Midwifery Res J. 2008;4:107-14.
9. Kutryk M, Fitchett D. Hill's sign in aortic regurgitation: enhanced pressure wave transmission or artefact? Can J Cardiol. 1997;13:237-40.
10. Danaei G, Finucane MM, Lin JK, et al. National, regional, and global trends in systolic blood pressure since 1980: systematic analysis of health examination surveys and epidemiological studies with 786 country-years and 5.4 million participants. Lancet. 2011;377:568-77.
11. O'Brien E, Asmar R, Beilin L, et al. European Society of Hypertension recommendations for conventional, ambulatory and home blood pressure measurement. J Hypertens. 2003;21:821-48.
12. Stergiou GS, Kollias A, Destounis A, et al. Automated blood pressure measurement in atrial fibrillation: a systemic review and meta-analysis. J Hypertens. 2012;30:2074-82.
13. Weisser B, Hartrumpf T, Mengden T, et al. Exercise blood pressure in the elderly – proposal for normal values in view of the 1999 WHO blood pressure classification. Dtsch Med Wochenschr. 2001;126 (suppl 3): S159.
14. Beevers G, Lip GHY, O'Brien E. ABC of hypertension. Part II. Conventional sphygmomanometry: technique of auscultatory blood pressure measurement. BMJ. 2001;322:1043-7.
15. Mancia G, Bombelli M, Cuspidi C, et al. Cardiovascular risk associated with white-coat hypertension: pro side of the argument. Hypertension. 2017;70:668-75.
16. Banegas JR, Ruilope LM, de la Sierra A, et al. High prevalence of masked uncontrolled hypertension in people with treated hypertension. Eur Heart J. 2014;35:3304-12.
17. Yano Y, Stamler J, Garside DB, et al. Isolated systolic hypertension in young and . middle-aged adults and 31-year risk for cardiovascular mortality: the Chicago. Heart Association Detection Project in Industry study. J Am Coll Cardiol. 2015;65:327-35.
18. Freeman R, Abuzinadah AR, Gibbons C, et al. Orthostatic hypotension. J Am Coll Cardiol. 2018;72:1294-309.
19. Naschitz JE, Slobodin G, Elias N, et al. The patient with supine hypertension and orthostatic hypotension: a clinical dilemma. Postgrad Med J. 2006;82:246-53.

CHAPTER 13

Precordium: Inspection, Palpation, and Percussion

INTRODUCTION

"Some wise man has said that one advantage of the stethoscope is that its use forces the physician to come within at least an 18-inch radius of the patient. Palpation reduces the remoteness to zero: The physician must touch the patient,"
–E Grey Dimond[1]

INSPECTION

Inspection prior to palpation of precordium makes palpation optimum. Precordial pulsation is better visible by a tangentially directed light beam on chest wall. Following precordial changes and pulsations should be noted.

Thoracic Structural Deformity

- Convex bulging in precordium indicates presence of heart disease in early childhood, when thoracic cage is malleable to accommodate dilated chamber in left-to-right shunt like ventricular septal defect (VSD), atrial septal defect (ASD) or congenital dilated cardiomyopathy. Bilateral prominence of the anterior part of chest along with bulging of upper segment of sternum and indrawing of the lower segment is present in large VSD due to dilated both ventricles and hyperkinetic pulmonary hypertension, whereas a unilateral bulge of second and third intercostal space parasternal may be due to ASD with volume overload of right ventricle.
- Both straight back syndrome and pectus excavatum can push the heart to the left and produce apparent cardiomegaly. The abnormal thoracic compression on heart can produce systolic and even diastolic murmur without any cardiac defect. Straight back syndrome is associated with ASD, whereas scoliosis is associated with cyanotic heart disease. Mitral valve prolapse is commonly associated with all the three thoracic deformities. Pectus carinatum is associated with Marfan syndrome (**Figs. 1** to **4**).
- In Turner syndrome, there is shield chest, hypoplastic breast along with neck webbing.

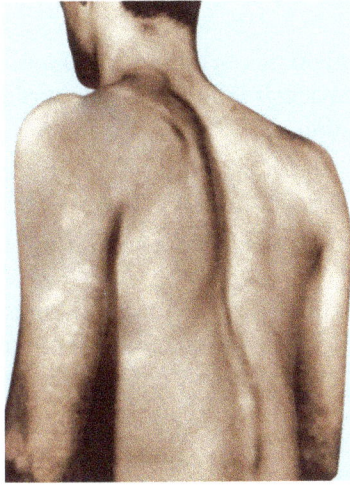

Fig. 1: Straight back syndrome.

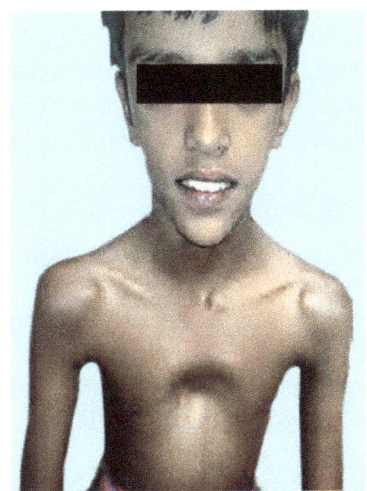

Fig. 2: Pectus excavatum.

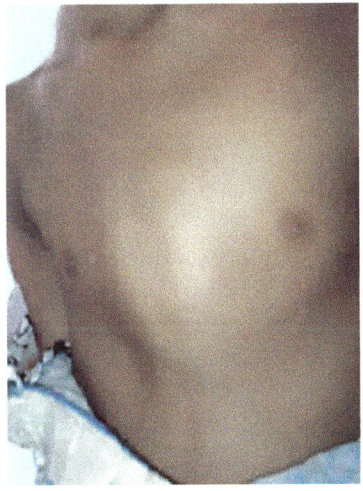

Fig. 3: Pectus carinatum.

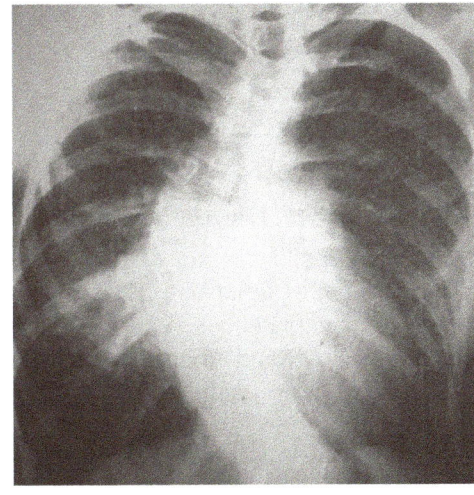

Fig. 4: X-ray feature of gross scoliosis.

Cardiac Pulsation

- Apical impulse
- Parasternal right ventricular impulse in left 3rd to 5th intercostal space
- Pulsation in mid precordium, in 3rd and 4th intercostal space at midclavicular line due to aneurysmal dilatation of left ventricle.
- Precordial retraction due to constrictive pericarditis or severe tricuspid regurgitation.

Arterial Pulsation
- Pulsation in left second intercostal space due to pulmonary artery pulsation.
- Right upper parasternal area or right sternoclavicular joint to look for aortic pulsation due to dilatation or aneurysm formation.

On Chest Wall
- Tortuous vessels on lateral chest wall and around scapula are suggestive of coarctation of aorta.
- Collateral venous channels on upper chest and bilateral distended neck veins are suggestive of superior vena cava syndrome. Unilateral venous distension of arm and adjacent chest may be due to subclavian venous thrombosis from device lead or dialysis fistula.

Beyond Precordium: Atherosclerosis
- Xanthelasmata
- Corneal arcus
- Frontoparietal baldness
- Crown-top baldness
- Diagonal earlobe crease

PALPATION

Apical Impulse

Palpation Tool: Hand
Ninety percent of cardiac motion vibration is in frequency range, which is subaudible and cannot be picked up by stethoscope.[1] Hand picks up some of them during palpation. Human hand has certain neurons, which are sensitive to positional change and others, which are sensitive to velocity. Fingers are relatively insensitive to movements, which are of large amplitude and low frequency (<5 Hz). Sensitivity increases with increasing frequency. Apical impulse is of high frequency, which is palpable, whereas low frequency filling sound is normally not palpable. Loud first heart sound from mitral stenosis and loud pulmonary component of second heart sound from pulmonary hypertension, and thrills, all being high frequency sound are palpable. The fingertips or its proximal area of the hand is the best site for picking up for relatively faint vibration.

Definition: Apical Impulse
Apical impulse is defined as the most lateral palpable ventricular movement on chest wall. The following physiological mechanisms have been proposed to explain the formation of apical impulse.

Basic Mechanism: Apical Impulse
- *Mechanical and angiographic correlation*: Long back, Haycraft[2] and Rushmer[3] suggested that apical impulse is formed by right rather than the left ventricle.

Apical impulse or apex beat is related to the apical portion of heart, but it bears no relation to the anatomical apex of ventricular cavity. Apex beat lies in the anteroseptal ventricular wall, around 3 cm anterior to left ventricular cavity and same distance lateral to right ventricular cavity in normal left ventricular angiocardiogram.[3] As septum is formed predominantly by left ventricular muscle, apex beat is formed by left ventricle in normal heart (**Fig. 5**).

Left ventricular systole consists of three parts. Pre-ejection period (from Q-wave in ECG to onset of carotid pulsation) consists of protosystole and isometric contraction phase. Ejection period consists of left ventricular ejection. Postejection period consists of protodiastole and isovolumetric relaxation period. In consequence, apical beat consists of two small outward impulse. First is the pre-ejection beat, beginning before and ending after first heart sound. Second is the ejection beat, beginning before the carotid upstroke and ending well before second heart sound. During the last part of systole and postejection period, there is an inward movement, which is due to apical retraction. Ventricle is wrapped by external and internal spiral fasciculi extending from base to apex, whereas circular fasciculi lie in between and they do not extend to the apex. Activation of circular fasciculi results in contraction of the upper part of the heart, whereas activation of spiral fasciculi results in apical retraction (**Fig. 6**).

- *Recoil theory*: According to Norman and Harrison,[5] apical impulse occurs at the very onset of left ventricular ejection, 0.08 second after onset of QRS complex and to precede carotid upstroke by 0.01–0.02 second and represents recoil movement which develops as left ventricular flow strikes on aortic resistance. During ventricular contraction, the heart rotates along its long

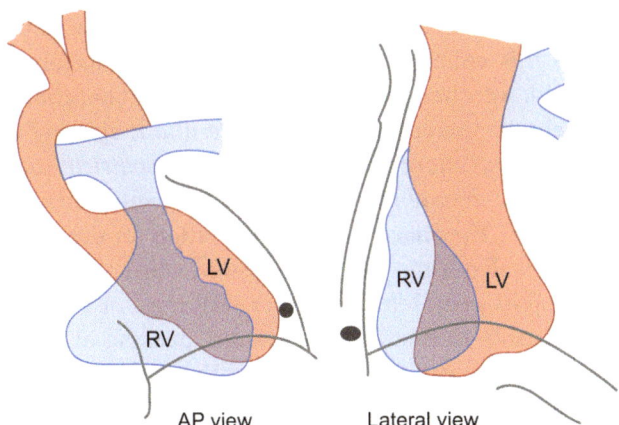

Fig. 5: Superimposed view of right and left ventriculogram in anteroposterior (AP) and lateral view. Apex beat (black dot) lies 3 cm anterior to left ventricular (LV) cavity and 2 cm lateral to right ventricular (RV) cavity, on anteroseptal ventricular wall.[4]

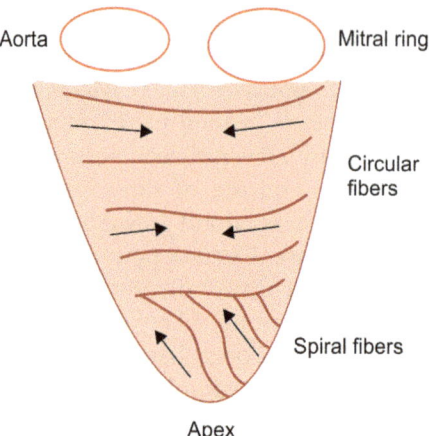

Fig. 6: Circular fasciculi wrapping the ventricle do not reach at apex, which is wrapped by spiral fasciculi responsible for apical retraction.

axis and makes the left ventricle swinging forward and striking on the chest wall.
- *Physical principle*: Ranganathan et al. proposed[6] physical principle of Newton's third law to explain the mechanism of apical impulse. During isovolumetric contraction phase, the force of contraction is equally distributed on all walls of left ventricle, including closed aortic valve and apex. As the forces balance each other, there occurs no effective appreciable movement of heart. Then aortic valve opens and ejection period begins. This upward flow of blood produces a force in opposite direction of flow, i.e., downward to apex of left ventricle, which moves downward. Aorta acts as coiled pipe, which is fixed posteriorly. Rapid ejection of blood from left ventricle into this coiled pipe produces an uncoiling force, which pulls aorta along with attached left ventricle upward and anterior. Ranganathan et al. comprehensively concluded—*"The resultant effect of the two forces described above will move the apex of the left ventricle toward the chest wall during systole despite the fact that the left ventricle is contracting and becoming smaller"*. They have further explanation for the retraction of apex beat from chest wall during rest part of systole. During outward and anterior movement of apex beat, left ventricular wall tension is maximum. Apical impulse is palpable in first third of systole, peaking at first heart sound, when left ventricular wall tension is high. The tension starts diffusing due to three factors. Major amount of blood is ejected from left ventricle within first third of ejection period. Left ventricle becomes smaller in volume. Left ventricular wall becomes thicker. Due to reduction of tension, apex beats starts moving away from chest wall well ahead of second heart sound.

Normal Apical Impulse (Fig. 7)

Normal apical impulse is defined as the thrust at the beginning of systole, small in amplitude and brief in duration, palpable in left 5th intercostals space on midclavicular line or within 10 cm from midsternal line. It occupies on chest wall an area with a diameter not >2.5–3 cm, width equal to two fingerbreadths horizontally and over one intercostal space vertically.[6]

Method

Palpation for apical impulse is done with patient in supine position. If not palpable, patient should lie in a partial left lateral position (in 50% of adult above 50 years, apical impulse is not palpable in supine position). Location of apical impulse should not be determined in left lateral position, as in this posture, apex is shifted laterally. However, nature of apical impulse and all diastolic events should be assessed in left lateral position. Sometimes elevation of the chest to about 30° may be helpful. The fingertips seem best to pick up faint brief movement. Most accurate way to appreciate apical impulse is with the patient sitting up and leaning forward in expiration and palpitation is done from behind.

Timing

Apical impulse begins before the first heart sound, continues over carotid upstroke and ends well before second heart sound. Timing should be done by keeping other hand on carotid artery or by simultaneous auscultation. This mechanism explains the fact that normal apical impulse recedes from the chest wall and becomes impalpable after the onset of the carotid upstroke or the

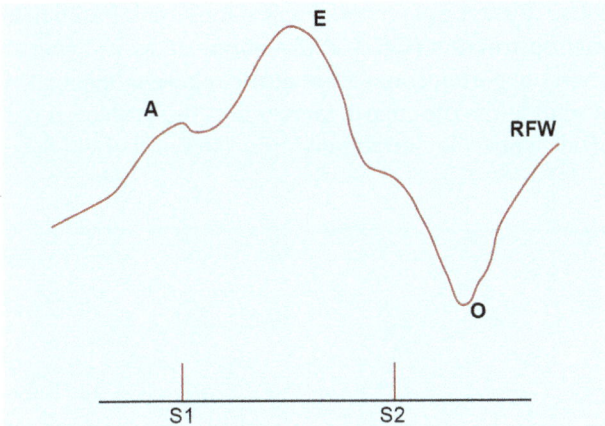

Fig. 7: Normal apex cardiogram. First outward movement, due to beginning of left ventricular systolic movement, begins after S1; isovolumetric contraction ends with aortic valve opening, shortly after, outer movement ceases (at E point). Then, the retraction begins, which ends at the nadir (O) point, where the mitral valve opens. From S2 to O point is the isovolumetric relaxation phase. Diastolic events, including the rapid filling wave (RFW), are not palpable in normal situation.

first heart sound and well before second heart sound, indicators of onset of ejection.

Point of Maximum

Point of maximum impulse is often used as a synonym for apical impulse. This should be avoided because maximum precordial pulsation may be due to right ventricular impulse, pulmonary arterial pulsation, or aortic aneurysm.

Abnormal Apical Impulse

Hyperdynamic or hyperkinetic apical impulse (forceful and ill-sustained) (**Figs. 8A to C**) is defined as a thrust of large amplitude and rapid rise. This pattern occurs in volume overload states with large stroke volume. The clinical conditions are hypermetabolic state, such as hyperthyroidism, anemia, pregnancy, and cardiac disease like mitral regurgitation, moderate to early part of not-too-severe aortic regurgitation, patent ductus arteriosus, and VSD with large left to right shunt. Immediate recoiling back due to apical retraction like normal apical impulse is an important sign. Once there is significant left ventricular hypertrophy, hyperkinetic apical impulse losses its character and becomes sustained one.

Hypokinetic apical impulse is found in conditions with reduced stroke volume, like in acute myocardial infarction and dilated cardiomyopathy.

Sustained apical impulse is defined as a thirst which persists throughout ejection period. As mentioned earlier,[6] persistent wall tension throughout ejection period is the mechanism of sustained apical impulse. There are two types of sustained apical impulse:
1. Heaving apical impulse (sustained and forceful) is defined as a thrust that is swift in upstroke, exaggerated in amplitude, and is sustained throughout the ejection phase. This type of powerful apical impulse is found in left ventricular outflow tract obstruction (LVOTO) like aortic stenosis, hypertrophic cardiomyopathy, and hypertension, severe aortic regurgitation—all conditions are associated with left ventricular hypertrophy. The sustained nature is due to absence of left ventricular retraction during later part of ejection period. In left

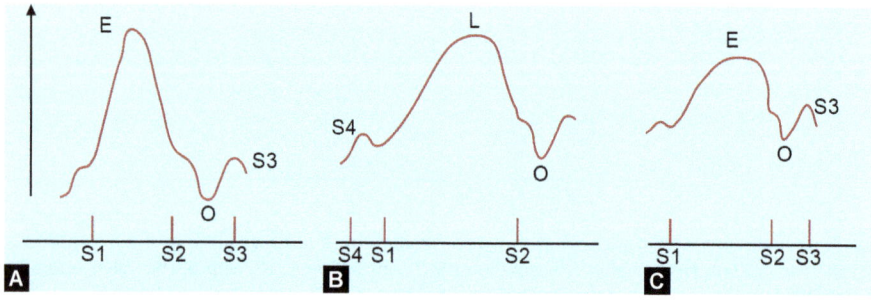

Figs. 8A to C: Various apical impulses: (A) Forceful and ill-sustained apex; (B) forceful and sustained apex; and (C) sustained, but smaller amplitude apex.

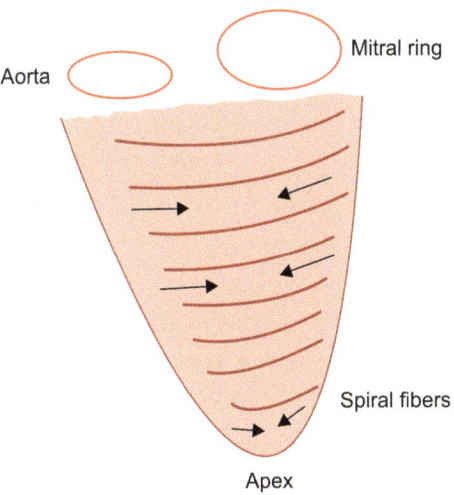

Fig. 9: Heaving apical impulse: In left ventricular hypertrophy, circular fasciculi reach at apex and prevent its retraction by spiral fibers.

ventricular hypertrophy, the circular fasciculi extend toward apex and during contraction prevent its retraction by the spiral fasciculi, as mentioned above (**Fig. 9**).[3]

2. Sustained apical impulse also occurs in left ventricular systolic dysfunction, where persistent wall tension due to poor emptying of left ventricle is the mechanism of sustained apical impulse rather than left ventricular hypertrophy. The thirst is here sustained but not forceful.

Left Ventricular Enlargement

Left ventricular enlargement is defined by:
- Apical impulse, in supine position, outside midclavicular line
- Apical impulse in supine position beyond 10 cm from midsternal line.
- An enlarged area of apical impulse (in longitudinal axis)—apical impulse palpable in more than one intercostal space.
- An enlarged area of apical impulse—a palpable area of >3 cm in diameter (roughly >2 fingerbreadths).

An apical impulse >3 cm in diameter is the most sensitive, specific, and predictive parameter in compare to apex-midsternal distance or midclavicular line criteria. In one study, these clinical parameters were compared to echocardiogram[7] to identify increased left ventricular end-diastolic volume. An apical diameter >3 cm was found 92% sensitive and 91% specific to detect left ventricular enlargement. The positive and negative predictive values were 86% and 95%, respectively (**Boxes 1** and **2**).

BOX 1	A displaced apical impulse to the left, in absence of left ventricular enlargement.
• Pectus excavatum • Straight back • Scoliosis	• Congenital absence of pericardium • Enlarged right-sided chambers pushing the left ventricle

BOX 2	Imperceptible apical impulse.
• Obesity • Emphysema • Pericardial effusion	• Constrictive pericarditis • Left-sided pleural effusion • Dextrocardia

Right Ventricular Impulse

Normal Right Ventricular Impulse

Right ventricular impulse is normally palpable beyond neonatal age as a systolic retraction in lower left parasternal area. Right ventricular inflow is in contact with anterior chest wall in 4th and 5th parasternal space, whereas the outflow is in contact with 3rd space. Thus, its area of contact with chest wall is wider than left ventricle. Even then, normal right ventricular impulse is not palpable. This is because normal right ventricular force of contraction is nearly one-fifth of that of left ventricle. Thus, right ventricle cannot produce the forces that left ventricle produces during isovolumetric contraction or ejection phase, which forces move the left ventricle anteriorly to chest wall. As right ventricle contracts, it becomes smaller and moves away from chest wall. In some children and adults with thin chest wall, a brief gentle systolic pulsation may be palpable in left lower parasternal area. A palpable right ventricular impulse indicates either right ventricular hypertrophy or enlargement.

How to Look for Parasternal Impulse? (Figs. 10A to C)
- By heel of the palm, in the 3rd and 4th left intercostals space at sternal edge, breath-holding at end-expiration.
- By placing three fingers in the 3rd, 4th, and 5th intercostal spaces, parasternally.
- Ulnar border of the hand can be placed in the parasternal area.
- Sometimes, the right ventricular impulse is better palpable from epigastric area particularly in emphysema. Here the downward thrust of the right ventricle is palpable by the pad of the upward pointing fingers at the end of deep, held inspiration. Right ventricular impulse strikes on the tip of the fingers, whereas pulsatile abdominal aortic aneurysm strikes on the finger pads. In a normal adult, any palpable subcostal right ventricular impulse indicates right ventricular enlargement.

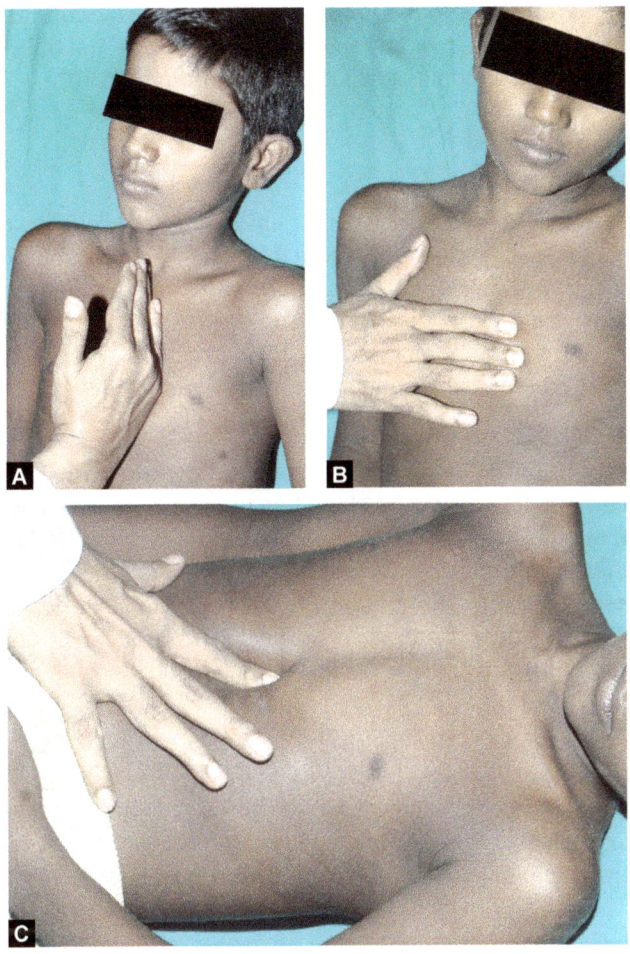

Figs. 10A to C: How to palpate right ventricle? (A) Ulnar side of the examining hand is placed over left parasternal area; patient is asked to hold breathe at end exhalation; (B) alternately, three fingers are placed over left 3rd, 4th, and 5th intercostal space, parasternally. Patient is asked to hold breath at end exhalation; and (C) hand is placed over subxiphoid area and tip of the index finger is pointed upward and left. Patient is asked to hold breathe in full inspiration.

Abnormal Right Ventricular Impulse

Hyperkinetic impulse is found in right ventricular volume overload like ASD, tricuspid regurgitation or pulmonary regurgitation. Location is usually 4th and 5th space.

Forceful and sustained impulse is found in right ventricular pressure overload. In infundibular stenosis, location is in 4th and 5th space, whereas in valvular stenosis, it is in 3rd–5th space. It may be associated with a palpable right ventricular S4.

Silent parasternal area is found in some congenital cardiac conditions affecting the right ventricle, characterized by absence of any parasternal pulsation such as Ebstein's anomaly and hypoplastic right heart syndrome (**Box 3**).

Medial, Lateral, and Median Apical Retraction

Medial Retraction

As mentioned earlier, only left ventricular apical segment touches chest wall in systole. Rest of the heart moves away from the chest wall in systole. Thus, normal apical impulse is associated with retraction medial to interventricular sulcus. During ejection period, anterior right ventricle moves away from chest wall. It is a localized zone, better seen than palpable (**Figs. 11** and **12**). Best way to perceive retraction is to place a palpating finger on apex beat and to put a mark lateral to it.

Lateral Retraction

A forceful right ventricular impulse is seen in right ventricular dominance, associated with either pressure overload like pulmonary stenosis or pulmonary hypertension or volume overload like ASD. Forceful right ventricular contraction produces anterior movement, which is felt as parasternal right ventricular pulsation. Enlarged right ventricle pushes left ventricle posterior and occupies apical area. There is a diffuse pulsation, which extends from reciprocal retraction, lateral to interventricular sulcus, further lateral to which, one can get the left

> **BOX 3**   **Grading parasternal impulse.**
> - *Grade 1*: Mild lift; can be perceived only by placing a pencil along the left sternal border; easily compressible by counter pressure; sustained less than one third of systole
> - *Grade 2*: Prominent lift; not easily compressible; sustained more than half of systole
> - *Grade 3*: Forceful, noncompressible by counter force; sustained throughout systole

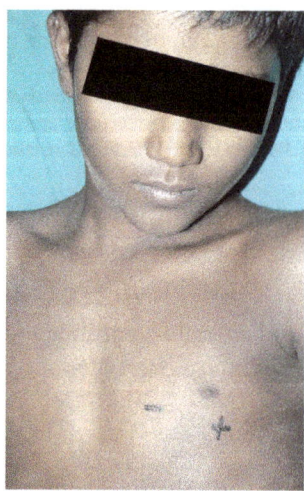

Fig. 11: Outward apical imputes is denoted by (+) and medial retraction is denoted by (−).

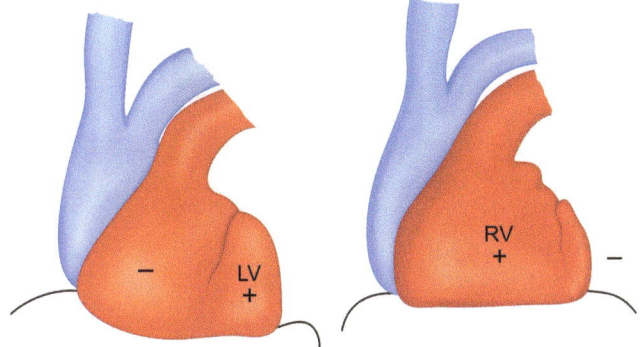

Fig. 12: Medial [dominant left ventricular (LV)] and lateral retractions [dominant right ventricular (RV)].

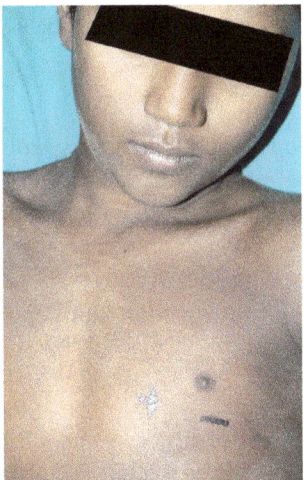

Fig. 13: Right ventricle forming apex (+) with lateral retraction (−).

ventricular impulse. A grossly enlarged right ventricle can push the left ventricle backward and takes its position as apex. Thus, left ventricle does not have any contact with chest wall. Relatively underfilled left ventricle moves away during systole, produces lateral retraction. Right ventricular apex is diffuse, extending from left parasternal area to apical area with lateral retraction (**Fig. 13**), as Gillam et al.[8] narrated in their experimental study—"Thus *the right ventricle may produce a widespread precordial impulse, extending from the left sternal edge to the apex*".

Median Retraction: Biventricular Hypertrophy (Fig. 14)

When both the left ventricular apical impulse and right ventricular parasternal impulses are palpable, there will be a zone of retraction in between, at the site of interventricular sulcus. This retraction is named as median retraction.

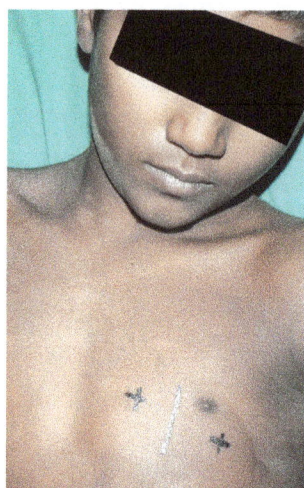

Fig. 14: Biventricular impulses (+) with retraction in between (–).

Arterial Pulsation

Pulmonary arterial pulsation is palpable as a systolic bulge in the left second intercostals space when the artery is dilated due to increased pressure or flow, poststenotic dilatation, and idiopathic dilatation of pulmonary artery. Similarly, aortic pulsation is palpable in upper right sternal edge or sternoclavicular junction when the aortic root is dilated, as in aortic arch aneurysm or right aortic arch. In malposed great artery, like L-transposition, aortic pulsation may be palpable in left second intercostal space.

Tracheal Tug

An aortic aneurysm, sometimes compresses the left bronchus with each pulsation and the bronchus pulls down the trachea. This downward pull of the trachea with each pulsation, can be appreciated by keeping the tip of the forefinger on the cricoid cartilage, standing behind the patient, and applying a steady upward pressure.

Heart Sound

In certain conditions, first heart sound (S1) and second heart sound (S2) become palpable. In mitral stenosis, S1 is loud and snapping and becomes palpable as a taping apical impulse (a misnomer because what palpable is the vibration, not the impulse). S2 is palpable when pressure is high in the great arteries. These closure sounds of the semilunar valves are also called diastolic shock due to their sharp vibrant quality. Aortic component of S2 is palpable in right second intercostals space in systemic hypertension and coarctation of the aorta, whereas pulmonary component is palpable in left second intercostals space in pulmonary hypertension. When aorta is anterior to pulmonary artery, as in any malposition of the great arteries, a palpable S2 in left second intercostals space is actually the aortic component. Third (S3) and fourth (S4) heart sound are never palpable sound.

Atrial Events

Normal atrial events are not palpable and detected only by apex cardiogram. When palpable, these are usually felt as double apical impulses—an additional outward impulse, either before or after the apical impulse. These movements are best felt by the fingertips with the patient in left lateral decubitus position. Using a wand as a lever at the apex beat, the impulses can be better demonstrable. More common is the palpable atrial contraction, which is basically a palpable *a* wave or presystolic wave (hump on the apical upstroke), normally not palpable and related to an accentuated atrial filling wave. This vigorous atrial contraction is found in patients with noncompliant left ventricle. The clinical conditions are LVOTO, hypertensive heart disease, and ischemic heart disease. A palpable atrial wave indicates that the patient is in sinus rhythm and there is no significant ventricular inflow obstruction. Palpable atrial wave may be the only evidence of ischemic heart disease (discussed further).

Ventricular Filling Occurs in Three Phases

Initial rapid filling phase, slow filling phase, when ventricular diastolic pressure and atrial pressure are equalized, and the third atrial contraction phase. Normally, rapid filling wave is not palpable. When large amount of blood enters ventricle during early rapid filling phase, it can produce a small wave after the downstroke of apical impulse, in early diastole. It occurs either in volume overload situations like mitral regurgitation or post-tricuspid left-to-right shunt or in heart failure.

Atrial Impulse

Right atrial impulse is sometimes palpable at right parasternal edge, when the aneurysm of the sinus of Valsalva ruptures in the right atrium or when the right atrium becomes ventricularized in Ebstein's anomaly.

Left atrial impulse is produced by chronic severe mitral regurgitation, due to expansion of the left atrium by the regurgitant blood. As left atrium is midline posterior chamber, its expansion produces the lifting of the whole heart in systole. This impulse may be confused with right ventricular impulse. A finger is placed each on apical and the parasternal impulse. The left atrial impulse begins and ends later than the apical impulse, whereas the right ventricular impulse begins and ends at the same time. The hemodynamic correlate of this impulse is the *v* wave of the left atrial pressure pulse (**Fig. 15**). Normally, left parasternal precordial tracing shows an early outward systolic movement, which begins before S1, peaks in early systole, and is followed by a major negative wave that is maximum at or near A2. In chronic mitral regurgitation, there is a late outward movement (LOM), which peaks around A2. More severe mitral regurgitation is, higher is the ratio of LOM/E ratio (**Fig. 16**) in apex cardiogram.[9]

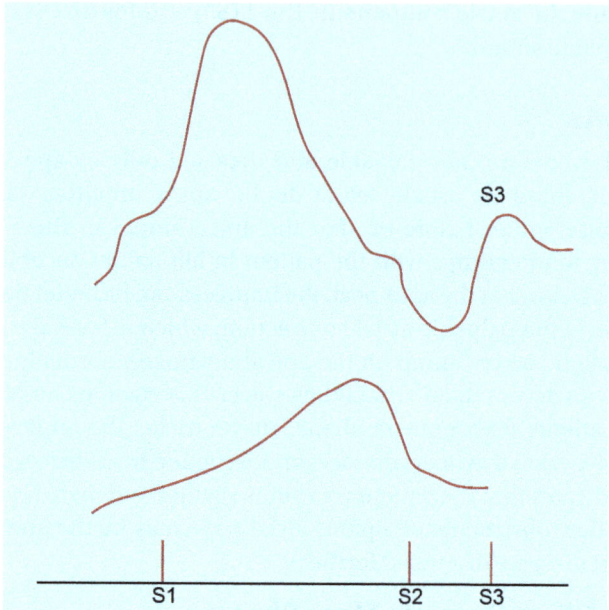

Fig. 15: Precordial impulse in severe mitral regurgitation. Upper curve is from left ventricular (LV) impulse. Lower curve is from left atrial impulse, which begins and ends later than LV apical impulse.

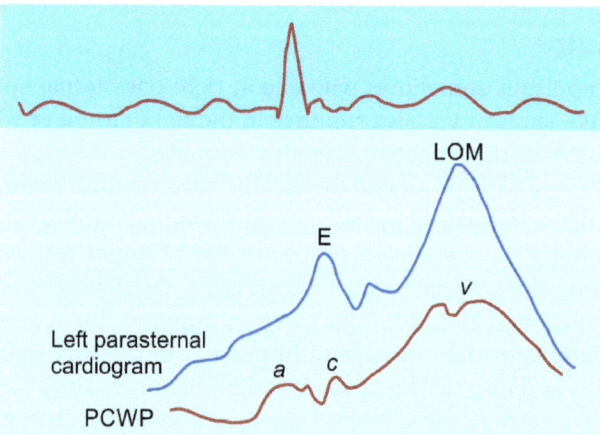

Fig. 16: Left parasternal cardiogram. Late outward movement (LOM)/early outward movement (E) ratio is high in severe mitral regurgitation. LOM corresponds to large *v* wave in pulmonary capillary wedge pressure (PCWP) tracing.

Inward Retractions (Fig. 17)
Constrictive Pericarditis[10]
Constrictive pericarditis, specifically the annular type specific, is associated with rocking movement. The tethering effect of constricted pericardium on atrioventricular groove and right ventricular outflow tract (RVOT) prevents the upward and downward movement of these regions in systole and diastole. During the steep right ventricular filling phase, the free segment of right ventricular anterior wall shows an outward movement in diastole, coinciding with diastolic knock. Systolic inward movement of the right ventricle may be due to adherent effect of pericardium to the anterior chest wall (**Fig. 17**).

Tricuspid Regurgitation[10]
In severe tricuspid regurgitation, dilated right ventricular forms the apex. During ejection phase, it empties very rapidly as it has two outlet namely right atrium and pulmonary artery. The right ventricle, which, like an overdistended balloon in diastole, empties rapidly in systole. This rapid emptying leads to an apical systolic retraction. Another explanation of the retraction is the palpable equivalent of the paradoxical motion of the septum. There is also right atrial systolic expansion due to large and rapid regurgitant blood rapidly pouring in right atrium. In early diastole, there is a large outward movement of the apical impulse due to greatly increased preload return to right ventricle. All these movements, systolic apical retraction, systolic left parasternal outward movement, and diastolic outward movement of right ventricle produce a right ventricular rock. The outward movement is due to expanding right atrium, which receives the regurgitant blood.

Thrill
It is the palpatory counterpart of a loud murmur (at least grade 4) and best palpable by the base of the fingers. A thrill does not bear any other clinical information.

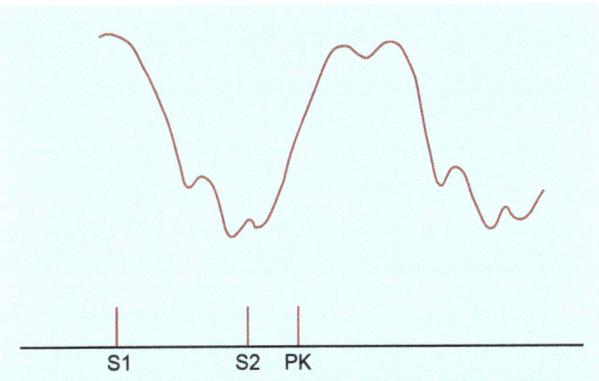

Fig. 17: Apical impulse in constrictive pericarditis. Systolic retraction and diastolic outward movement, which coincides with pericardial knock (PK).

Apical Impulse in Special Clinical Conditions
Mitral Stenosis
Apical impulse is classically described in mitral stenosis as tapping, which is the palpatory vibration of first heart sound, during its abrupt closure of mitral leaflet. Duroziez in 1862 first described the tapping impulse in mitral stenosis. Cossio in 1941 first described that apical impulse in mitral stenosis consists of two very closely sequential phenomenon—a slow-rising impulse due to ventricular systole and the tapping vibration of S1.[11] This sign is not present in all the patients with mitral stenosis, because in some patients a definite apical impulse may not be present and in some others, S1 may not be palpable due to leaflet calcification. More delayed is the palpable vibration of S1 from apical impulse, more severe is the stenosis. This delay cannot be assessed at bedside, because the interval from the ventricular impulse to the palpable vibration is <0.12 second. This can be assessed by combined recording of apex cardiogram, phonocardiogram, and ECG (**Fig. 18**).[12] What was happening actually to the cardiac movement were studied[10] by Boicourt et al. they found three types of apical impulses in mitral stenosis:
1. *Dominant mitral stenosis*: Apical impulse is normal along with associated tapping S1.
2. *Dominant mitral stenosis with pulmonary hypertension*: Apical impulse is sustained. Right ventricular hypertrophy secondary to pulmonary hypertension can occupy the apical area and produces sustained apical impulse.
3. Dominant mitral stenosis with tricuspid regurgitation produces apical retraction and outward sustained movement of parasternal area.

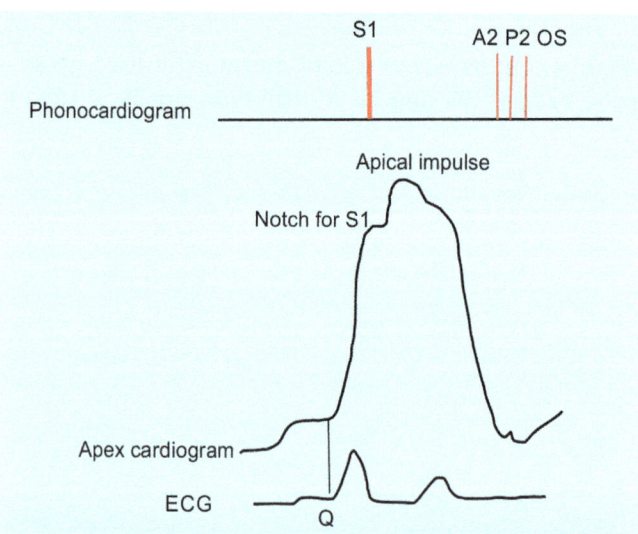

Fig. 18: Apex cardiogram in mitral stenosis. Vibration of S1 produces a notch on the upslope. More severe the stenosis, more nearer the notch is toward the peak. The "notch" ratio is calculated by the vertical distance from the onset of apex cardiogram to the level of the notch and the height of the entire apex cardiogram. Higher the ratio, severe is the stenosis.[12]

Hypertrophic Cardiomyopathy

Hypertrophic obstructive cardiomyopathy may be associated with triple apical impulse. Here, the forceful and sustained apical impulse is interrupted by the mid-systolic obstruction and creates the impression of double apical impulse. Both the humps are thus in systole. Third component is the palpable atrial wave, produced by the vigorous atrial contraction which occurs in late phase of diastole (**Fig. 19**).

Ischemic Heart Disease

Ranganathan et al. did an exhaustive study[13] on pattern of apical impulse in ischemic heart disease. They concluded:
- Palpable atrial wave may be the only clinical sign of ischemic heart disease.
- A sustained apical impulse indicates associated left ventricular dysfunction.
- A sustained apical impulse along with preceding atrial wave indicates significant left ventricular dysfunction.
- A sustained apical impulse and absence of atrial wave indicate loss of atrial pump along with severe left ventricular dysfunction.
- A normal apical impulse indicates ischemic heart disease with normal left ventricular function.

Left ventricular aneurysm causes a sustained systolic bulge in between the apex and the parasternal area, usually associated with a palpable atrial sound. The similar impulse, in the same location, is found during an ischemic episode as a result of transitory dyskinesia of the anterior segments of the ventricular wall.

Cyanotic Heart Disease

Tetralogy of Fallot

Tetralogy of Fallot (TOF) is usually characterized by an apical impulse which is not palpable, as it is underfilled (**Fig. 20**). A well palpable apical impulse may occasionally be found in pink TOF with good pulmonary flow or in association

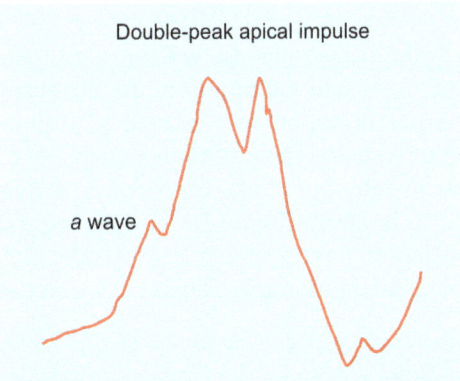

Fig. 19: Apex cardiogram in hypertrophic cardiomyopathy. Triple apical impulse-presystolic *a* wave and bifid apical impulse.

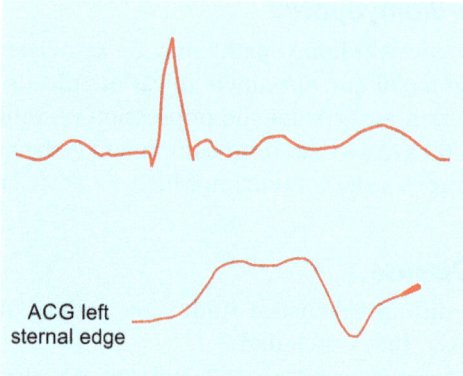

Fig. 20: Apex cardiogram (ACG) in tetralogy of Fallot. Sustained right ventricular impulse, which can extend from left parasternal area to apical area. There is no presystolic *a* wave, as right ventricle is decompressing through nonrestrictive ventricular septal defect.

with multiple major aortopulmonary collateral arteries (MAPCAs). Hypertrophied right ventricle contracts against systemic resistance in TOF. Thus, it should recoil back on chest wall and imparts a gentle impulse, like a normal left ventricle does. This may be described as a grade 1 parasternal impulse. As the obstruction is at infundibular level, impulse is best palpable in left 4th intercostal space and downward at subxiphoid area. A grossly hypertrophied right ventricle may displace left ventricle and occupies the normal apical area, imparting a diffuse apical impulse, continuous with the parasternal pulsation along with a lateral retraction. A right sternoclavicular pulsation may be found due to dilated right-sided aortic arch. In severe form of TOF, A2 may be palpable, whereas in mild to moderately severe form, including pink TOF, a systolic thrill may be palpable across RVOT.

Severe Pulmonary Stenosis with Stretched PFO/ASD (Fallot's Trilogy)

Fallot's trilogy is the cyanotic heart disease with most prominent right ventricular impulse, often a grade 3 parasternal pulsation. In classical valvular pulmonary stenosis, the parasternal pulsation may extend to 3rd intercostal space. In secondary infundibular stenosis, the pulsation is palpable on 4th and 5th intercostal space, whereas in subinfundibular obstruction, it is restricted to only 5th intercostal space. Thrill is always found in left 2nd intercostal space. Neither pulmonary artery pulsation, nor P2 should be palpable. Right atrial contraction as presystolic vibration and pulmonary valvular click vibration may be palpable.

Tricuspid Atresia

Tricuspid atresia is the prototype of cyanotic heart disease with left ventricular dominance associated with silent left parasternal area. In tricuspid atresia with increased pulmonary flow, apical impulse may be overactive. In presence of large VSD, when right ventricle is well formed, a gentle left parasternal impulse may be present.

Ebstein's Anomaly

Ebstein's anomaly is accompanied by normal left ventricular apical impulse. A silent left parasternal area is characteristic negative point. This is because of small functional right ventricle. Atrialized right ventricle may produce an undulating rippling motion in parasternal area. Remodeled dilated right ventricular infundibulum may impart a parasternal pulsation in left 3rd intercostal space.

Single Ventricle

Single ventricle may be left ventricular or right ventricular. Left ventricular type produces a normal apical impulse. Increased pulmonary flow may produce a hyperkinetic apical impulse. Outlet chamber pulsation may be palpable parasternal at left 3rd intercostal space. If there is subaortic obstruction, a thrill may be palpable at this location. As aorta is anterior, A2 may be palpable. Right ventricular type produces a diffuse apical impulse and outlet chamber pulsation is absent.

The d-transposition of the Great Arteries

The d-transposition of the great arteries (d-TGA) produces a prominent right ventricular impulse, as right ventricle bears the systemic vascular resistance. In presence of VSD, as large grossly unsaturated blood recirculated in systemic circulation, right ventricular impulse becomes prominent. Left ventricular pulsation is usually absent, as it ejects against pulmonary vascular resistance. However, in presence of VSD or significant pulmonary hypertension, apex may be formed by left ventricle and features of biventricular hypertrophy may be present. As aorta in anterior, A2 may be palpable.

Congenitally Corrected TGA, VSD and PS

Congenitally corrected TGA, VSD and PS presents with largest right ventricular impulse amongst congenital cyanotic heart disease, due to disposition of ventricular septum, which is oriented anteroposterior. Interventricular sulcus is just behind left border of sternum and inverted left ventricle is behind sternum. Hence, left ventricular movements cannot be appreciated on palpation staring from left parasternal region to apical area. In presence of left atrioventricular valve regurgitation, right ventricular impulse may be hyperdynamic. As ascending aorta is left and anterior, aortic pulsation and A2 may be palpable in left second intercostal space.

TABLE 1: Difference between right and left ventricular apical impulse.

RV apex	LV apex
Diffuse, palpable over wider area and continuous with parasternal pulsation	Localized
Lateral retraction (retraction is best appreciated in lateral decubitus position)	Medial retraction
Found in: • All diseases under tetralogy physiology umbrella • TGA	Found in: • Tricuspid atresia • Single (left ventricle) ventricle • DORV, PS, restrictive VSD • Ebstein's anomaly • Pulmonary atresia, intact septum • Vena cava to left atrial communication

(DORV: double outlet right ventricle; PS: pulmonary stenosis; TGA: transposition of great arteries; VSD: ventricular septal defect; RV: right ventricular; LV: left ventricular)

Truncus Arteriosus

Truncus arteriosus is typically associated with biventricular enlargement: A left ventricular apical impulse due to truncal regurgitation and right ventricular impulse due to increased pulmonary vascular resistance. Right sternoclavicular pulsation is common due to right-sided aortic arch.

Vena caval connection to left atrium is another cyanotic heart disease, where cyanotic heart disease is associated with left ventricular apical impulse. Basic difference between left and right ventricular apex is summarised in **Table 1**.

PERCUSSION

Auenbrugger introduced cardiac percussion in 1761.[14] Then over two centuries, percussion of the heart loses its relevance in modern cardiac practice. Excepting in situation like situs abnormalities and dextrocardia, cardiac percussion is not done routinely. There are various clinical methods suggested for percussion, most of which have not been standardized or compared to other imaging (**Figs. 21** and **22**).

Heckerling introduced precordial percussion to diagnose cardiomegaly and compared the percussion data with CT (computed tomography) image of heart.[15] Heckerling's percussion method[16] is described here.

Percussion Method

There are three methods of percussion—direct, indirect, and auscultatory percussion. Indirect percussion is the commonly followed method. The basic purpose is to identify left and right heart border. Remembering the surface anatomy of the heart, percussion is carried out in the following steps:

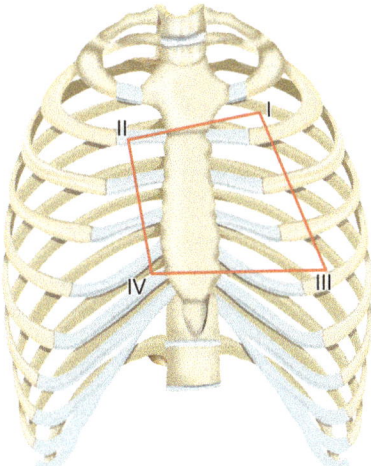

Fig. 21: Surface anatomy of heart. I: 1.5 inch from midline on the lower border of the 2nd left costal cartilage; II: 1 inch from the midline on the upper border of the 3rd right costal cartilage; III: 3.5 inch from midline on the lower border of the left 5th intercostal space; and IV: 0.5 inch from the midline on the right 6th costal cartilage.

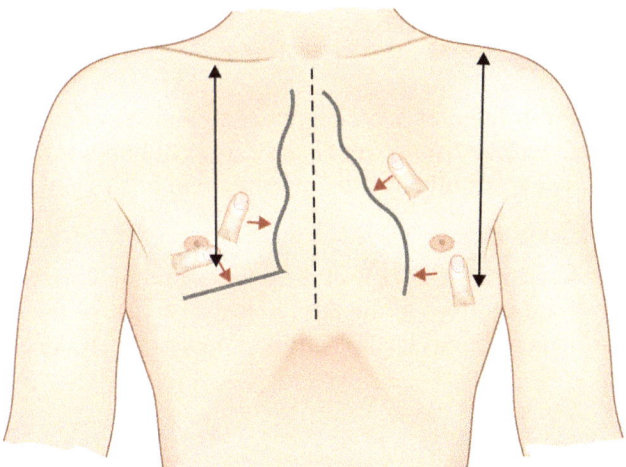

Fig. 22: Percussion point and zones.

- Patient is placed in supine position.
- Light indirect percussion is done in the left 2nd through 6th intercostal space and the right second through 5th intercostal space.
- Left middle finger is gently pressed against chest wall in each intercostal space, with its long axis parallel to ribs and the tip of the right middle finger delivers a light blow to the distal interphalangeal joint of the pleximeter finger.
- To delineate left heart border, percussion starts on each left intercostal space from mid-axillary line and to delineate right heart border, percussion starts

on each right intercostal space from mid-clavicular line. The pleximeter finger is moved medially along each space at 1 cm increment, until a dull percussion note is detected. Then the finger is moved lateral to the dull point and percussion restarted at 0.5 cm increment until a dull point is detected. Each dull point is marked by skin pencil.
- To delineate right heart border, percussion starts on each right intercostal space from midclavicular line to midline. In place of percussion on 5th intercostal space to detect dullness of the right cardiophrenic border, upper border of liver dullness can be detected first by percussion on midclavicular line and then one space above the liver dullness is chosen and percussion done along this space from midclavicular line to midline.

Percussion in Special Situation

Left Parasternal 2nd Intercostal Space
The space is usually resonant. A dull note indicates dilated pulmonary artery or malposed dilated aorta.

Right Parasternal 2nd Intercostal Space
When this space is dull on percussion, probabilities are aortic aneurysm, dilated ascending aorta or pericardial effusion.

Situs
In situs inversus, liver dullness is on left upper abdomen and fundal tympany is on right upper abdomen. In situs ambiguous, liver dullness extends from right upper, mid- and left upper quadrant of upper abdomen.

Pericardial Effusion
In 1878, Rotch described[17] this sign of dullness extending from 2 to 3 cm from the right edge of the sternum in the 5th intercostal space, at the cardiohepatic angle in pericardial effusion (**Fig. 23**). This is known as Rotch sign. He described

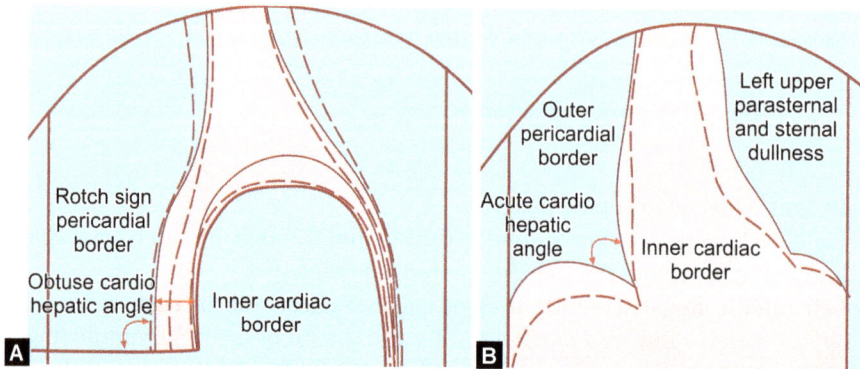

Figs. 23A and B: (A) Pericardial effusion and Rotch sign: dullness extends laterally, as cardiohepatic angle becomes obtuse; (B) Pericardial effusion and Morris sign: Cardiohepatic angle is acute, and dullness extends upward on sternum and left and right upper intercostal space, parasternal.

that the angle became obtuse in pericardial effusion and produced the dullness. Subsequent work by Morris and Bader[18] disagreed to Rotch. Pericardial effusion in recumbent posture depresses diaphragm and the cardiohepatic angle becomes more acute. Moreover, in early pericardial effusion, dullness extends to upper sternum including left 2nd or even 1st parasternal intercostal space, all of which become dull on percussion.

CONCLUSION

To remind you, your hand is more sensuous than transducer!

REFERENCES

1. Dimond EG. Precordial vibration: clinical clues from palpation. Circulation. 1964;30:284.
2. Haycraft JB. The movements of the heart within the chest cavity and the cardiogram. J Physiol (Lond). 1891;12:438.
3. Rushmer RF. Cardiovascular Dynamics, 2nd edition. Philadelphia and London: Saunders; 1961.
4. Deliyannis AA, Gillam PMS, Mounsey JPD, et al. The cardiac impulse and the motion of the heart. Br Heart J. 1964;26:396.
5. Norman J, Harrison T. Movement and forces of human heart. IV. Precordial movement (kinetocardiogram) in relation to ejection and filling of ventricles. Arch Intern Med. 1958;101:582.
6. Ranganathan N, Sivaciyan V, Saksena FB. The art and science of cardiac physical examination. Humana Press, Springer; 2006. p. 115.
7. Eilen SD, Crawford MH, O'Rourke RA. Accuracy of precordial palpation for detecting increased left ventricular volume. Ann Intern Med. 1983;99:628-30.
8. Gillam PMS, Deliyannis AA, Mounsey JPD. The left parasternal impulse. Br Heart J. 1964;26:726.
9. Basta LL, Wolfson P, Eckberg DL, et al. The value of left parasternal impulse recording in assessment of mitral regurgitation. Circulation. 1973;48:1055-65.
10. Boicourt OW, Nagle RE, Mounsey JPD. The Clinical Significance of Systolic Retraction of the Apical Impulse. Br Heart J. 1965;27:379.
11. Cossio P. Choquoe de la punta mitral. Rev Argent Cardiol. 1943;10:145-61.
12. Floyed J. Willis PW, Craige E. The apex impulse in mitral stenosis: Graphic explanation of the palpable movements at the cardiac apex. Am J Cardiol. 1983;51:311-4.
13. Ranganathan N, Juma Z, Sivaciyan V. The apical impulse in coronary heart disease. Clin Cardiol. 1985;8:20-33.
14. Bedford DE. Auenbrugger's contribution to cardiology: history of percussion of the heart. Br Heart J. 1971;33:817-21.
15. Heckerling PS, Wiwner SL, Christopher J, et al. Accuracy and reproducibility of precordial percussion and palpation for detecting increased left ventricular End-diastolic volume and mass. JAMA. 1993;270:1943-8.
16. Heckerling PS, Wiener SL, Moses VK, et al. Accuracy of precordial percussion in detecting cardiomegaly. Am J Med. 1991;91:328-34.
17. Rotch TM. Absence of Resonance in the Fifth Right Intercostal Space Diagnostic of Pericardial Effusion. Boston Med Surg J. 1878;99:389, 421.
18. Morris RS, Bader ER. A comparison of the percussion and roentgen-ray findings after injection of pericardium. JAMA. 1917;LXIX:450-3.

CHAPTER 14

First Heart Sound

INTRODUCTION

Hippocrates (460 to 370 BC) used to auscultate by the direct application of the ear to the patient's chest. Using this technique, Hippocrates described—"*You shall know by this that the chest contains water but not pus, if in applying the ear during a certain time on the side, you perceive a noise like that of boiling vinegar.*" Hippocrates began auscultation, but he did not describe first heart sound! After centuries, Charles JB Williams (1805–1889) coined the term "LUBB-DUPP" and then began the journey of first heart sound as LUBB!

COMPONENTS OF FIRST HEART SOUND

In cardiac cycle, after late atrial contraction, the stretched ventricle starts its contraction. When ventricular pressure crosses atrial pressure, atrioventricular valve leaflets get apposed and closed. As contraction continues, semilunar valves open, once ventricular pressure crosses great artery pressure and blood is accelerated in the great vessels. First heart sound (S1) comprises all these four events, which used to occur in a quick succession. They are named as:

- Atrial component is the small frequency vibration that occurs when blood column strikes on and dissipates from the ventricular wall. In normal condition, this atrial sound is too soft to be audible and does not contribute in S1. In short PR interval, it occurs very closely to S1 and contributes in its sound.[1]
- Mitral component is the high frequency vibration of mitral valve closure (M1) and is effectively the first component of S1. Merely apposition of mitral leaflets does not produce M1. Mitral valve apparatus actually acts as parashot. The moving column of blood pushes the mitral leaflets toward left atrium, whereas papillary muscle and chordae prevent its eversion. As chordae reach its limit, the leaflets become tense and prevent the moving column of blood. The sudden deceleration of the column of blood produces the high frequency vibration or M1.
- Tricuspid component is the vibration of tricuspid valve closure (T1) and is the second component (T1) of S1. Mechanism of its origin is same as M1.

However, its frequency is relatively lower in compare to M1 because flow is from relatively lower pressure right ventricle. Its maximum intensity at left lower sternal edge and enhancement of its intensity on inspiration and immediately after Valsalva indicate the tricuspid valve origin of this sound. Because of its relative low frequency, T1 normally is not audible. It only enhances the duration of S1.

- Aortic component (A1) is the small frequency vibration component, which occurs when ventricle ejects blood in great vessels. Deceleration of ejecting blood column on the aortic wall produces this component. When deceleration is significant, aortic component may be audible.[2] When audible, aortic component is heard at apex and does not vary with respiration or Valsalva like T1.

In many of the patients, S1 is single. Only when the split between M1 and T1 or A1 exceeds 20 ms, then the other components are audible. In children and younger persons T1 and in adult A1 is more audible. S1 is medium to high frequency sound and its pitch is lower than second heart sound (S2).

HEMODYNAMIC CORRELATION

Mitral valve closure does not occur immediately at the point, where left ventricular pressure crosses left atrial pressure. This is because of mitral valve inertia, forward flow continues for 20–30 ms, after which the valve closes at the downstroke of the *c* wave of left atria pressure curve. This is also applicable for T1, which occurs not at the right ventricular-right atrial pressure crossover but at the *c* wave (**Fig. 1**).

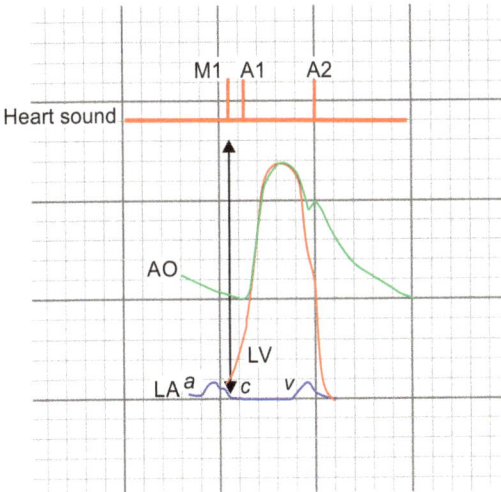

(AO: aorta)

Fig. 1: Pressure curve of left ventricle (LV) and left atrium (LA) along with apex phonocardiogram. mitral valve closure (M1) is coincident with the downstroke of the left atrial *c* wave and separated from left ventricular left atrial pressure crossover by an interval of 30 ms. Aortic component of S1 can be seen.

MECHANISM

The debate between atriogenic and ventriculogenic valve closure theories continued for century, after the first atriogenic theory of mitral valve closure was proposed by Baumgarten in 1843.[3] As mentioned, S1 occurs not at the apposition of the valve leaflets but rather the tensing of the leaflets and sudden deceleration of blood resulting from this event that could lead to vibrations of the cardiohemic system and audible sound. Aortic component occurs due to aortic valve opening and sudden acceleration of blood in the root of the aorta.

TIMING

One must use the diaphragm to pick up this high frequency sound at the apex and the left lower sternal area. M1 occurs before the carotid upstroke because M1 precedes left ventricular ejection. But this delay between M1 and upstroke is too short to be appreciated at bedside. T1 coincides with the carotid upstroke.

SPLITTING

Physiological

Mitral valve closure occurs 20-50 ms earlier than the T1 of first heart sound. Normally, the gap is nearing 20 ms and two components cannot be differentiated on auscultation. M1 occurs earlier than T1 because of two factors. Left ventricular contraction starts earlier than the right ventricle, hence mitral valve closes earlier than the tricuspid valve. Besides, left atrial contraction is more effective than the right atrium in exerting the closing force, as a result of which the mitral valve is in closing position at the onset of systole and closes earlier. M1 is best appreciated at the apex and T1 is at the left lower sternal area.

Pathological

Right bundle branch block (RBBB) is the most common cause of wide split of the S1. However, in many cases of RBBB, T1 is not delayed because the block is at the arborization level (peripheral) causing a delayed right ventricular upstroke, but right ventricular contraction starting at usual time. In Ebstein anomaly, the right bundle is stunted with poor growth of the peripheral parts, causing a delayed right ventricular contraction. More important here is the delayed movement of the abnormal anterior tricuspid leaflet. Tricuspid stenosis and atrial septal defect (ASD) are the other causes of delayed T2.

Reversed splitting of S1 is very rare. Severe mitral stenosis or left atrial myxoma can cause the reversed splitting. Left bundle branch block should cause reversed splitting, but here also the block is at the peripheral level and onset of left ventricular contraction is not delayed.

INTENSITY (BOX 1)

The intensity of S1 is predominantly decided by the mitral component. It can be compared to S2 to assess its intensity. When S1 is softer than S2 at the apex, it can be described as soft. When it is louder than S2 at the base, it can be described as loud S1.

INCREASED INTENSITY (BOX 2)

Pathophysiology

- Position of the mitral valve at the onset of systole is the most important determinant of S1 amplitude or intensity. More open the valve remains at the onset of ventricular systole, more the leaflets have to travel from the open to closed position. This long travel results in the valve closure during the steeper part of the left ventricular pressure pulse, producing loud S1. As the PR interval is progressively decreased from 130 to 30 ms, there is progressively increase in intensity of M1. At an interval of 30-75 ms, mitral valve is maximally separated by atrial contraction at the onset of ventricular contraction, resulting in loud S1. At a PR interval <10 ms, left atrium and left ventricle contract simultaneously and S1 becomes soft. On the other hand, at a very long PR interval, atrium starts relaxing and the mitral valve comes to a closing position at the onset of ventricular contraction. Mitral stenosis and atrial myxoma (high transmitral pressure gradient), post-tricuspid left to right shunt (increased transmitral flow), produce loud M1 by keeping the mitral valve wide open at the onset of ventricular systole.
- Left ventricular contractility and rate of rise of ventricular pressure are other important determinants of S1 intensity. In normal volunteer, isotonic exercise or catecholamine infusion increase S1 intensity by increasing left ventricular contractility, whereas beta-blocker reduces the intensity by opposing effect.[4]

BOX 1   **Factors determining the intensity of first heart sound.**

- Position of the valve at the onset of systole
- Left ventricular contractility and rate of rise of ventricular pressure
- Valve pliability
- Valve cusp adequacy

BOX 2   **Loud first heart sound.**

- Mitral stenosis
- Atrial myxoma
- Post-tricuspid left-to-right shunt
- Short PR interval
- Tachycardia
- Mitral valve prolapse syndrome
- Tricuspid stenosis
- Atrial septal defect

In conditions like anemia, fever, pregnancy, and arteriovenous (AV) fistula increased rate of rise of left ventricular pressure enhances the intensity of S1 and conditions like myxedema, cardiomyopathies, and acute myocardial infarction reduced rate of left ventricular pressure development reduces S1 intensity. Beat-to-beat variation of S1 intensity in patient with pulsus alternans is due to same mechanisms.

S1 in Mitral Stenosis

Loud and sharp S1 is synonymous with mitral stenosis. Two factors play role in the mechanism. First factor is increased left atrial pressure, which delays the pressure crossover between left ventricle and left atrium. Second factor is presystolic gradient between left atrium and left ventricle, which prevents the preclosure of mitral valve. Thus, at the onset of ventricular contraction mitral valve closure starts from a domed position and traverses a longer excursion. In consequence of these two factors, S1 occurs at the time of steep ventricular pressure pulse and causes loud and sharp S1 (**Fig. 2**).

S1 in Mitral Valve Prolapse[5]

In mitral valve prolapse (MVP) syndrome, M1 is loud in spite of mitral regurgitation. The major mechanism is increased amplitude of mitral valve excursion beyond the line of closure, resulting in increased tension of the mitral chordal apparatus. Other explanations are merging of click sound with M1 and increased adrenergic activity in this pathology. Prolapse should be pansystolic for the merging of prolapsing sound with S1, otherwise in mid- or late-systolic prolapse, S1 intensity is usually normal. On the other hand, in case of flail mitral valve, failure of coaptation and ineffective valve closure result in reduced or absent M1 (**Fig. 3**).

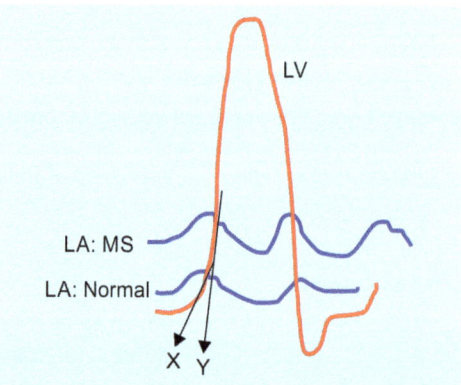

Fig. 2: Pressure curve of left ventricle (LV) and left atrium (LA) in normal mitral stenosis. In later, mitral valve closes at a point of steeper left ventricular pressure pulse (Y slope). In normal left atrial pressure curve, mitral valve closes at an early part of left ventricular pressure pulse (X slope).

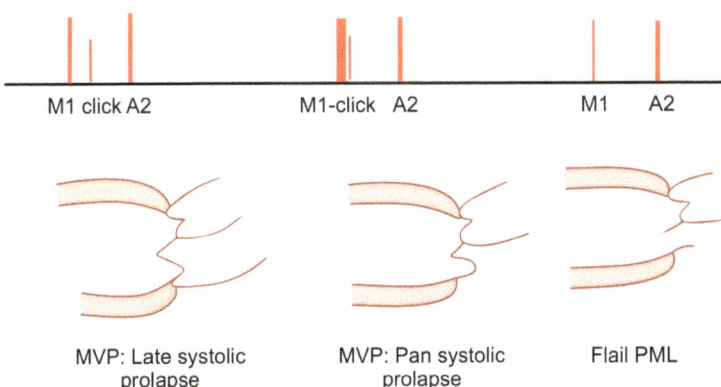

(PML: posterior mitral leaflet)

Fig. 3: In mitral valve prolapse (MVP): Mid to late systolic prolapse, mitral valve closure (M1) is normal; in pansystolic prolapse, M1 is loud; in flail mitral valve, M1 is either soft or absent.[5]

S1 in Tricuspid Stenosis and ASD

Tricuspid valve closure component is loud in tricuspid stenosis due to high transtricuspid pressure gradient. In ASD, large left-to-right shunt keeps the tricuspid valve cusps in the position found in rapid right ventricular filling throughout diastole. Thus, the velocity of tricuspid valve closure with the onset of right ventricular systole is rapid and results in loud T1. Another mechanism is the better audibility of T1, because apex is formed by right ventricle.

S1 in Ebstein Anomaly

Mitral valve closure-tricuspid valve closure (M1-T1) split is wider. T1 occurs when the large anterior leaflet of tricuspid valve reaches its limit of anterior excursion, gets maximally tensed and produces a sharp sound similar to that of a sail snapping the wind, known as sail sign. This sound not exactly due to tricuspid valve closure, which is mostly ineffective due to presence of significant tricuspid regurgitation.

Decreased Intensity (Box 3)

First heart sound is soft or absent in severe rheumatic mitral or tricuspid regurgitation. Reduced rate of left ventricular pressure due to mitral valve leak during isometric contraction phase is the most plausible explanation. Ineffective valve closure is another mechanism. Stenosed mitral or tricuspid valve with gross calcification causes loss of valve pliability with a soft S1. Semiclosing position of the mitral valve at the onset of ventricular systole, as happens in prolonged PR interval or chronic severe aortic regurgitation may cause soft S1, because the valve halting occurs at the beginning part of ventricular systole, when pressure rise is not steep. Similarly, in acute severe aortic regurgitation with increased left ventricular

> **BOX 3** **Soft first heart sound.**
> - Severe mitral regurgitation or tricuspid regurgitation
> - Grossly calcified, nonpliable valve
> - Prolonged PR interval
> - Chronic or acute severe aortic regurgitation
> - Severe aortic stenosis
> - Left ventricular systolic dysfunction
> - Pericardial effusion, obesity, and chronic obstructive pulmonary disease

end-diastolic pressure, S1 becomes soft, sometimes inaudible. In severe aortic stenosis, S1 is soft, probably because of powerful left atrial contraction causes a rapid rise of ventricular end diastolic pressure causing semiclosing position of the mitral valve at. In left ventricular systolic dysfunction, poor rate of rise of pressure as well as increased end diastolic pressure causes soft S1. Pericardial effusion, obesity and COPD are other obvious causes of soft S1.

Varying Intensity

Complete heart block, Mobitz type I block, and ventricular tachycardia with atrioventricular dissociation cause variable intensity of S1. In complete heart block, the intensity of S1 varies with the changing PR interval and is maximum at the PR interval of 0.11 second.

Atrial fibrillation[6] is the most common cause of variable intensity of S1. Loud S1 occurs after a short RR interval. During short RR interval, left ventricular filling is less and its contractility should be less forceful. On the other hand, during short RR interval, left atrial pressure cannot fall at a lower level. These two factors play opposite role on the S1 intensity. The second factor usually dominates, leading to loud S1 after short cycle. After a longer RR interval, S1 is down because the valve leaflets remain partially closed. Though preceding RR interval controls S1 intensity, the RR interval prior to preceding RR interval plays an important role by postextrasystolic potentiation. Shorter the RR interval preceding the preceding RR interval, louder is the S1.

Alternate loud and soft S1, auscultatory alternans, may be found in cardiac tamponade and severe left ventricular dysfunction.

Sound Surrounding S1 (Fig. 4)

M1-T1 versus S1-ejection Click[7]

First heart sound-ejection click interval is wider than the interval between M1-T1. T1 is best audible at tricuspid area. Aortic ejection click is widely distributed on precordium, whereas pulmonary valvular click is best heard in left second or third intercostals space. M1 is usually louder than T1, whereas click is louder than S1. Inspiration increases the intensity of T1, reduces intensity of pulmonary valvular click and does not affect aortic click significantly.

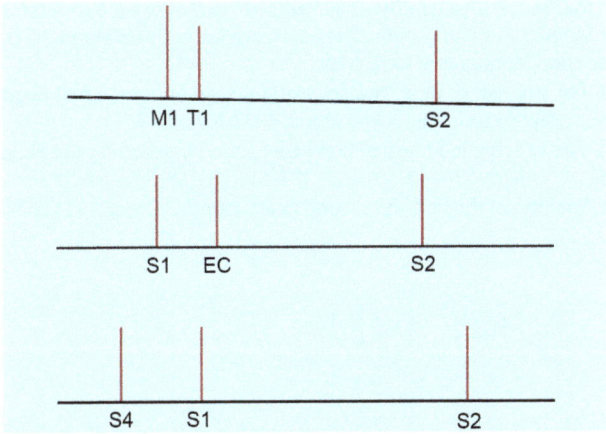

(EC: ejection click; M1: mitral valve closure; S1: first heart sound; S2: second heart sound; S4: fourth heart sound; T1: tricuspid valve closure)

Fig. 4: Events around S1.

M1-T1 versus S1-nonejection Click

First heart sound-mitral valve prolapse click interval is similarly wider than the M1-T1 interval. Dynamic auscultation results in shifting of the click in relation to S1. The effect is less obvious for M1-T1 relation.

M1-T1 versus S4-S1

Fourth heart sound is low frequency sound and preceds S1. It is localized at the apex and best audible with the bell of the stethoscope.

CONCLUSION

Rouanet, in 1830 first described first heart sound. What he did pumping water through an animal heart, which was held to his ear, as there was no stethoscope. He could hear two major noises from each side of the heart, one at the beginning and another at the end of systole. He described them as tensioning of atrioventricular and semilunar valves. After nearing two centuries, we have developed so many instrumentations to hear first heart sound. Unfortunately, we have lost our interest to hear it anymore.

REFERENCES

1. Kincaid-Smith P, Barlow J. The atrial sound and the atrial component of the first heart sound. Br Heart J. 1959;21:470-8.
2. Waider W, Craige E. First heart sound and ejection sounds. Echocardiographic and phonocardiographic correlation with valvular events. Am J Cardiol. 1975;35:346.
3. Baumgarten A. Ueber dem mechanismus durch welchen die venosen herzklappen geschlossen werden. Arch Anat Physiol Lpz. 1843;463.

4. Thompson ME, Shaver JA, Leon DF, et al. Patho-dynamics of the first heart sound. In: Leon DF, Shaver JA (Eds). Physiologic Principles of Heart Sounds and Murmurs. Dallas, American Heart Association Monograph. 1975;46:8.
5. Tei C, Shah PM, Cherian G, et al. The correlation of an abnormal first heart sound and in mitral valve prolapse syndrome. N Eng J med. 1982;307:334-9.
6. Rytand DA. The variable loudness of first heart sound in auricular fibrillation. Am Heart J. 1949;37:187.
7. Leatham A. Splitting of the first and second heart sounds. Lancet. 1954;267:607.

CHAPTER 15

Second Heart Sound

INTRODUCTION

Rouanet in 1832[1] first described that second heart sound (S2) resulted from the closure of semilunar valve. S2 is sharper, shorter, and higher pitched than S1. Leatham, one of the masters on cardiac auscultation, described[2] S2 as "the key to auscultation to heart."

MECHANISM OF SECOND HEART SOUND PRODUCTION

During the closure of the semilunar valves, clapping of the leaflets does not produce the sound. Sudden deceleration of the retrograde flow of the blood column in the aorta or pulmonary artery (PA) by the closed tensed valves set the vibration of the cardiohemic system. The high frequency components of this vibration produce S2.

PHYSIOLOGICAL SPLITTING (FIG. 1)

In 1865, Potain[3] first described clinically the splitting of normal S2 and its respiratory variation. S2 shows splitting on inspiration and narrowing on expiration. This is known as physiological splitting. Right and left ventricular (LV) mechanical systole are nearly equal in duration. However, right ventricular (RV) ejection starts prior to LV ejection, has longer in duration, and ends after LV ejection. Thus, the pulmonary component (P2) occurs 10-20 ms after aortic component (A2) of S2.[4] One cannot appreciate two components unless the split is >30-50 ms. This causes the S2 single during expiration in 90% of normal persons, where the split is <15-20 ms. Inspiratory splitting in normal persons is in the range of 20-60 ms. The range depends on the age of the patient and depth of inspiration. In person over 40 year of age, S2 may be single in both phase of respiration.

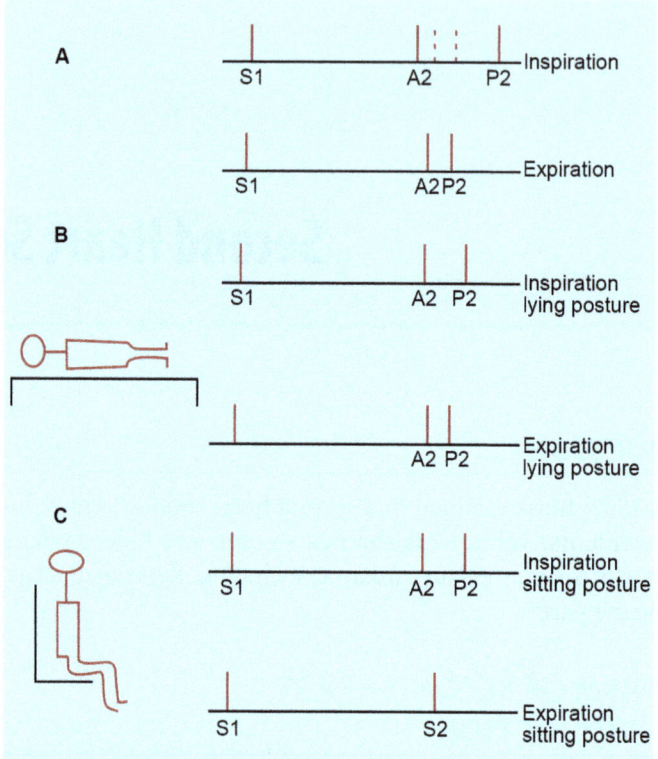

(S1: first heart sound; S2: second heart sound)

Fig. 1: Physiological splitting of S2. (A) During inspiration, P2 is delayed and A2 occurs earlier. Inspiratory shifting of P2 is more than shifting of A2; (B) in lying down posture, due to increased preload, S2 may appear as persistently splitted, due to audibly wide expiratory splitting; and (C) in sitting posture, expiratory splitting narrows down and becomes audibly single. Thus, proper assessment of S2 splitting should be done with patient in sitting posture.

Traditional Explanation

Traditional explanation of the physiological splitting of S2 is the difference of right and LV ejection time. Inspiration augments RV preload, effective filling pressure, and end-diastolic volume and stroke output of the right ventricle. It has an opposite effect of all the above parameters on left ventricle. The result is the prolongation of Q-P2, shortening of Q-A2, and an increase in A2-P2 gap during inspiration. 86% of the increase is contributed by prolongation of RV systole and 14% is contributed by shortening of LV systole (**Fig. 2**).[5]

Shaver later showed that physiological splitting was due to complex interplay between dynamic changes in pulmonary vascular resistance and to changes in pulmonary and systemic venous return during respiration.[4] Hang-out time was the basis of this complex interplay.

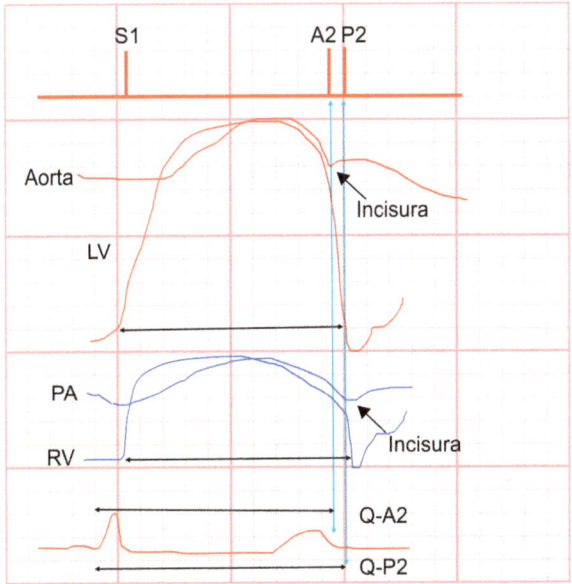

(LV: left ventricular; RV: right ventricular)

Fig. 2: Duration of mechanical systole of both ventricles are more or less equal; RV ejection starts prior to LV ejection, has longer in duration and ends after LV ejection; Q-P2 > Q-A2.

Hang-out Time

Hang-out time is defined as the interval between the end of the ventricular ejection and closure of the semilunar valve. This time is longer in PA than the aorta. Pulmonary hang-out time may be up to 60–70 ms, whereas aortic hang-out time may be below 20–30 ms. Semilunar valve is closed only when the PA or aortic diastolic pressure crosses that of the respective ventricle. Pulmonary vasculature is more compliant than the systemic vasculature; pulmonary vascular resistance is one-tenth of that of aorta and PA has less elastic recoil power than that of the aorta. Thus, it takes a longer time for the diastolic pressure building up in the PA than in the aorta for this crossover (**Fig. 3**).

Incisura

Point of crossover of aorta or PA over its respective ventricle in the pressure curve is called incisura, which coincides with S2. Hang-out time can also be defined as the distance between the ventricular pressure curve and the aortic or pulmonary incisura. Actual cusp apposition occurs before the incisura. Due to inertia, the forward flow continues. Duration of this forward flow determines the hang-out time and depends on the vascular capacitance, vascular resistance, and the recoil property of the aorta versus PA.

During inspiration, there is increased pulmonary vascular capacitance resulting in longer PA hang-out time and increased venous return resulting in longer RV ejection time. P2 is delayed by both of these factors, more important

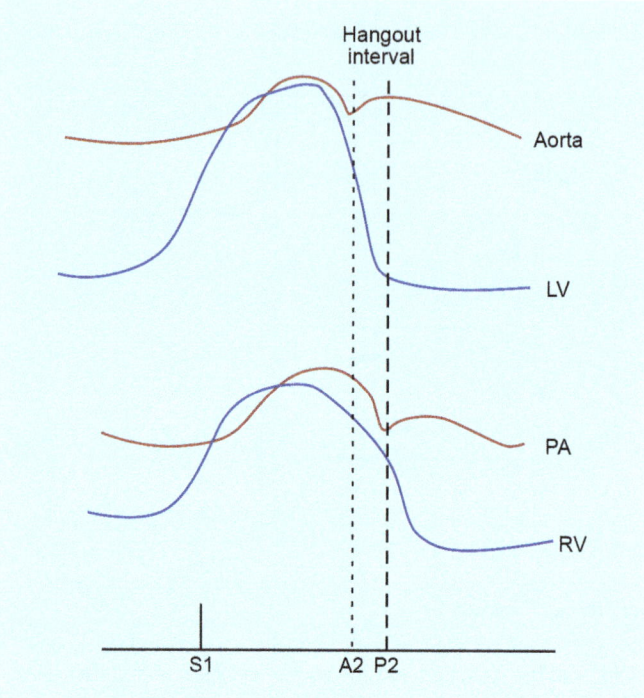

(LV: left ventricular; PA: pulmonary artery; RV: right ventricular)

Fig. 3: Hang-out interval, which is defined as the interval between the end of the ventricular ejection and closure of the semilunar valve. It is up to 70 ms for P2 and 30 ms for A2.

being the hang-out time. Inspiration causes decreased intrathoracic pressure, which is transmitted in the pulmonary veins with a pulling effect, without any change in the aortic capacitance. LV stroke volume is decreased with shortening of ejection time, resulting in early A2.

PATHOLOGICAL/PERSISTING SPLITTING (BOX 1)

Pathological splitting of S2 is defined as any audible expiratory splitting (>30 ms) at bedside, both in supine and upright posture.[6] The term persisting splitting appears to be more meaningful.[7]

Wide Persisting Splitting (Box 2)

Second heart sound is said to be widely splitted:
- When both of its components can be appreciated in expiration, particularly in standing position; there may be further widening during inspiration.
- Inspiratory widening >60 ms; may be single on expiration.

Most common causes are the electrical abnormalities including right bundle branch block (RBBB), Wolff-Parkinson-White (WPW) syndrome with LV pre-excitation. There is late activation of the right ventricle resulting in delayed P2.

> **BOX 1   Pathological/persisting splitting of second heart sound.**
> - Wide persistent splitting
> - Wide fixed persistent splitting
> - Narrow persistent splitting
> - Reverse splitting

> **BOX 2   Wide splitting of second heart sound.**
>
> **Electrical causes:**
> - RBBB
> - WPW syndrome.
> - LV paced beat
> - LV ectopic
>
> **Mechanical causes:**
> - Delayed P2 (moderate-to-severe pulmonary stenosis, acute pulmonary embolism)
> - Early A2 (severe MR, large VSD, constrictive pericarditis)
>
> **Prolonged hang-out time:**
> *Mobile*:
> - Idiopathic dilatation of PA
> - Mild pulmonary stenosis
>
> *Fixed*:
> - ASD (fixed)
> - RV systolic dysfunction (fixed)

(ASD: atrial septal defect; MR: mitral regurgitation; RBBB: right bundle branch block; RV: right ventricular; WPW: Wolff–Parkinson–White; VSD: ventricular septal defect ; LV: left ventricular; PA: pulmonary artery))

Mechanical causes include pulmonary valvular stenosis, infundibular stenosis, and peripheral PA stenosis, all of which prolong RV activation time resulting in delayed P2. In pulmonary valvular stenosis, severity is directly proportional to expiratory splitting. When the splitting is 70-80 ms, RV systolic pressure approximates 70-80 mm Hg. Severe mitral regurgitation (MR) and large ventricular septal defect (VSD) cause wide expiratory splitting due to early A2 by shortening LV mechanical systole. Wide inspiratory splitting due to early A2 occurs in constrictive pericarditis. Inspiration causes decreased intrathoracic pressure as well as decreased pulmonary venous pressure, which is an extracardiac structure. But this thoracic pressure swinging is not reflected on cardiac chambers due to constricted pericardium. Thus, left atrial pressure remains normal during inspiration. This diminished pulmonary vein—left atrial pressure gradient during inspiration causes reduced LV venous return and ejection time. Wide split is found in idiopathic dilatation of PA due to prolonged hang-out time.

Wide Fixed Splitting

Atrial Septal Defect

The split is defined fixed when the respiratory variation is <20 ms. This is one of the most consistent auscultatory finding and hallmark of all forms of atrial septal defect (ASD). There are two theories: Traditional and hang-out interval theory.

Traditional theory[8] states that right and left atrium act as a common reservoir in ASD, receiving blood from systemic and pulmonary venous system. From this common reservoir, blood passes to either of the ventricle, depending on the compliance of the two ventricles, and amount of blood remains constant throughout the respiratory cycle. However, the composition of blood varies with respiration. On inspiration, right ventricle gets more systemic venous blood and in consequence, less pulmonary venous blood is shunted to right atrium. On expiration, as right ventricle gets less systemic and more pulmonary venous flow. Reciprocal change occurs in LV stroke volume and ejection time. In consequence, right or LV filling and output ratio show little of changes with respiration. As RV compliance is more than left ventricle, it receives more blood across ASD, and its output exceeds that of left ventricle by an amount which is determined by the RV compliance ecceeding LV compliance. As a result, RV event and P2 are delayed in compare to LV event without any respiratory variation (**Fig. 4**).

Hang-out interval theory[9] states in other way. Right ventricle uses to adapt chronic volume overload and ejects the increased volume load without any significant increase in ejection time. Thus, wide split cannot be explained by the prolongation or shortening of electromechanical systole of right or left ventricle alone. Then came the hang-out interval theory. Due to long-standing volume overload of right side of circulation, pulmonary arteries become significantly dilated. Pulmonary vascular bed becomes a high capacitance low-resistance system with wide prolonged hang-out interval. Coupled with normal and low systemic vascular hang-out interval, wide pulmonary hang-out interval leads to wide persistent split of S2. Wideness persists even after ASD closure indicating high pulmonary vascular capacitance rather than theory of electromechanical systole or shunt reciprocation is responsible for wide splitting of S2 (**Fig. 5**). Wide splitting found in idiopathic dilatation of PA is another evidence of this theory. As capacitance is already increased, inspiration does not cause any additional increase. This fixed hang-out time in both phases of respiration causes the fixed splitting.

In ASD, the split may be <60 ms. Grade of shunt, probably is not related with degree of splitting.

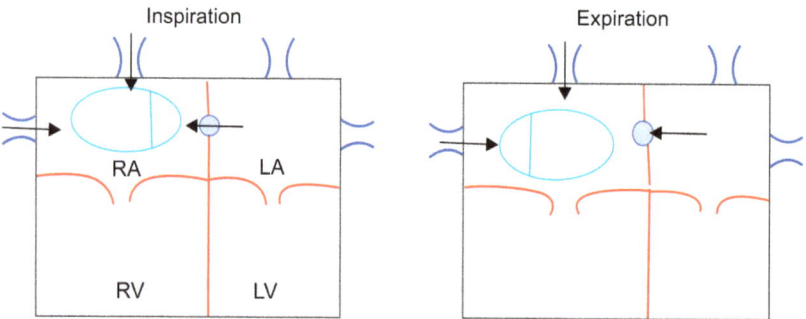

Fig. 4: On inspiration, more venous return to right atrium with reciprocal reduced left-to-right shunt across atrial septal defect (ASD). During expiration, the reverse happens with less venous return to right atrium and more left-to-right shunt across ASD.

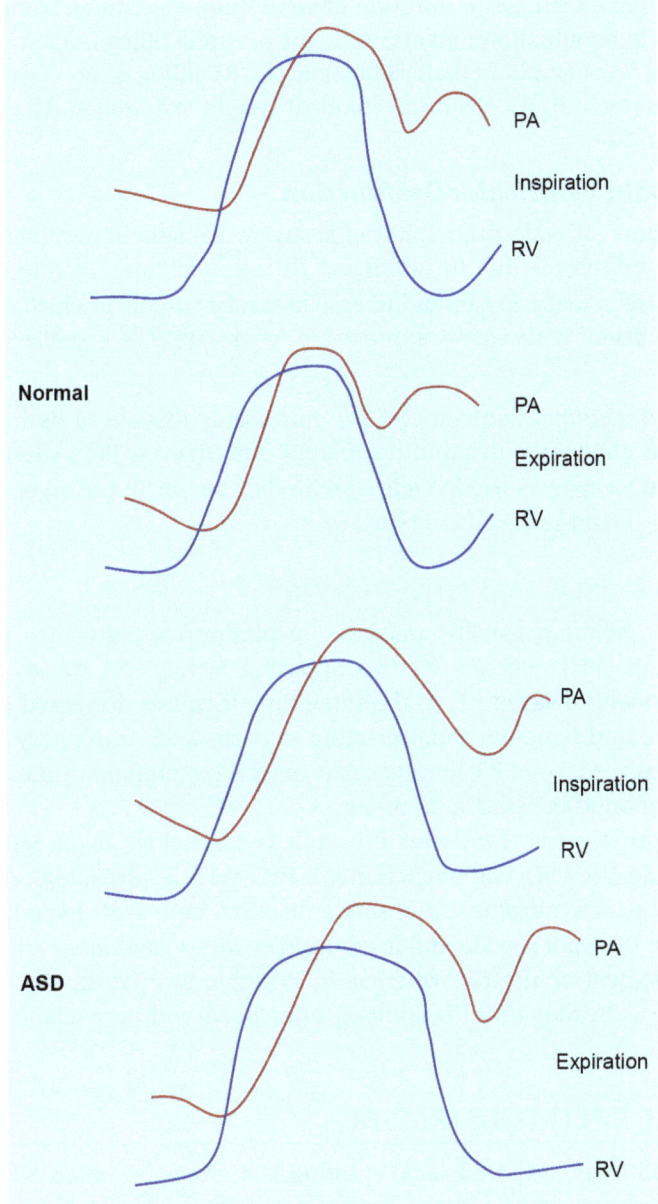

(LV: left ventricular; PA: pulmonary artery; RV: right ventricular; ASD: Atrial septal defect)

Fig. 5: ASD: In normal situation, pulmonary hang-out interval widens more in inspiration, which is responsible for inspiratory split. In ASD, hang-out interval is fixed in both phases of respiration, causing the fixed splitting of S2.

Atrial Septal Defect with Atrial Fibrillation[9]

Longer the RR interval is in atrial fibrillation, wider will be the splitting in ASD. This is because QP2 progressively increases with increasing cycle length due to selective increase in duration of ventricular electromechanical systole. Longer cycle length allows greater time for diastolic filling. As left ventricle is thicker and less compliant than right ventricle, RV filling is more, which causes selective increase in RV electromechanical systole resulting in delayed P2 and widening of S2.

Severe Right Ventricular Dysfunction

Another cause of wide fixed splitting is severe RV systolic dysfunction. Wide expiratory splitting is due to prolonged RV ejection time. During inspiration the failing right ventricle cannot increase its stroke volume or ejection time and S2 remains fixed. Wide split is appreciable when RBBB is associated with RV failure.

Pseudofixed splitting: Sometimes S2 is mistakenly diagnosed as having fixed splitting. In children with rapid respiratory rate, there is little variation of RV volume and S2 appears fixed. A late systolic click before S2 and an opening snap after S2 may be mistaken as wide fixed S2.

Splitting in Pulmonary Hypertension[10]

Expiratory splitting usually persists. Inspiratory splitting in pulmonary hypertension (PH) depends on two opposing factors. PH causes prolonged RV ejection with delayed P2. At the same time it causes decreased pulmonary capacitance and hang-out time resulting in narrow S2. Inspiratory splitting is usually preserved. Loud P2, however, may mask A2 in pulmonary area, for which split can better be assessed at the apex.

In mitral stenosis (MS) with PH, split is physiological. In MR with PH, split is wide. In VSD with hyperkinetic PH, split is physiological, whereas in Eisenmenger syndrome, S2 is single. In ASD, both with hyperkinetic and obstructive PH, split is wide and fixed. In PDA with hyperkinetic PH, split may be physiological or reverse, whereas in Eisenmenger syndrome, splitting is physiological. In idiopathic PH, splitting is persistent with appreciable expiratory splitting.

REVERSE SPLITTING (FIG. 6)

Reverse splitting[11] or paradoxical splitting is appreciable when S2 is splitted during expiration and becomes narrow or single during inspiration. During expiration, A2 shifts beyond P2. Inspiration have its usual effect on S2, i.e., P2 is delayed. That results in either closely splitted or single S2 during inspiration. Common cause of reverse splitting is delayed electrical activation of the left ventricle, like left bundle branch block (LBBB), RV pacing, and pre-excitation of the right ventricle. Prolonged LV ejection time is another cause of reverse splitting. Increased LV stroke volume, like severe AR and large PDA, and LV outflow obstruction, like AS and HCM, cause prolonged LV ejection time (**Box 3**).

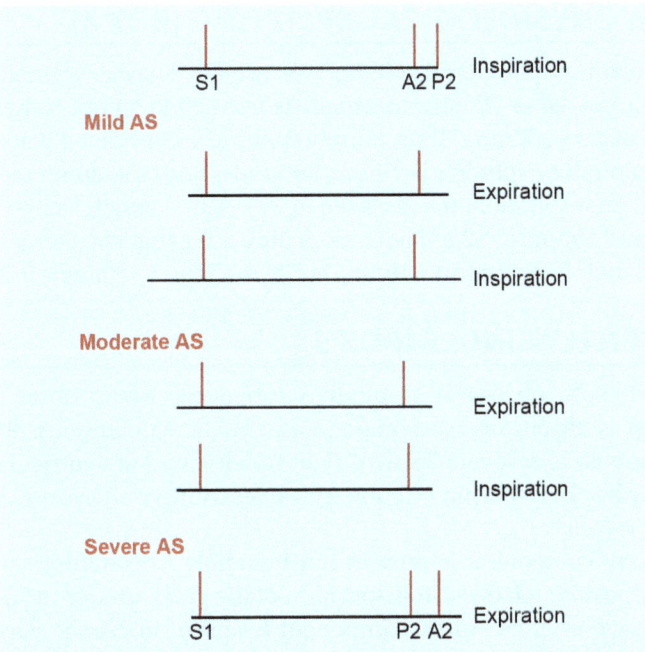

Fig. 6: Reverse split: S2 in aortic stenosis (AS). Here, A2 is delayed. In inspiration, P2 is delayed. Thus, A2 merges to P2 in severe AS in inspiration. In expiration, P2 occurs earlier as usual, and A2 is delayed, resulting in wider split.

BOX 3	Reverse splitting.
Electrical causes:	**Mechanical causes:**
• LBBB	• Increased LV stroke volume (severe AR, large PDA)
• RV pacing	• LVOT obstruction
• WPW syndrome	• Ischemic episodes
	• LV systolic dysfunction

(AR: aortic regurgitation; LBBB: left bundle branch block; LVOT: left ventricular outflow tract; PDA: patent ductus arteriosus; WPW: Wolff–Parkinson–White; LV: left ventricular)

Reverse splitting can be classified as:
- *Type 1:* S2 is usually single during inspiration, and reversely splitted in expiration.
- *Type 2:* S2 shows normal inspiratory splitting and reverse splitting in expiration.
- *Type 3:* S2 is single in inspiration, as well as in expiration, though A2-P2 sequence is reverse in expiration. This is because, during reverse splitting, P2-A2 separation is <20 ms.

Reverse splitting can be occasionally found in ischemic heart disease, during acute ischemic event. Severe LV systolic dysfunction is another cause of reverse splitting, particularly when it is associated with LBBB.

NARROW PHYSIOLOGICAL SPLITTING (BOX 4)

The term narrow physiological splitting was used by Shaver. Normal inspiratory splitting is from >20 to 70 ms and usually is from 30 to 40 ms. If the splitting is <30 ms it is narrow splitting. Thus, narrow splitting is considered between 20 and 30 ms. If inspiratory splitting is closed to 30 ms, both the components can be appreciated on inspiration. If it is closed to 20 ms, one may get single clear S2 in expiration and "impure" S2 in inspiration, indicating that two components have just opened up.[12] If inspiratory splitting is <20 ms, then S2 is single in inspiration.

PERSISTENTLY SINGLE (BOX 5)

Single S2 in both phases of respiration can occur when either of the two components is absent or two components remain synchronous. P2 is absent in pulmonary atresia, severe PS with right to left shunt at ventricular septal or atrial septal level, dysplastic pulmonary valve, truncus arteriosus, and absent pulmonary valve.

Pulmonary component is present but inaudible in conditions where PA is abnormally positioned, like d-transposition of the great arteries (dTGA) or other malposed great arteries. Aortic component is absent in calcific aortic stenosis or aortic atresia. Both the components occur simultaneously in VSD with bidirectional shunt, having equal pulmonary and systemic vascular resistance.

BOX 4 — Narrow physiological splitting.

- Due to delayed A2:
  - LVOT obstruction
  - LBBB
  - PDA, AR
- Due to early P2
  - Early PAH

(AR: aortic regurgitation; LBBB: left bundle branch block; LVOT: left ventricular outflow tract; PDA: patent ductus arteriosus; PAH: pulmonary arterial hypertension)

BOX 5 — Single second heart sound.

Absent P2:
- Pulmonary atresia
- Severe PS and dysplastic pulmonary valve
- Truncus arteriosus
- Absent pulmonary valve
- Occasionally in old age

Inaudible P2:
- d-TGA
- MPGA

Absent A2:
- Calcific AS
- Aortic atresia

Inaudible A2:
- Loud P2 in pulmonary area
- Loud pansystolic murmur (VSD, MR)
- Prolonged ejection systolic murmur (PS)

Synchronous A2 and P2:
- VSD with bidirectional flow
- Single ventricle

(AS: aortic stenosis; PS: pulmonary stenosis; d-TGA: d-transposition of great arteries; MPGA: malposed great arteries; VSD: ventricular septal defect; MR: mitral regurgitation)

Sometimes, P2 is inaudible in old age with increased anteroposterior diameter of chest.

How to Identify A2 or P2 When S2 is Persistently Single?

Most important point is clinical association. In a situation of cyanotic heart disease with low-flow situation, a loud single S2 means that it should be A2 and not P2. On the other hand, in a clinical situation of severe aortic stenosis, a single S2 means that it is more probable P2. Another technique is to auscultate by the traditional "inching technique". P2 is audible across a zone of pulmonary valve, PA and right ventricle, whereas A2 is audible across aortic valve, ascending aorta and left ventricle. Thus, a loud P2 may be audible at left 2nd–4th intercostal space and apex with same intensity, when it is formed by right ventricle. However, P2 is barely audible at right 2nd intercostal space and downward (**Fig. 7**). This clinical technique is applicable to identify A2 versus P2, only when great arteries are normally related.

INTENSITY

Loudness or intensity of S2 depends on the closing force, which is the diastolic gradient across the aortic and pulmonary valve. This gradient between aorta and left ventricle is much higher than between PA and right ventricle. For this reason, A2 is louder than P2. This loudness makes A2 audible both at the base as well as apex, whereas P2 is audible at the left second or third intercostals space. That left ventricle forming the apex can be another contributing factor for the transmission of A2 at the apex. A2 is louder than P2 in 95% cases, even at left 2nd intercostal space. Normally, P2 is not audible down to the third left intercostal space and only in 5% cases, it is audible at apex.

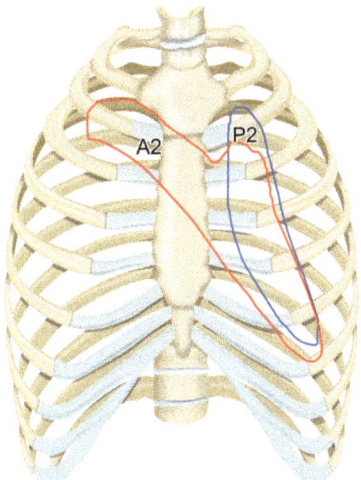

Fig. 7: A2 is audible in sites, where loud P2 is audible; however, P2, even loud is not audible in certain site, where A2 is audible.

Most common cause of loud A2 is hypertension, hyperkinetic circulation, and aneurysm of the ascending aorta. Hyperkinetic flow causes stretching of the aorta by increased volume during systole with vigorous recoiling during diastole contributing to loud A2. Diminished intensity of A2 is calcific AS and severe AR.

Most common cause of louder P2 is PH. Left to right shunt by increasing flow along with dilatation of PA and hyperkinetic circulation by increasing flow also cause loud P2. P2 is equal to A2 in mild PH; louder than A2 in moderate PH; it becomes audible all through the precordium in severe PH. Apical transmission of loud P2 in PH caused by MS and VSD, is somehow rare. A very loud P2 can mask A2 in pulmonary area. P2 without PH is usually not audible at apex. When apex is formed by the right ventricle as in ASD or primary tricuspid regurgitation, P2 is audible at the apex with normal PA pressure. Depressed sternum may cause louder S2, due to the closer proximity of the chest wall with the heart.

CONCLUSION

We are very confident with our clinical second heart sound. When we get a wide and fixed S2 on a clinical background, but echocardiogram is not showing any echo-dropout, we know something is missing. Certainly, we do a transesophageal echocardiogram as next step. When we get a loud and booming P2, but echocardiogram is not showing any significant tricuspid regurgitation, we do a contrast echocardiogram or even cardiac catheterization to confirm our clinical diagnosis of significant pulmonary artery hypertension.

REFERENCES

1. Rouanet J. Analyse des bruits du coeur. Paris Thesis, No. 252; 1832.
2. Leatham A. The second heart sound, key to auscultation of the heart. Acta Cardiol. 1964;19:395.
3. Potain M. Note sur les dedublements normaux des bruits du coeur. Bullt Mem Soc Med Hop Paris. 1866;3:138.
4. Curtis EL, Mathews RG, Shaver JA. Mechanism of normal splitting of the second heart sound. Circulation. 1975;51:157.
5. Aygen MM, Braynwald E. The splitting of the second heart sound in normal subjects and in patients in congenital heart disease. Circulation. 1962;25:328-45.
6. Shaver JA, O'Toole JD. The second heart sound: Newer concepts. Part 1: Normal and wide physiological splitting. Mod Concepts Cardiouasc Dis. 1977;46:7.
7. Felner JM. The second heart sound. In: Walker HK, Hall WD, Hurst JW (Eds). "Clinical Methods: The History, Physical, and Laboratory Examinations", 3rd edition. Boston: Butterworths; 1990. page 122.
8. Harris C, Wise J, Oklay CM. Fixed splitting of second heart sound in ventricular septal defect. British Heart J. 1971;33:428-31.
9. O'Toole JD, Reddy PS, Curtis EI. The mechanism of splitting of the second heart sound in atrial septal defect. Circulation. 1977;56:1047-53.
10. Sutton G, Harris A, Leatham A. Second heart sound in pulmonary hypertension. Br Heart J. 1968;30:743-56.
11. Gray I. Paradoxical splitting of the second heart sound. Br Heart J. 1956;18:21.
12. Constant J (Ed). Bedside Cardiology, 2nd edition. Boston: Little Brown and Company; 1976.

CHAPTER 16

Third Heart Sound

INTRODUCTION

Pierre-Carl Potain, the French physician described third heart sound in 1876 as,—"*the sudden cessation of distention of the ventricle in early diastole**". This ventricular theory of third heart sound still exists.

PHYSIOLOGY

Third heart sound (S3) is a low frequency, low-pitched ventricular filling sound. There are many theories regarding the mechanism of S3. The term ventricular filling sound implies that the sound is due to—"*gallop sound was produced as the dilating ventricle quickly reached the point where the fibrous resistance of its walls limits its distension, and the sharp arrest of the ventricle caused a tension, a shock, and a gallop sound*" and this ventricular theory was proposed first by Potain.[1] This theory was discarded and then came the mitral valve premature-closing theory,[2] which stated that during rapid filling, mitral leaflets came prematurely in closing position and produces S3. However, atrioventricular pressure pattern and echocardiographic features showed that mitral valve remains in intermediate position, i.e., halfway between fully open and fully closed position during production of S3 (**Fig. 1**).

The most acceptable theory[3] is the valve-open theory, which states that during rapid ventricular filling, the apex of the ventricle descends, and mitral valve moves rapidly upward. The descent ceases as soon as the mitral valve apparatus is placed under tension, which sets the cardiohemic system under vibration and produces S3. Rapid ventricular filling followed by sudden cessation or reduction of filling is the most important contributing factor.

---

* Potain, P. Du rhythme cardiaque appelee bruit de galop. Bull Mem Soc Med Hop. 1876;12: 137-66.

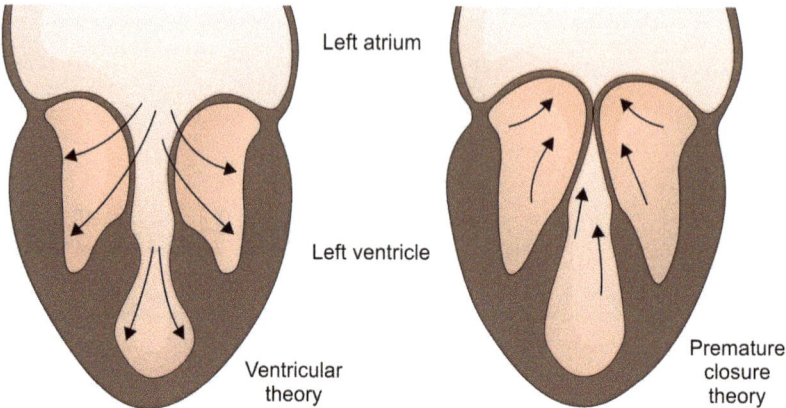

Fig. 1: Ventricular theory of third heart sound (S3): Rapid ventricular filling producing vibration of left ventricular muscle. Premature closure theory of S3: During rapid filling, mitral leaflets came prematurely in closing position.

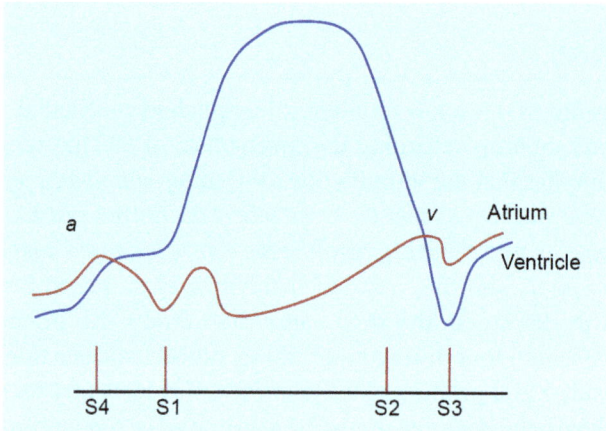

Fig. 2: Hemodynamic correlation and timing of third heart sound (S3): During rapid ventricular filling phase, higher atrial-ventricular gradient, due to higher v wave causing higher atrial pressure and rapidly expanding ventricle with lower filling pressure causes S3.

HEMODYNAMIC CORRELATION

- Left atrial-left ventricular pressure-flow interaction in early ventricular diastole plays the important role in genesis of S3.
- A pathological S3 occurs, when left atrial pressure crosses 18–20 mm Hg.
- Rate of V and Y descents, which reflects rate of left atrial emptying is very rapid, when S3 is present (**Fig. 2**).

HOW TO DETECT IT?
Third heart sound is relatively a faint sound and often can be missed. It can be best picked up by the bell of the stethoscope lightly pressing on the skin exactly at the apex, the patient lying in left lateral decubitus in a quiet room. Coughing a few times or a few sit-ups can make a S3 better audible. This sound waxes and wanes with respiration and postures and may be present on every second third or fourth beat. This is an event around the S2. It follows A2 by 120–200 ms in the ventricular early rapid filling phase and coincides with *y* descent of the atrial pressure pulse.

CHARACTERISTICS
Left-sided versus Right-sided S3
Right ventricular S3 is best heard at left parasternal area in supine position and is increased in intensity with respiration and passive leg rising.

Physiologic S3
Third heart sound is physiologically heard in normal children and in 25% of young adult. In children, there is small size of the heart and rapid inflow. Small size offers resistance to early filling, along with rapid inflow produces the effect for S3. Physiologically, 80% filling occurs during rapid ventricular filling. It is rarely heard in normal person above the age of 40 years. This is because, on aging diastolic relaxation becomes impaired due to stiffening effect of aging, hypertrophy or fibrosis. Diastolic filling is shifted to later in diastole and 35–40% of diastolic volume is flowed during atrial contraction phase. As filling is less during rapid ventricular period, physiological S3 is rare at this age.

Gallop Sound
Third heart sound associated with pathological condition of heart is called as a ventricular diastolic gallop or protodiastolic gallop sound. Presence of S3 or S4 causes tripling or quadrupling of sound and creates an auscultatory impression of the canter of a horse. This effect is more impressive in presence of tachycardia. When both S3 and S4 are present, they produce a diastolic rumble.

Summation Gallop
When atrium contracts during rapid filling phase, the flow is enhanced and produces S3, known as summation gallop. This to happen requires normal atrial contraction and abnormal atrial depolarization during ventricular depolarization. Most common condition is mild sinus tachycardia with shorten diastolic period, prolonged PR interval, and atrioventricular dissociation. When pathological S3 or S4 is reinforced together, then it is known as augmented gallop.[4]

How to Differentiate Physiologic S3 versus Pathologic S3?

Clinical situation is the most important factor. Physiologic S3 is softer and disappears completely on sitting or standing. A palpable S3 is usually pathological which is louder and sharper (higher pitch) than physiological S3.

THIRD HEART SOUND IN SPECIAL SITUATION

High Flow State

High-output states like pregnancy, anemia, thyrotoxicosis, and arteriovenous fistula produce high flow across the atrioventricular valves at a high speed and may produce S3. In these conditions, heart is hyperkinetic, receiving increased diastolic flow at a high rate, and ejecting increased blood during systole. In presence of rapid movement of large inflow, the transition of rapid expansion to slow expansion of ventricle can produce S3. S3 is not any indicator of ventricular dysfunction.

Physiological S3 in Mitral Stenosis

When S3 is present in patients with mitral stenosis, it is thought that either mitral stenosis is not severe or associated significant mitral regurgitation is present. In one study[5] of 100 patients with mitral stenosis, S3 was found in 18% of patients, most of whom were relatively younger in age and it was physiological S3. The study concluded that although stenotic valve can impede ventricular filling, it does not prevent occurrence of physiological S3.

Third Heart Sound in Ventricular Dysfunction

In patients with ventricular dysfunction, heart is not hyperkinetic, and rate of filling is not increased. Ventricular dysfunction, either systolic or diastolic, leading to increased ventricular end-diastolic pressure, may cause S3. One explanation is the noncompliant ventricle in which rapid early diastolic flow causes S3. Another explanation is that the distended ventricle with increased preload causes a suction effect and a rapid inflow in early diastole. Its presence in these conditions indicates ventricular end-diastolic pressure more than 15 mm Hg, ejection fraction less than 20%, and high serum brain natriuretic peptide (BNP).[6] Presence of S3 in chronic aortic regurgitation is an important hallmark of left ventricular dysfunction. In chronic mitral regurgitation, S3 might be an indicator of either increased flow or left ventricular dysfunction. S3 may be the earlier marker of left ventricular dysfunction. A persistent, loud S3 along with sinus tachycardia even after optimal medications for heart failure is a poor prognostic sign.

Ventricular Volume Overload due to AV Valve Regurgitation and Left-to-right Shunt

- Ventricle is enlarged due to increased preload and it contracts forcefully. In consequence, its relaxation is also rapid.
- Regurgitation volume increases atrial V wave height.
- Thus, increased preload enters ventricle with rapid force. This rapid expansion of ventricle followed by halting results in S3.

Third heart sound in these situations like mitral and tricuspid regurgitation is longer in duration and may simulates a short murmur. It is just an indicator of high flow across atrioventricular valve. However, S3 may also be an indicator of ventricular dysfunction.

Aortic Regurgitation

In chronic aortic regurgitation, end-diastolic volume is increased. However, end-systolic volume is increased only after development of systolic dysfunction. S3 appears in chronic aortic regurgitation only after development of increased end-systolic volume due to left ventricular dysfunction. S3 is more common in acute aortic regurgitation, where acute volume overload generates a hyperdynamic apical impulse with an S3.

CONCLUSION

The clinical importance of third heart sound lies not in diagnosis, but in prognosis. In fact, third heart sound is one of the most important clinical prognostic marker in cardiovascular disease.

REFERENCES

1. Potain PCE. Les bruits de galop. Sem Mid (Paris). 1990;20:175.
2. Gibson AG. The significance of a hitherto undescribed wave in the jugular pulse. Lancet. 1907;2:1380.
3. Abrams J. The third and fourth heart sound. Primary Cardiol. 1982;8:47.
4. Grayzel J. Gallop rhythm of the heart. I. Atrial gallop, ventricular gallop and systolic sounds. Am J Med. 1960;28:578-92.
5. Gamble WH, Reddy PS. Preservation of the third heart sound in mitral stenosis. N Engl J Med. 1983;308:498.
6. Marcus GM, Michaels AD, DeMarco T, et al. Usefulness of the third heart sound in predicting an elevated level of B-type natriuretic peptide. Am J Cardiol. 2004;93:1312.

CHAPTER 17

Fourth Heart Sound

INTRODUCTION

Pierre-Carl Potain, the French physician described fourth heart sound in 1876 as,- *"the abruptness with which the dilatation of the ventricle takes place during the presystolic period, a period which corresponds to the contraction of the auricle*".*

PHYSIOLOGY

Charceley in 1838 first described[1] fourth heart sound (S4). Normally, atrial contraction does not produce any palpable precordial vibration or audible sound. When becomes audible, it is known as atrial diastolic gallop, presystolic gallop or S4, which like third heart sound (S3) is a low frequency low-pitched ventricular filling sound during atrial contraction. Potain[2] described S4 as— *"dull, much more so than normal sound. It is a shock, a perceptible elevation; it is hardly a sound. If one applies the ear to the chest, it is affected by tactile sensation perhaps more so than the auditory one.... An elevation felt by the hand usually coincides with this sound."*

Presystolic expansion of left ventricle, during atrial contraction, produces this sound. Pressure-overloaded or noncompliant ventricle with raised end-diastolic pressure requires a vigorous atrial support to maintain an optimal preload. There are two theories regarding mechanism of S4.

1. *Pressure-volume relation*: The accelerated flow in the ventricle in end-diastole followed by sudden cessation sets the cardiohemic system in vibration, which produces S4. A functionally competent atrium and nonstenotic atrioventricular (AV) valve are prerequisite for the S4. It occurs at the same time of *a* wave in atrial pressure pulse and after the P wave of electrocardiogram (ECG) (**Fig. 1**).
2. Cardiac motion rather than pressure or volume change is responsible for the genesis of externally audible S4. S4 corresponds to the A wave in apex cardiogram. A large *a* wave may not produce an audible S4 unless it has a

---

*Potain, P. Du rhythme cardiaque appelee bruit de galop. Bull Mem Soc Med Hop. 1876;12: 137-66.

very sharp rise or fall. Shaver quoted[3] the cardiac motion theory as—"*the displacement of the chest wall with atrial contraction is not due to simple passive transmission of pressure changes inside the ventricle but is caused by the impact of the whole heart on the chest wall through the intervening structures*" (**Fig. 2**).

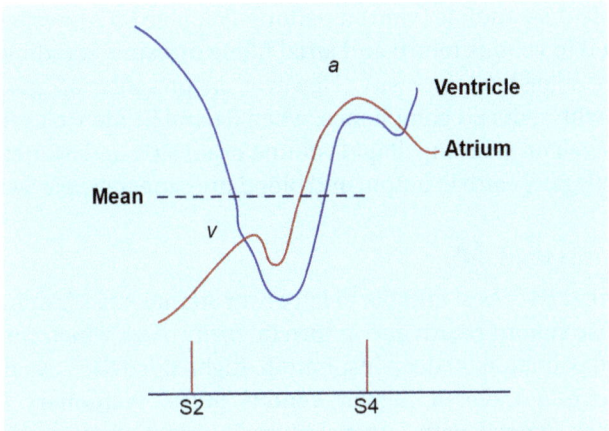

(S2: second heart sound; S4: fourth heart sound)

Fig. 1: Physiology of S4: Pressure-volume theory; during presystolic phase, higher atrial-ventricular pressure gradient, due to higher *a* wave causes S4. Mean atrial pressure is not very high.

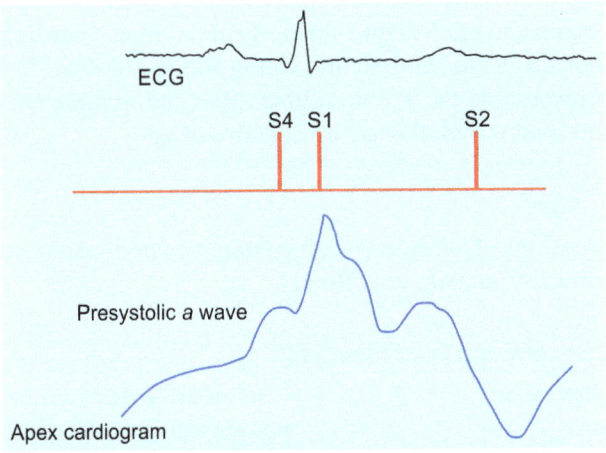

(ACG: apex cardiogram; ECG: electrocardiogram)

Fig. 2: Physiology of S4: Cardiac motion theory; S4 occurring at the time of *a* wave (after P wave in ECG) in ACG.

HOW TO DETECT IT?

Left Ventricular S4

It can be best picked up, like S3, by the bell of the stethoscope lightly pressing on the skin at the apex, the patient lying in left lateral decubitus in a quiet room. S4 is coupled with first heart sound (S1) in its timing. A functionally competent atrium and nonstenotic mitral valve are prerequisite for the S4. It occurs at the same time of *a* wave in left atrial pressure pulse and after the P wave of ECG. Sometimes, it is better palpable than audible (vide palpation). Palpable S4 is always pathological. As S4 is related to venous return and atrial filling pressure, standing significantly reduces even abolish S4 intensity. However, in presence of gross ventricular hypertrophy with reduced compliance, when S4 and S1 are well separated, S4 is well audible even on standing. Rapid volume expansion and isometric hand grip by raising heart rate, cardiac output and blood pressure increase S4 intensity.

Right Ventricular S4

Right ventricular S4 is best audible at left lower sternal edge. Inspiration and leg raising increase venous return and in turn intensity of S4, which can be palpated by subxiphoid palpation on deep inspiration. Right-sided S4 is usually associated with prominent *a* wave in jugular venous pulse. Pulmonary hypertension and pulmonary stenosis with intact septum are most common causes of right ventricular S4.

FOURTH HEART SOUND IN SPECIAL SITUATION

Physiologic S4

Many of the phonocardiographic studies[4] have shown that S4 occurs in 70% of older population with or without heart disease and as such, a recorded S4 should not play any significant clinical role in elderly population. In elderly population, it is as physiologic as S3 in children and young adults. However, in most of these elderlies, the recordable S4 is not audible. Thus, an audible S4 along with a palpable counterpart is pathological irrespective of age.

Pressure Overload

Most common causes of left sided S4 are systemic hypertension, aortic stenosis, and hypertrophic cardiomyopathy (**Box 1**).

BOX 1	Causes of fourth heart sound (S4).
• Systemic hypertension • Aortic stenosis • Hypertrophic cardiomyopathy • Acute ischemic episode • Dilated cardiomyopathy	• Restricted cardiomyopathy • Acute regurgitant lesions • Pulmonary arterial hypertension (right-sided S4) • Pulmonary stenosis (right-sided S4)

Aortic Stenosis

Goldblatt and Braunwald[5] showed that presence of S4 in aortic stenosis correlated with a peak systolic gradient ≥70 mm Hg or greater and left ventricular end-diastolic pressure ≥12 mm Hg and tall *a* wave in left atrial pressure pulse ≥14 mm Hg. May be S4 is more significant in patients with aortic stenosis below 40 years of age. Palpable presystolic *a* wave is more important than audible S4 to decide the severity of aortic stenosis.

Hypertrophic Cardiomyopathy

Fourth heart sound is so consistent with both obstructed as well as nonobstructed hypertrophic cardiomyopathy, that its absence casts doubt in the diagnosis of hypertrophic cardiomyopathy.

Raised End-diastolic Pressure (Fig. 3)

Acute coronary syndrome, during the ischemic episode, is consistently associated with S4. Dilated cardiomyopathy, restrictive cardiomyopathy, and acute mitral or aortic regurgitation can cause S4, due to raised left ventricular end-diastolic pressure. These conditions are also associated with S3.

AV Block

Fourth heart sound is better audible in presence of first-degree AV block due to its separation from S1 (S4 sound occurs after the completion of atrial contraction, around 0.16 second after the beginning of the P wave in the ECG). In 2:1 AV block, S4 is audible on every missed beat. In complete heart block, S4 is intermittently heard and at a faster rate than S1 or S2.

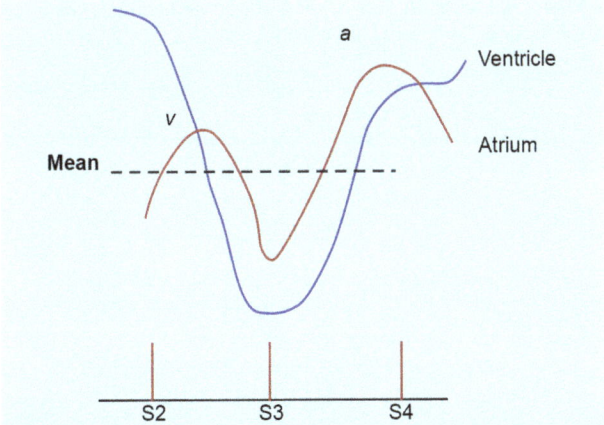

(S2: second heart sound; S3: third heart sound; S4: fourth heart sound)

Fig. 3: Acute mitral regurgitation and S3, S4: Both *a* wave (causing S4) and *v* wave (causing S3) are high and mean left atrial pressure is high.

Mitral Stenosis

Fourth heart sound is never found in isolated mitral stenosis, in spite of forceful atrial contraction. As Shaver described[5]—"*The force of the atrial contraction is primarily conserved as kinetic energy by increased velocity of the blood across the mitral valve.*" Rather, forceful atrial contraction produces the presystolic murmur—"*the galloping noise with a gasp*" as described by Potain. However, in presence of left ventricular hypertrophy due to concomitant aortic valve disease, atrial contraction sound may be audible.[6]

Others

Increased stroke volume and cardiac output like thyrotoxicosis, anemia, and large arteriovenous fistula can cause S4 along with S3.

CONCLUSION

Fourth heart sound is the clinical counterpart of echocardiographic diastolic dysfunction.

REFERENCES

1. Charcelay LJ. Memoire sur plusieurs cas remarquables de d6faut de synchronisme des battements et des bruits des ventricules du coeur. Arch Gen de Med Paris. 1838;3:393.
2. Potain PC. Du rhythme cardiaque appelee bruit de gallop. In: Ruskin A (Ed). Classics in Arterial Hypertension. Springfield, Illinois: Charles C Thomas Publisher; 1956.
3. Reddy PS, Meno F, Curtis EI, et al. The genesis of gallop sounds: Investigation by quantitative phono and apex cardiography. Circulation. 1981;63:922.
4. Spodick DH, Quary-Pigotti VM. Fourth heart sound as a normal in older persons. N Engl J Med. 1973;288:140.
5. Goldblatt A, Aygen MM, Braunwald E. Hemodynamic phonocardiographic correlation of the fourth heart sound in aortic stenosis. Circulation. 1962;26:92.
6. Reddy PS, Salarni R, Shaver JA. Normal and abnormal heart sounds in cardiac diagnosis: Part II. Diastolic sound. Curr Probl Cardiol. 1985;10:1-55.

CHAPTER 18

Ejection Sound

INTRODUCTION

Ejection sounds are high-pitched sound occurring in ventricular systole at the onset of ejection phase. They are pulmonary or aortic in nature and either valvular or vascular in origin. Valvular clicks are due to sudden halting of the diseased semilunar valve at the end of its maximal excursion. It occurs at the end of the isovolumic contraction phase, around 40–60 ms after S1. Vascular click occurs during ejection of blood commonly in a dilated pulmonary or aortic root. The clinical significance of a valvular click is that the obstruction across the right or left ventricular outflow tract is at the valvular level and not at the supra or subvalvular level and the leaflets are relatively pliable. Vascular click does not have much clinical significance.

PULMONARY VALVULAR CLICK

Pulmonary click (**Fig. 1**) occurs 0.09 second after q wave on electrocardiogram (ECG). Mild to moderate pulmonary stenosis is the most common cause of pulmonary valvular click. It is a high-pitched sound, localized in the pulmonary area. Its most important characteristic is that *it is the only right-sided event, which is decreased in intensity in inspiration*. This nature of click is called phasic or inconstant. During inspiration, the increased inflow of blood in right ventricle increases the right ventricular end-diastolic pressure, which equilibrates pulmonary artery end-diastolic pressure, which is already low in the setting of pulmonary stenosis to right ventricular end-diastolic pressure gradient, which causes forward movement of the pulmonary valve and its partial presystolic opening. At the onset of right ventricular systole, there is less excursion of the partially opened valve, thus decreasing the intensity of the ejection click (EC). When there is complete presystolic opening, EC may be absent. The classical echocardiographic study by Weyman[1] demonstrated this nature of pulmonary valvular click. In mild pulmonary stenosis, the respiratory variation may be absent, because inspiratory right ventricular pressure does not equilibrate pulmonary artery end-diastolic pressure. On the other hand,

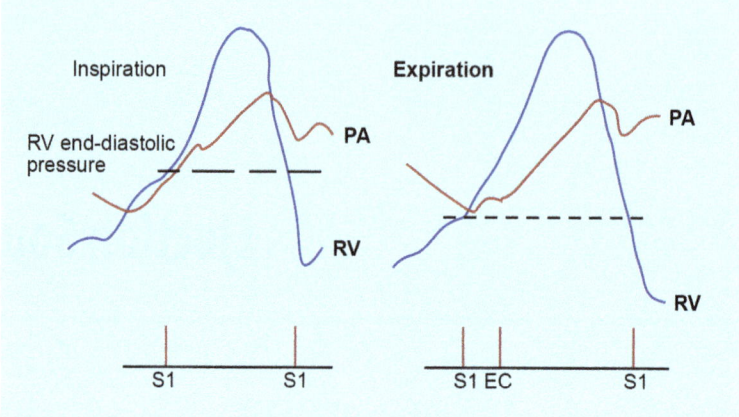

Fig. 1: Pulmonary valvular ejection click (EC): During inspiration, increased preload causes higher right ventricular end-diastolic pressure (RVEDP) resulting in lower pulmonary artery (PA) end-diastolic to RVEDP gradient. This leads to absent EC during inspiration. During expiration, RVEDP comes down, with higher pulmonary artery to RVEDP and EC can be heard.

in severe pulmonary stenosis, vigorous right atrial contraction can preopen the pulmonary valve in end-diastole, causing a presystolic EC.[2] More severe is the stenosis, more the click is shifted to S1. As pulmonary stenosis progresses over time, valve becomes scarred. At the same time, right ventricular isometric contraction time shortens. In effect, click moves toward S1. They may be merged together on inspiration and produce a loud summated sound at the apex.[3] Click indicates obstruction at valvular level and usually is absent in infundibular stenosis.

PULMONARY VASCULAR CLICK

Pulmonary vascular click is also named as pulmonary root ejection sound. Pulmonary hypertension, idiopathic dilatation of pulmonary artery, and other conditions with dilated pulmonary artery produce an EC, which is vascular in origin. It is also a localized high pitch sound, best audible at left 2nd or 3rd intercostal space. Leatham and Vogelpoel initially described[4] that the vascular click is enhanced on expiration, but Shaver later showed[3] the constant nature of pulmonary vascular click. The click occurs at the full opening of the pulmonary valve, during the upstroke of pulmonary artery pressure curve. The sound is produced due to sudden halting of the rapidly accelerating column of blood by the pulmonary artery when its elastic limit is reached. Whether click is arising from the aortic wall or from the pulmonary valve at its full opening is not yet settled. Vascular click is delayed than valvular click in case of pulmonary hypertension due to a longer isovolumic contraction period of the right ventricle working against a higher pressure. Pulmonic click can be related to ejection of blood into a pulmonary artery through a normal pulmonic valve under normal pressure, as

TABLE 1: First heart sound (S1)-vascular click versus MI-T1.

	Pulmonary vascular click	Second component of split S1
Position in early systole	Later (wide splitting of S1)	Earlier (narrow splitting of S1)
Site of maximum intensity	Pulmonary area	Tricuspid and mitral area
Quality	High pitched, clicking	Abrupt
Effect of respiration	Constant	Enhanced on expiration

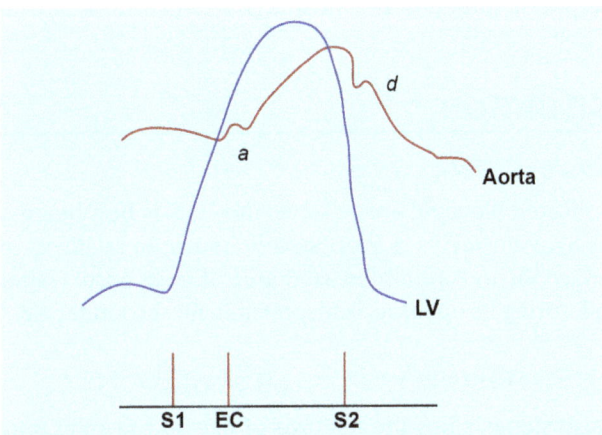

Fig. 2: Aortic valvular click: It occurs at the end of isovolumetric contraction, once left ventricular (LV) pressure pulse crosses over the aortic pressure pulse, only when it can open the aortic valve against aortic pressure.

in idiopathic dilatation of the pulmonary artery, in which click occurs earlier in systole (**Table 1**).

AORTIC VALVULAR CLICK

Aortic click (**Fig. 2**) occurs 0.12 second after q wave on ECG, i.e., it occurs later than pulmonary click. It typically occurs in valvular aortic stenosis and bicuspid aortic valve. The click sound is coincident with the maximum excursion of the bicuspid leaflet or domed valve when its elastic limit is reached. The sudden deceleration of ejected column of blood sets the cardiohemic system in vibration. The low-frequency vibration is recorded as anacrotic notch in the pressure pulse and the high-frequency sound is recorded as aortic valvular click. Thus, it corresponds in timing with the anacrotic notch in the upstroke of the aortic pressure curve. The click is often better heard at the apex, rather than the base and does not show any variation with respiration (constant click). In case of aortic stenosis, severe the stenosis, earlier will be the click in relation to

S1. Intensity of the click has no relation to severity of aortic stenosis. Rather, it is related to the mobility of the cusp. Click will be diminished or absent in calcific aortic stenosis with nonpliable leaflets.

AORTIC VASCULAR CLICK

Aortic vascular click or root ejection sound occurs in situations with dilated aortic root, like systemic hypertension, ascending aortic aneurysm, coarctation of aorta, and Fallot's physiology. Its timing is after the anacrotic notch of the aortic pressure pulse. Its mechanism is similar to pulmonary vascular click. Vascular click is localized in nature, poorly transmitted from aortic area, and inaudible at the apex.

SPECIAL SITUATION

Bicuspid Aortic Valve

In an uncomplicated bicuspid aortic valve, the click is best heard at the apex. It is louder than S1, followed by a short systolic murmur, relatively louder A2 and a short early diastolic murmur. Increased area of large cusp, responsible for the ejection sound during its opening, is responsible for the louder A2.

Pulmonary Stenosis versus Atrial Septal Defect

Mild pulmonary stenosis has the features of ejection systolic murmur, normal intensity of P2 and a persistent split of S2. Sometimes it is difficult to differentiate it from small atrial septal defect. Valvular click is the clue in favor of pulmonary stenosis.

Tetralogy of Fallot

In tetralogy of Fallot (TOF) with severe pulmonary stenosis or pulmonary atresia, aorta is dilated and dextroposed and aortic vascular click is commonly found. In fact, presence of aortic click is suggestive of severe form of TOF. Click is best heard at right upper sternal border and may be appreciated at left upper sternal border and apex (**Box 1**).

All the above points are not consistent. Pulmonary click in presence of pulmonary hypertension may be loud enough to be audible over a wider area and

---

BOX 1 Mechanism of aortic click in tetralogy of Fallot.

- Aorta is dilated
- It is dextroposed
- Pulmonary artery going across aorta is narrower than normal
- More severe the right ventricular outflow tract obstruction, more is the flow across aortic valve

may occur later in systole. Many a times, pulmonary click may show less variation with respiration. Moreover, Perloff described aortic click intensity selectively decreasing with inspiration, i.e., phasic rather than constant.

Pulmonary valvular click may be present in less severe form of TOF with valvular stenosis, where the stenotic valve is still mobile. However, the click here is constant and does not decrease in intensity on inspiration. Martin and Shaver in their study[5] offered the explanation—*"The large ventricular septal defect provides a runoff for the increased venous return into the left ventricle, thereby preventing a significant inspiratory increase in right ventricular end-diastolic pressure. Palliative shunting procedures which direct flow into the pulmonary artery may also prevent an obvious inspiratory drop in pulmonary artery pressure in some patients. Either or both of these factors could explain the lack of respiratory variation which was evident in this group of patients".*

CONCLUSION

A simple ejection click provides information on the level of obstruction, severity of obstruction, and valve mobility.

REFERENCES

1. Weyman AE, Dilin JC, Feigenbaum H, et al. Echocardiographic patterns of pulmonary valve motion in valvular pulmonary stenosis. Am J Cardiol. 1974;34:644.
2. Leatham A, Weitzman D. Auscultatory and phonocardiographic signs of pulmonary stenosis. Br Heart J. 1957;19:303.
3. Shaver JA. Salarni R, Reddy PS. Normal and abnormal heart sounds in cardiac diagnosis: Part I. Systolic sound. Curr Probl Cardiol. 1985;10:1-68.
4. Leatham A, Vogelpoel L. The early systolic sound in dilatation of pulmonary artery. Br Heart J. 1951;16:21.
5. Martin CE, Reddy PS, Donald FL, et al. Genesis, frequency and diagnostic significance of ejection sound in adults with tetralogy of Fallot. Br Heart J. 1973;35:402-12.

Nonejection Sound

INTRODUCTION

As mentioned earlier, early systolic click, occurring within 80 ms of first heart sound (S1), is generally considered to be related to ejection phenomena, which include opening of aortic or pulmonary valve and ejection of blood in aorta or pulmonary artery. Click however may occur due to nonejection phenomena, known as nonejection sound. Most common nonejection sounds are midsystolic click and opening snap (OS).

MIDSYSTOLIC CLICK (FIG. 1)

Mitral Valve Prolapse

Levine first described[1] midsystolic click as "systolic gallop rhythm". He believed that the click is extracardiac in origin. Barlow later described[2] the click-late systolic murmur as a cardiac syndrome.

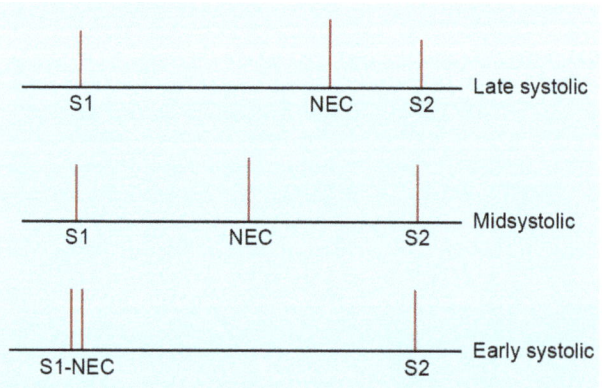

Fig. 1: Nonejection click (NEC) of mitral valve prolapse. Depending upon the severity and dynamic maneuvers, click may be classically midsystolic, late systolic or early systolic.

Physiology

Mitral valve prolapse is the most common cause of nonejection click. It occurs due to sudden tensing of the prolapsing atrioventricular (AV) valve during systole. A long, redundant leaflet, too large for the contracting ventricle is prolapsed in mid to late part of systole when the *click dimension* (ventricular volume at which leaflet cannot be accommodated) is reached.

Location

This high frequency, sharp clicking sound, best heard at the apex, is audible over a wider area on the precordium. There might be multiple clicks, which, depending on the degree of malcoaptation, may or may not be associated with murmur. Multiple clicks are due to different area of large, scalloped, redundant leaflets prolapsing at different time.

Dynamic auscultation bears a very important application on this click. Any maneuver, which reduces the ventricular volume like standing, Valsalva phase 2, causes an early prolapse of the mitral valve followed by a long murmur. Supine posture and Valsalva phase 4 by increasing ventricular volume cause late prolapse and late systolic murmur. Click may even merge with S1, making it louder in very early prolapse. By this hemodynamic maneuver, S1-nonejection click can be differentiated from S4-S1, S1-ejection click and M1-T1. Beat-to-beat variation of click occurs in patients with atrial fibrillation.

Clinical Significance

Isolated click does not have much clinical relevance. Associated mitral regurgitation determines the overall prognosis.

Other Causes of Nonejection Click (Box 1)

Left-sided pneumothorax, adhesive pericarditis, complete absence of pericardium, left ventricular aneurysm, atrial and ventricular septal aneurysm, and left atrial myxoma may cause systolic nonejection click, which does not change appreciably on hemodynamic maneuvers.

PSEUDOEJECTION SOUND

Hancock first described[3] the term "pseudoejection" sound in hypertrophic cardiomyopathy. The sound begins 40–100 ms after the upstroke of indirect carotid pulse. Either the anterior mitral leaflet (AML) abutting on the septum during

---

BOX 1 | **Causes of nonejection click.**

- Mitral valve prolapse
- Left-sided pneumothorax
- Adhesive pericarditis/complete absence of pericardium
- Left ventricular aneurysm
- Atrial and ventricular septal aneurysm
- Atrial myxoma

systolic anterior motion or sudden deceleration of blood in the left ventricular outflow tract causes this apparent ejection sound. Provocative maneuvers like Valsalva strain, standing or amyl nitrite inhalation increase the intensity of the pseudoejection sound and make it earlier to occur.[4]

OPENING SNAP

Mitral Opening Snap

Rouches in 1888 described[5] the diastolic sound in relation to mitral stenosis (MS)—"le claquement d'ouverture de la mitrale". Opening of a normal AV valve is acoustically silent. Sudden tensing of the stenosed mitral valve at its full opening produces the mitral OS. It is like S1, mostly contributed by AML. It occurs 40–120 ms after S2, well after isovolumic relaxation time. This is because OS is occurring not exactly with mitral valve opening, rather after its full excursion. Thus, transmitral flow begins before OS with maximum flow occurring after OS.

Opening snap is a high-pitched sound, which is best-heard medial to the apex. As it is a loud sound, can be heard over a wide area of the precordium. Occasionally, it may be palpable.

An audible OS indicates the valve is pliable and probably suitable for valvuloplasty. More importantly, it is the most important indicator of severity of MS. Severe the stenosis, higher will be the left atrial pressure. Left atrial pressure crossover the left ventricular pressure pulse, which indicates opening of mitral valve, will be earlier. A2-OS interval varies from 40 to 140 ms. Shorter the A2-OS interval, severe will be the MS (usually below 80 ms). One should focus during expiration, when two components are S2 and OS. If the cadence simulates a closed split, it indicates early OS and severe MS. If the cadence simulates S3, it indicates late OS and mild MS (**Fig. 2**).

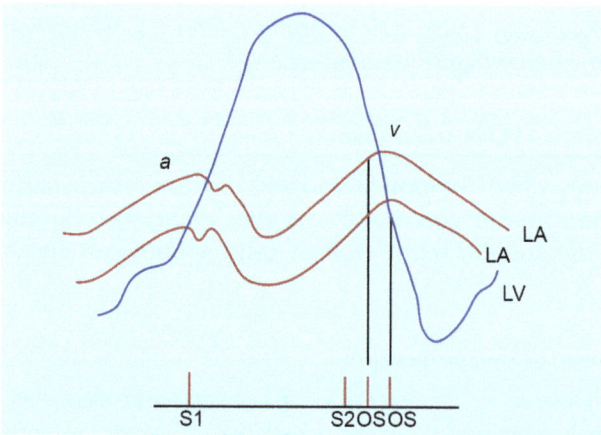

Fig. 2: Severity assessment of mitral stenosis (MS): Severe the MS, higher will be the left atrium–left ventricular (LA–LV) diastolic pressure gradient and shorter will be the S2-OS (opening snap) distance.

However, this interval may be affected by other factors, such as tachycardia (shortened diastole, shorter time for left atrium for emptying leading to shorter interval), bradycardia (longer diastole and increased interval), aortic stenosis (delayed A2 and shorter interval), mitral regurgitation (early OS and shorter interval), low cardiac output (low atrial pressure, delayed OS, and longer interval), and high left ventricular end-diastolic pressure (low gradient across mitral valve, delayed OS, and longer interval).

Light exercise shortens A2-OS interval by tachycardia and increased preload. Thus, exercise may unmask severity of MS in otherwise doubtful case. Atrial fibrillation does influence S2-OS interval. After short cycle, as left atrium gets lesser time and its pressure remains high, OS occurs earlier with lesser A2-OS interval than after long cycle (**Fig. 3**).

Opening snap is absent when stenosed mitral valve is grossly calcified and nonpliable. Only tip calcification does not affect, but its extension to the body affects OS. This sound is often absent in congenital MS as because the leaflets are not pliable. Concomitant aortic regurgitation or presence of significant pulmonary hypertension with loud P2 can mask the softer OS. Even after mitral valvuloplasty, OS may persist.

Mitral OS may be present in situations, other than MS. In an elegant study[6] with echocardiogram and phonocardiogram correlation, mitral OS was found in many other situations (**Box 2**).

Increased flow across mitral valve may produce an opening sound. It typically occurs 90–110 ms after A2, of lesser intensity and correlates to full descent of AML opening and before rapid filling phase, i.e. third heart sound (**Table 1**).

Tricuspid Opening Snap

Tricuspid OS[7] is associated with a rare entity like tricuspid stenosis, severe tricuspid regurgitation, large atrial septal defect (ASD), and Ebstein's anomaly.

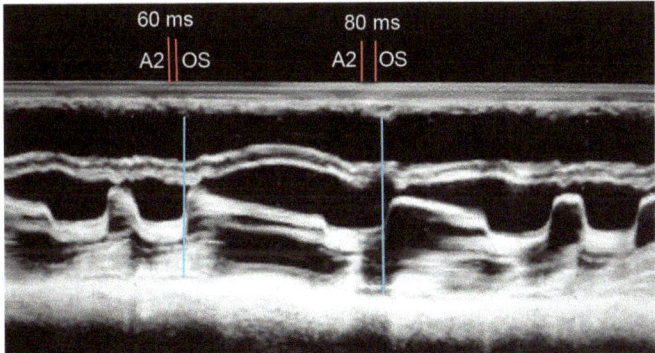

Fig. 3: A2-OS (opening snap) gap in atrial fibrillation (AF) with variable R-R interval. Following a short cycle in complex 2 the A2-OS interval is 60 ms. After the longer diastolic emptying time in complex 3 the A2-OS interval is 80 ms because of a decrease in left atrial pressure.

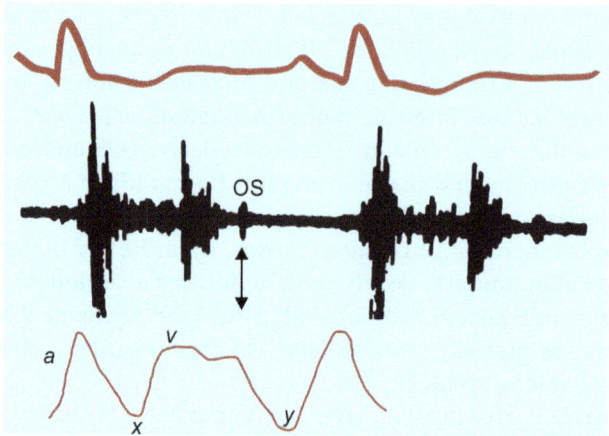

Fig. 4: Tricuspid opening snap (OS) in severe tricuspid regurgitation. Jugular venous pulse demonstrates prominent *a* wave, large *v* wave, and deep *y* trough; OS occurs at the peak of *v* wave. Pulse demonstrates prominent "a" wave (A) consistent with right ventricular hypertrophy and broad systolic wave ("v" wave; V) of tricuspid insufficiency. Opening snap occurs just before beginning of descent of "y" wave (Y).

BOX 2: Causes of mitral opening snap, other than mitral stenosis.

- Mitral regurgitation
- Ventricular septal defect
- Patent ductus arteriosus
- Tricuspid atresia with a large atrial septal defect
- Tetralogy of Fallot occurring after BT shunt
- Thyrotoxicosis

(BT: Blalock-Taussig)

TABLE 1: Mitral opening snap (OS) versus third heart sound (S3).

	OS	S3
Frequency	High	Low
Location	Wider area	At apex
Best heard	With diaphragm, any body position	Left lateral decubitus position with bell
Interval: A2 to:	40–140 ms	100–200 ms
Character	Sharper and louder	Dull and softer

Like any right-sided event, its intensity is increased with inspiration. Its timing is reflected in jugular venous pulse. OS occurs simultaneously with the peak of *v* wave. In case of tricuspid regurgitation or ASD, right ventricular S3 is common. S3 occurs at the end of steep descending limb, i.e., *y* trough (**Fig. 4**). Events around S2 are described in **Figure 5**.

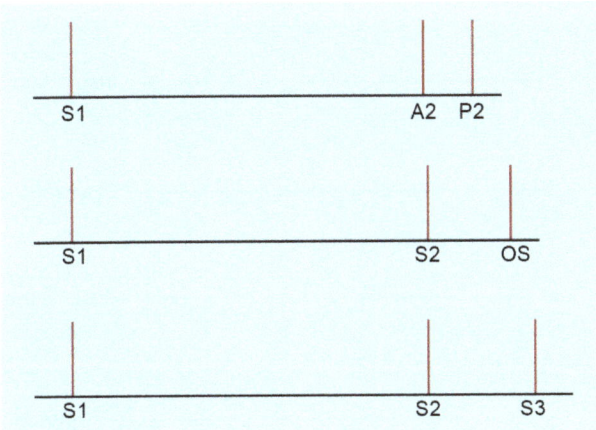

(OS: opening snap)

Fig. 5: Events around S2.

TABLE 2: Mitral stenosis (MS) versus atrial septal defect (ASD).

	MS	ASD
Similarities		
S2-OS/A2-P2	S2-OS MS	A2-P2
Diastolic murmur		Flow murmur
Differences		
Inspiration	A2-P2-OS	A2-P2
	S2-OS narrows	A2-P2 widens P2 intensity ups A2-P2 narrows
Standing	OS intensity downs S2-OS widens	

(OS: opening snap)

Special Situation: Mitral Stenosis and Atrial Septal Defect

Opening snap can often be heard at the left upper parasternal area and can be confused as pulmonary component of widely splitted S2. In ASD, there can have a diastolic flow murmur; S1 can also be loud due to T1 component. Assuming A2-OS as widely splitted S2, MS can wrongly be diagnosed as ASD. But during inspiration, MS should have three high frequency components at pulmonary area—A2, P2, and OS. Other points in favor of second component being OS are: It is equally loud at the apex as well base; its intensity is decreasing with inspiration; split is getting narrowed on inspiration and wider on standing (**Table 2** and **Fig. 6**).

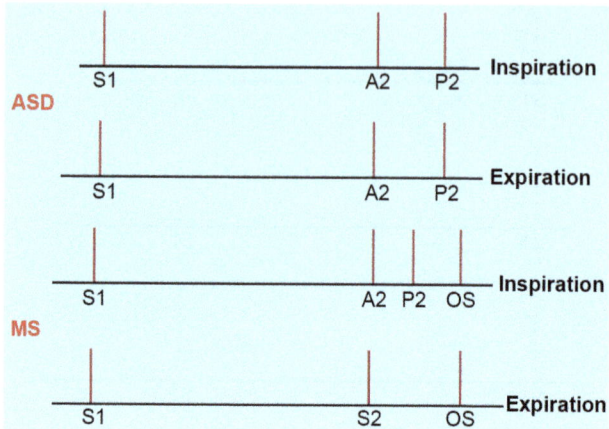

Fig. 6: Mitral stenosis (MS) versus atrial septal defect (ASD). In ASD, in both phases of respiration, there will be two components around S2 (A2 and P2). In MS, whereas during inspiration, there will be three components, A2, P2, and opening snap (OS) and during expiration, only one component, S2.

PERICARDIAL SOUND

Pericardial Knock

Physiology

Pericardial knock is a pathognomonic sign in constrictive pericarditis. Knock is more frequently found in more advanced disease and in calcified constrictive pericarditis. Pericardial knock is a low frequency early diastolic filling sound, which is heard over a wider area between left parasternal spaces to apex. It often has a snapping quality. Its intensity is increased on inspiration.

In an elegant work on constrictive pericarditis, Patrick Mounsey[8] first demonstrated the mechanism of pericardial knock. He recorded phonocardiogram and right heart catheterization. As per his work, pericardial knock was originated from right ventricle. Rapid early diastolic filling is abruptly halted by the restrained pericardium, due to fixed space. Rapid halting is followed by steep rise of ventricular pressure. Pericardial knock is synchronous with the onset of steep upstroke, coinciding with the abrupt halting of rapid diastolic filling. Pericardial knock remains absent in a good number of patients, in whom early diastolic filling is slower and halting is not that abrupt.

Shaver explained in other ways. During ventricular contraction, some of the released energy is stored in two forms: In the spatial rotation of the heart and contraction of the myofibrillar elements and their supporting structures. In constrictive pericarditis, less energy is stored in first form and more energy is stored in the second form due to deformation of the adherent pericardium. At the end of contraction—"the ventricular wall and adherent pericardium may spring back with greater than usual force, causing a diastolic wave as well as pericardial knock".[9]

In constrictive pericarditis, there is high filling pressure with large atrial v wave. It occurs in ventricular rapid filling phase. During this phase, there is sudden halting of the expanding ventricle, due to the constricted, restrained pericardium, causing the pericardial knock or S3.

Timing
It occurs 100–120 ms after S2, later than mitral OS, but earlier to left ventricular S3. It corresponds with the rapid y descent.

Clinical Significance
Features of constrictive pericarditis may simulate those of congestive heart failure. Pericardial knock may be confused as S3. That the knock occurs earlier and higher in frequency than S3 may be a differentiating point. As pericardial knock is early diastolic event, it may be confused with very closed S2. Pericardial knock is snapping in character and widely heard over pericardium. Its interval from S2 is >A2-P2. On inspiration, three components can be identified: A2-P2-pericardial knock.

Pericardial Rub

Physiology
It is a leathery, high frequency sound and is scratchy in quality. They are best heard in the left parasternal second and third intercostal space, the bare area of heart, patient leaning forward or knee-chest position, and on breath-holding at expiratory phase.

Timing
It occurs in three phases of cardiac cycle—in atrial systole, in ventricular systole, and in ventricular rapid filling phase. However, mostly it is biphasic: During atrial systole and ventricular systole.

Clinical Significance
It may be found in acute pericarditis of any etiology. However, all the three components are found in idiopathic pericarditis, post-traumatic pericarditis, and pericarditis associated with chronic renal failure. Some systolic murmurs, as in hyperthyroidism (Means–Lerman sign) and in Ebstein anomaly, due to its scratchy superficial nature, may be simulated as pericardial rub. Pericardial rub is best heard with patient in sitting forward with held expiration.

Mediastinal Crunch (Hamman Sign)

Physiology
It consists of multiple scratchy sounds in various phase of cardiac cycle, due to presence of air in pericardial and mediastinal spaces.

Clinical Significance

It may be found after cardiac surgery with open pericardium. Associated mediastinal emphysema, with crepitations in the neck, is the clue.

PROSTHETIC VALVE[10,11]

Prosthetic valves produce characteristic auscultatory sound due to its component motion and altered flow pattern. They alter the normal laminar flow, themselves are potentially stenotic and interfere with normal auscultatory landmarks. Prosthetic valves are implanted in a background of altered hemodynamic. The residual ventricular dysfunction, pulmonary hypertension, and rhythm abnormalities—all the factors alter the auscultatory feature of prosthetic valve sound. In most of the cases, there is patient-prosthesis mismatch, i.e., potentially stenotic. Considering all these factors, identifying normal and abnormal prosthetic sound is clinically very relevant for identifying prosthetic valve dysfunction including obstruction, incompetence, thrombosis, and other complications (**Box 3**) (**Fig. 7**).

Ball and Valve

Ball and cage valves are no more in use. However, many patients are still living with these valves. These valves produce loud low frequency opening and closing sound due to excursion and seating back of the ball. They are high pitch, clicking metallic sound.

Aortic ball valve produces a loud opening sound, around 60 ms after S1. At the onset of systole, the ball reaches at the apex of the cage. The to-and-fro movement of the ball may produce multiple clicks. The closing sound is less prominent. It precedes A2 component, maintain the physiological splitting. Commonly associated left ventricular dysfunction and LBBB produce paradoxica splitting. Both the components are best audible at the apex and lower left sternal area. The normal ratio of opening and closing sound on phonocardiogram is >0.5. Any ratio significantly lower or absent opening sound indicates prosthetic valve dysfunction. A grade 2, 3 ejection systolic murmur is audible at aortic area with radiation to carotid, indicating normal mismatch or residual gradient. Any audible diastolic murmur indicates valve dysfunction.

BOX 3	Types of prosthetic valve.

• Mechanical valve:
   ○ Monoleaflet valve
   ○ Bileaflet valve
   ○ Ball and cage valve
	• Bioprosthetic valve:
	   ○ Stented
	   ○ Stentless
	   ○ Percutaneous bioprosthetic valve

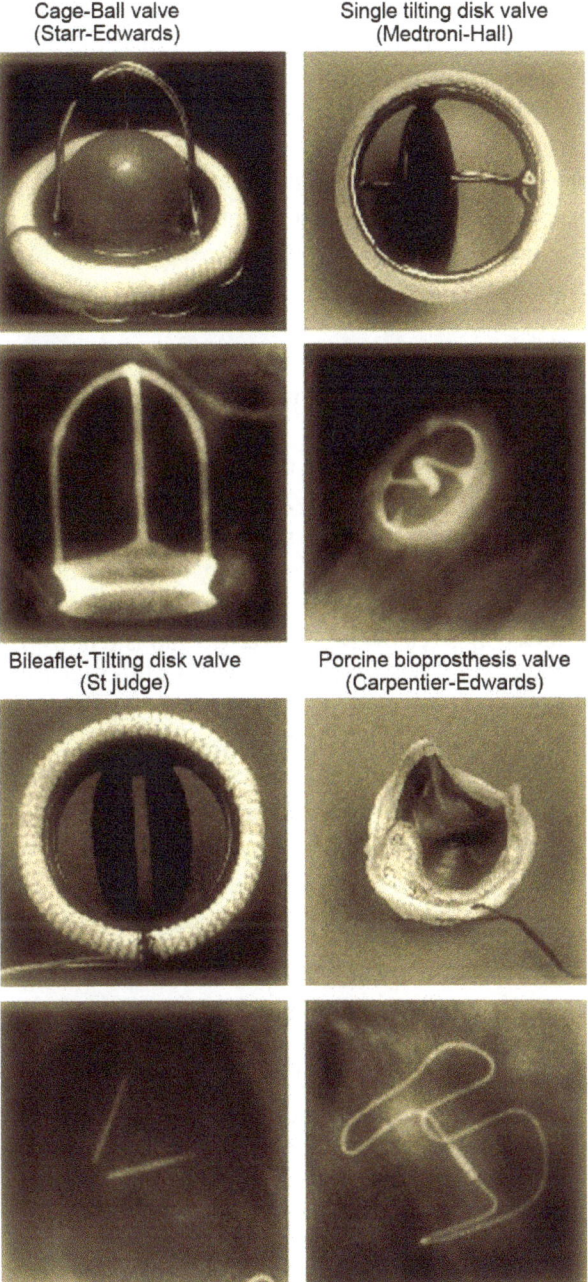

Fig. 7: Different prosthetic valves.

Mitral ball valve produces a loud OS 70–110 ms after A2. It is best audible at the apex. A2-OS gap does not show much beat-to-beat variation in atrial fibrillation. A very short A2-OS gap, <50 ms, indicates significant prosthetic valve dysfunction. A long A2-OS interval, >170 ms, indicates interference of normal valve excursion. Closing sound is less prominent and occurs obscuring normal S1 and is best audible at left lower sternal area. A smaller grade early to mid-systolic murmur is audible between apex to left lower sternal edge, produced by the rigid valve cage projected in the left ventricular outflow tract. Any diastolic murmur indicates valve dysfunction.

Tilting-disk Valve

Disk valve produces clicking sound of high frequency, less prominent than the ball valve, mostly closing sound.

Aortic disk valve does not produce audible opening sound. It occurs 40 ms after M1. Closing sound is prominent. Any reduced intensity of closing sound indicates reduced movement due to thrombus. Low-grade ejection systolic murmur and occasional diastolic murmur may be present even in a normally functional valve.

Mitral disk valve OS is relatively faint. A2-OS gap is relatively shorter, within 40–80 ms. Its closure sound at apex is prominent. Any hindrance in the movement of the valve by thrombus leads to diminished intensity of the opening sound. Normally functioning disk valve is associated with ejection systolic murmur, due to same mechanism as like aortic ball valve. As any prosthetic valve is "stenotic", the disk valve also is, and a diastolic murmur is common.

Bileaflet, tilting disk valve produces same pattern of sound, excepting that in aortic area, it does not produce any diastolic murmur.

Clinical Significance

Malfunction of the mechanical valve prosthesis includes ball degeneration, strut fracture, thrombus and pannus formation, infection or dehiscence. Multiple clicks may indicate a malfunctioning valve. Both early and late opening of the valve, in relation to S2, indicate valve obstruction. Absence of valve sound indicates dehiscence of the prosthetic valve. Appearance of new sound or murmur indicates valve malfunction.

Bioprosthesis

Both opening and closing sounds are soft and do not clinically help much to identify valve malfunction. This is applicable both to surgical and transcatheter valve replacement. In aortic area, they produce soft closing sound and in mitral area, opening sound. Degeneration of this sort of valve may produce multiple clicks and musical murmur. Appearance of new murmur or increase in grade of existing murmur, either systolic or diastolic may help to assess valve dysfunction (**Fig. 8**).

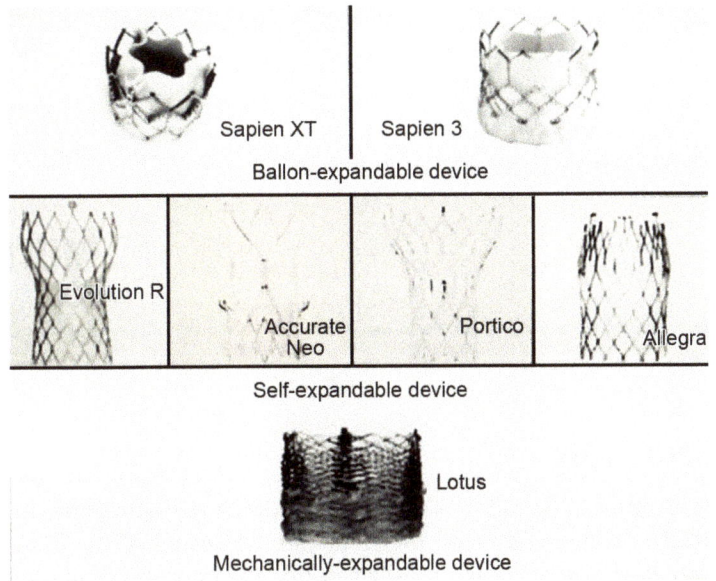

Fig. 8: Different transcatheter aortic prosthetic valve.

CONCLUSION

Mitral valve click plays a vital diagnostic role. Echocardiogram may overdiagnose mitral valve prolapse. Presence of click confirms the diagnosis. In prosthetic valve, disappearance of opening or closing sound helps to diagnose sudden valve dysfunction and to proceed further imaging and intervention.

REFERENCES

1. Thompson WP, Levine SA. Systolic gallop rhythm: A clinical study. N Engl J Med. 1935; 213:1021.
2. Barlow JB, Bosman CK. Aneurysmal protrusion of the posterior leaflet of the mitral valve. An auscultatory-electrocardiographic syndrome. Am Heart J. 1966;71:166.
3. Hancock EW. The ejection sound in aortic stenosis. Am J Med. 1966;40:569.
4. Sze KC, Shah PM. Pseudoejection sound in hypertrophic subaortic stenosis. An echocardiographic corelative study. Circulation. 1976;54:504-9.
5. Rouches FJM. Du claquement d'ouverture de la mitrale. Theses pour le Doctorat en Medecine, Paris, Faculte De Medecine De Paris. 1888.
6. Millward DK, McLaurin LP, Craige E. Echocardiographic studies to explain opening snaps in presence of nonstenotic mitral valve. Am J Cardiol. 1973;31:64.
7. Pyhel HJ, Noble RJ, Tavel ME. Graphic technique in cardiology. Tricuspid opening snap in tricuspid insufficiency. Chest. 1977;72:651-3.
8. Mounsey P. The Early Diastolic Sound of Constrictive Pericarditis. Br Heart J. 1955;17(2):143-52.
9. Reddy PS, Salarni R, Shaver JA. Normal and abnormal heart sounds in cardiac diagnosis: Part II. Diastolic sound. Curr Probl Cardiol. 1985;10:1-55.
10. Smith ND, Raizada V, Abrams J. Auscultation of the normally functioning prosthetic valve. Ann Intern Med. 1981;95:594.
11. Vongpatanasin W, Hillis LD, Lange RA. Prosthetic heart valves. N Engl J Med. 1996;335:407.

Murmur

INTRODUCTION

Murmur is a series of vibration of variable duration, originating from heart or its vessels. RTH Laennec first heard murmurs and he described them on 1819[1] as file, grate, bellow or saw. After almost a century, the importance of murmur was resurfaced during World War I, when 4 million American shoulder were recruited, in whom routine examination detected systolic murmur with unexpected frequency. Samuel A Levine was then an army medical officer, who studied those systolic murmurs very meticulously and eventually graded systolic murmur. He[2] described—*"Systolic murmurs do occur but are not common in normal individuals. The louder ones are always associated with some form of cardiovascular disease."*

PHYSIOLOGY

Turbulence

Normal blood flow in the cardiovascular system is laminar in nature and usually inaudible. When laminar flow is disrupted, turbulent flow occurs. The critical point at which laminar flow is converted into turbulent flow is decided by the diameter of the channel, mean velocity of the flow, density, and viscosity of fluid, i.e., blood.[3] Turbulence is directly proportional to velocity of flow. Higher the flow velocity, more is the turbulence. Larger the diameter of vessel, higher is the turbulence. Relation of turbulence is complex with density and viscosity. It is directly related to density and inversely related to viscosity. In anemia, viscosity is reduced, and flow of velocity is high, whereas in cyanotic heart disease with polycythemia, viscosity is increased along with reduced flow velocity.

Vortex Shedding[4]

How turbulence produces sound? Turbulence does not produce enough acoustic force to produce audible sound. Actual mechanism is vortex shedding. When laminar flow gets obstructed, they produce minute eddies, which are the vortices. These vortices are shed in the direction of flow and leave wake in their original place. Blood rushes to fill up those left out wakes and produce vibration strong enough to create acoustically audible sound. At a critical level of amplitude and frequencies, vibrations can be appreciated as series of sound or murmur.

DETERMINANTS

Frequency

The most important determinant of murmur is frequency. Most of the cardiovascular murmurs are distributed on a wide scale of frequency, from 0 to 700 Hz. Pitch is the audible equivalent to frequency. Frequency determines the pitch and accordingly, murmur may be high-pitched or low-pitched. Pitch depends upon the flow and gradient. High gradient with low flow produces high-pitched murmur. In mitral and aortic regurgitation, there is high gradient between left ventricle and left atrium and aorta and left ventricle, respectively. In both situations, flow is only regurgitant amount. Thus, both lesions produce high-pitched blowing murmur. When both the lesions are severe and the flow is excess, the murmur may be medium to low frequency and relatively harsher. High flow with low gradient produces low and medium frequency murmur. In mitral stenosis, even if critical, the diastolic pressure gradient between left atrium and left ventricle cannot be very high. However, as entire stroke output passes through stenotic valve, it is a high flow situation. This high flow low gradient physiology produces a low to medium frequency rumbling murmur. High gradient and large flow produce mixed frequency murmur. In significant aortic or pulmonary stenosis (PS), gradient is high. At the same time, entire cardiac output passes through the obstructed valve. This high gradient, high flow physiology produces mixed (both high and low) frequency, harsh murmur (**Table 1**).

Intensity (Box 1)

As mentioned, Levine graded intensity of systolic murmur only because he was following up systolic murmur for a longtime.

Diastolic murmur is conventionally not graded, because grade does not convey any added hemodynamic information for diastolic murmur. However, grading of diastolic murmur has recently been mentioned in a monogram by European Society of Cardiology[4] as grade 1–4.

TABLE 1: Relation between gradient, flow, and frequency.

Gradient	Flow	Frequency	Lesion
High	Low	High	MR, AR
Low	High	Low to medium	MS, TS
High	High	Mixed (low and high)	AS, PS
Low	Low	Low	MS, TS with low cardiac output

(AS: aortic stenosis; AR: aortic regurgitation; MR: mitral regurgitation; MS: mitral stenosis; PS: pulmonary stenosis; TS: tricuspid stenosis)

> **BOX 1** **Levine grading system of systolic murmur.**
> - *Grade 1:* Faint murmur, often missed and better audible in a quiet room
> - *Grade 2:* Murmur is more prominent and easily appreciable
> - *Grade 3:* Murmur is loud without thrill
> - *Grade 4:* Murmur is associated with thrill
> - *Grade 5:* Is very loud; can be heard with part of the stethoscope raised off the chest wall
> - *Grade 6:* Can be heard even with stethoscope completely raised off chest wall

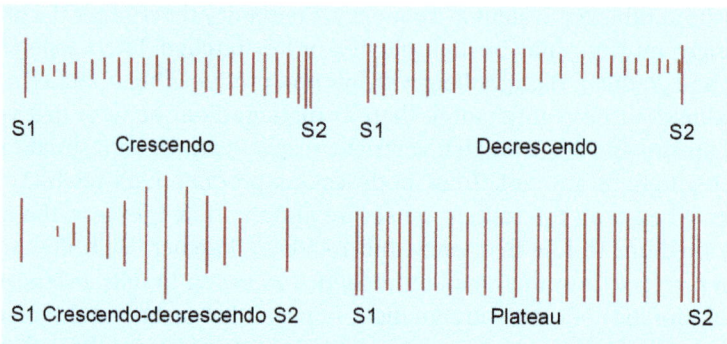

(S1: first heart sound; S2: second heart sound)
Fig. 1: Different shapes of murmur.

Shape (Fig. 1)

Crescendo murmur is the murmur, which is increasing in intensity (murmur of mitral stenosis), whereas decrescendo murmur is the murmur, which is decreasing in intensity (aortic regurgitation murmur). Crescendo-decrescendo murmur or diamond-shaped murmur is the increasing and decreasing intensity (murmur of aortic and PS). Plateau murmur is the murmur, which remains unchanged in intensity.

Character

A murmur may be blowing, harsh, rumbling, musical, scratchy or squeaky in nature.

Timing, Duration Location, and Radiation (Fig. 2)

In relation to cardiac cycle, the murmur may be systolic, diastolic or continuous. It may be a long or short murmur. The site where it is best heard and its radiation must be mentioned.

Dynamic Auscultation

Described separately.

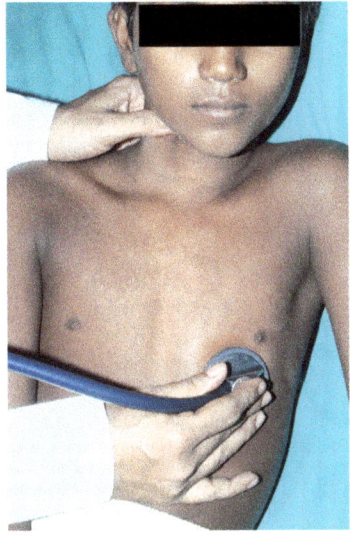

Fig. 2: Timing of the murmur with carotid artery.

BOX 2	Types of systolic murmur.

- Ejection systolic or midsystolic murmur
- Regurgitant systolic murmur:
  - Pansystolic murmur
  - Early systolic murmur
  - Late systolic murmur

SYSTOLIC MURMUR (BOX 2 AND FIG. 3)

Murmur is called systolic, when it is confined in systolic phase. Systolic murmur is either due to ejection of blood from ventricle to great vessels, or regurgitation of blood from high pressure chamber to low pressure chamber or shunting of blood from high to low pressure chamber. According to the time frame, it may be early, mid or late systolic. According to the frequency, it may be harsh or blowing. According to shape, it may be diamond or kite shaped.

EJECTION SYSTOLIC MURMUR (BOX 3)

Normally ejection of blood from ventricular chamber to great vessel does not produce any turbulence. Laminar flow pattern is disturbed, when there is either obstruction to flow or increased velocity of flow or large amount of blood flow, leading to ejection systolic murmur (ESM).

Physiology (Fig. 4)

Ejection systolic murmur with its crescendo-decrescendo nature, starts after first heart sound (S1) and ends before second heart sound (S2). This

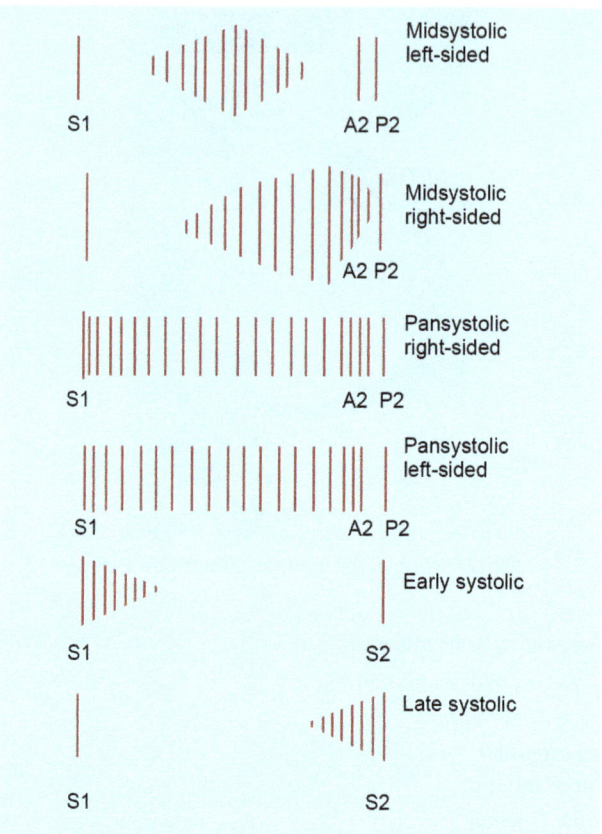

(A2: aortic componenet; P2: pulmonary component; S1: first heart sound; S2: second heart sound)

Fig. 3: Different systolic murmur.

| BOX 3 | Causes of ejection systolic murmur. |

Obstruction at outflow:
- Aortic stenosis (AS) (valvular, supravalvular, and subvalvular)
- Hypertrophic cardiomyopathy
- Pulmonary stenosis (PS) (valvular, supravalvular, and subvalvular)

Increased velocity:
- Rapid circulatory state such as anemia, thyrotoxicosis, and pregnancy
- Some of the innocent murmur
- Thoracic structural abnormalities

Increase volume of flow:
- Functional AS in presence of severe aortic regurgitation
- Functional PS in presence of large atrial septal defect

Dilated aortic or pulmonary root

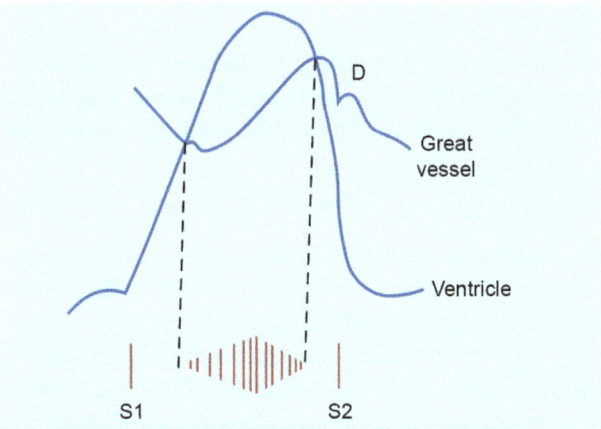

(S1: first heart sound; S2: second heart sound)

Fig. 4: Physiology of midsystolic murmur: After the isovolumetric contraction phase, when the ventricular pressure pulse crosses over arterial pressure pulse, ejection begins. Thus, the murmur stars after S1. It is followed by the slow ejection phase when the decrescendo part of the ejection systolic murmur (ESM) occurs. Then the ejection ceases followed by the hangout interval, which ends with S2. This explains why ESM ends before S2.

can be explained by the hemodynamic of ejection. S1 occurs at the onset of isovolumetric contraction phase after which the ventricular ejection starts, explaining the onset of ESM after S1. Initial part of the ejection is the rapid ejection phase when the crescendo part of the ESM occurs. It is followed by the slow ejection phase when the decrescendo part of the ESM occurs. Then the ejection ceases followed by the hangout interval which ends with S2. This explains why ESM ends before S2. When S1 and S2 are relatively soft, it becomes difficult to differentiate between ESM and pansystolic murmur.

Characteristics[5,6]

- *Frequency*: As mentioned earlier, as total stroke output passes through the semilunar valve, ESM is low to medium frequency and harsh in nature. This happens in case of ESM due to hyperkinetic flow or functional murmur or innocent murmur. In severe aortic and PS with very high-pressure head, i.e., high flow, high gradient physiology, the murmur may have additional high frequency tone.
- The peak is usually at early to midsystole in hyperkinetic and high flow state. In obstructive lesions, peak may be delayed.
- *Postectopic beat/post long R-R gap in atrial fibrillation (AF) potentiation*: Long diastolic gap in these situations increases preload and eventual stroke volume; hence the intensity of ESM is enhanced. Secondly, during the long diastolic gap, aortic diastolic pressure gets time to fall further and during ejection, ventricle faces lesser resistance. Last, during long diastole, ventricular contractile elements recover more calcium.

Aortic Stenosis (Fig. 5)

Aortic stenosis (AS) murmur is best heard at the base on right second intercostal space. However, it may be loud at the base on left second intercostal space or even at the apex. Actually, any aortic event can be heard anywhere on the area starting from right 2nd intercostal space to apex.

Grade

More loudly the murmur, more severe is the stenosis. A grade 4 murmur indicates severe stenosis, whereas a grade 1 murmur indicates mild stenosis. However, a murmur of grade 2, 3 cannot be correlated to AS severity. In low cardiac output situation, severe AS may not produce loud murmur. Longer the duration of murmur, severe is the stenosis. Classically, it is an ESM. More severe the stenosis, more the peak shifts toward S2. The late peaking is the hallmark of severity. When the peak is on first half of systole, it is mild AS. If the peak is on second half of systole, it is severe stenosis. However, in presence of associated conditions, which produces high transaortic flow, such as aortic regurgitation, ejection murmur may not be late peaking in spite of severe AS.

Point of interest is that AS murmur is produced by the high-velocity jet effect, not on the valve but on the ascending aorta. The high-velocity vibration produces a mixed-frequency, harsh murmur. Due to the superiorly directed jet in ascending aorta, murmur is conducted toward carotid artery. Radiation occurs in both the carotid artery, may be more on left than right.

Gallavardin phenomenon is more common in calcific AS of elderly. The high-frequency component is transmitted at the apex. This has a distinct musical quality. Due to its apical location, the murmur may be confused with mitral regurgitation murmur. However, the murmur is crescendo-decrescendo in nature and carries that distinct musical quality. As there is no commissural fusion in

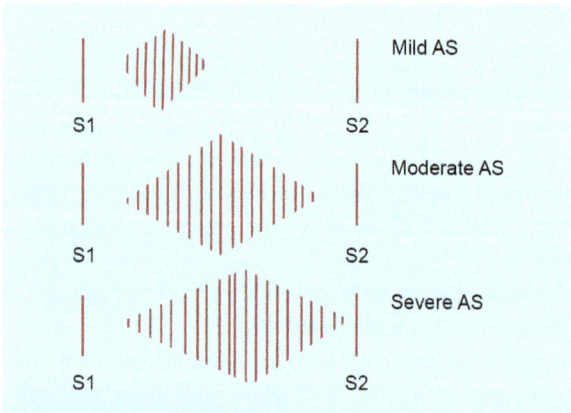

(S1: first heart sound; S2: second heart sound)

Fig. 5: Aortic stenosis (AS): Severe the AS, longer will be the murmur with the peak shifting toward A2, but it does not envelope A2. In its severe form, it retains its diamond shape.

calcific AS and bases are fixed, the cusps vibrate on jet effect. The vibration may produce the high-frequency component.[7]

In rheumatic AS, due to commissural fusion, A2 is down in intensity; ejection click is uncommon.

In calcific AS, due to absence of commissural fusion, leaflet movements are preserved. This probably explains the occasional musical property of the murmur. As mentioned, Gallavardin phenomenon is common. A2 is also preserved, unless valve is grossly calcified. Ejection click is usually absent.

In congenital valvular AS, ejection click is common; A2 is relatively preserved, even may be prominent. Aortic regurgitation is absent in early childhood and appears later.

In subvalvular stenosis, murmur is best heard in mid or left parasternal area; aortic regurgitation can be found in 50% cases. Click is absent; A2 is preserved; murmur may be in a lower down position.

In supravalvular stenosis, murmur is best heard in right first intercostal space; click is absent; A2 may be loud; aortic regurgitation which is often present in valvular or subvalvular AS, is absent in supravalvular stenosis; carotid conduction is more prominent.

Severity of AS can be judged with confidence by clinical examination alone. An anacrotic notch, slow rise, small volume and delayed peak of carotid pulse, forceful well-sustained apical impulse, diminished S1, single or paradoxical split of S2 are indicators of significant AS. More harsh and long murmur with delayed peak, severe is the AS. As mentioned earlier, presence of fourth heart sound (S4) in a younger patient indicates severe AS with a gradient >70 mm Hg.

Hypertrophic Cardiomyopathy

There is different opinion regarding the mechanism and character of the murmur. The murmur most commonly has been described as ESM. The murmur shows a late peaking in obstructive hypertrophic cardiomyopathy (HCM) and early peaking in nonobstructed HCM. The early peaking of the murmur is produced by the flow in left ventricular outflow tract due to hypercontractile left ventricular. The late peaking is due to obstruction. The murmur may be very short or absent in mild obstruction or in nonobstructed HCM. The murmur is usually grade 2, 3. Occasionally, the murmur may be associated with thrill, which indicates severe obstruction.

The murmur has also been described as combination of early ejection systolic and mid-late systolic murmur; the later is caused by mitral regurgitation (MR).[8] The evidence in favor of its being regurgitation murmur rather than ESM are:
- A mid-late systolic murmur is recorded in left atrium by intracardiac phonocardiography, while the typical ejection murmur peaking in early systole is recorded in aortic root.
- Its best location is between left lower sternal border and apex. The murmur may be heard or may radiate to base, but carotid transmission is unusual.

Ejection Systolic Murmur in Presence of Severe AR

This is a flow murmur, which is low to medium frequency, thus is less harsh in nature. Late peaking and Gallavardin's effect are usually not present. Associated findings of severe aortic regurgitation should be present.

Aortic Valve Sclerosis

Aortic valve sclerosis (AVS) is very common, almost 1 in every 4 people above the age of 65 years.[9] AVS is associated with calcification of leaflet without any interference of leaflet excursion of significant transvalvular pressure gradient. ESM here is less rasping, conduction is not widespread and A2 is normal in intensity. Calcific aortic valve disease encompasses a range of disease severity from mild leaflet thickening without valve obstruction, called aortic sclerosis, to severe AS. AVS is associated with many of the risk factors as coronary artery disease including age, male gender, hypertension, smoking, diabetes, and elevated low-density lipoprotein and lipoprotein (a). Aortic sclerosis is diagnosed on echocardiography, as focal areas of increased echogenicity on the valve leaflets with normal valve motion. Velocity across the valve may be normal, or only mildly elevated. Velocity <2.5 m/s or <2.0 m/s is sclerosis, if more is mild stenosis.

Pulmonary Stenosis (Fig. 6)

In valvular PS, the ESM is best heard at left second and third intercostals space, parasternal, which overlies the pulmonary trunk, with conduction toward neck. In infundibular and subinfundibular stenosis, murmur is best heard one or two

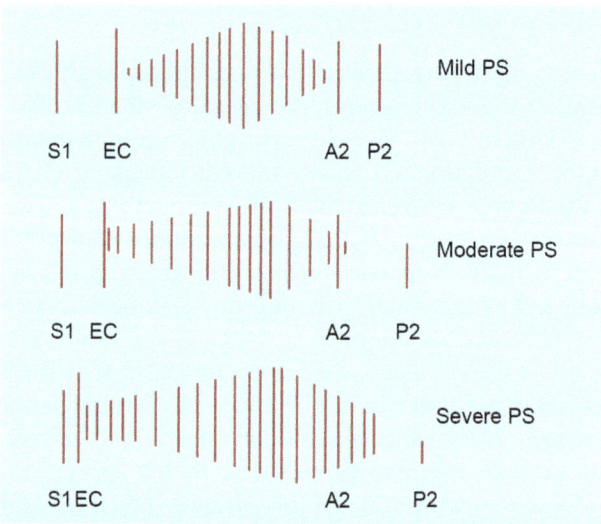

(A2: aortic component; EC: ejection click; P2: pulmonary component; S1: first heart sound)

Fig. 6: Pulmonary stenosis (PS): Severe the PS, longer will be the murmur with the peak shifting towards P2, thus enveloping A2. In its severe form, it will become kite shaped.

space down. The length and harshness of the murmur depend upon the severity of the murmur. In mild PS, the ESM starts after S1, with ejection click, and ends before A2. In moderate PS, the murmur extends to A2, which is still audible. In severe stenosis, the murmur extends beyond A2, which is masked by the murmur. The peak of the murmur also changes in accord with the severity of stenosis and in severe PS, the peak is closed to A2. Thus, a crescendo-decrescendo diamond-shaped murmur in mild PS becomes a kite-shaped murmur in severe PS.

Severity of Pulmonary Stenosis

Large *a* wave in jugular venous pulse (JVP), a left parasternal grade 3 pulsation, pulmonary ejection click either very closed to S1 or absent, widely splitted, sometimes fixed S2, down to absent pulmonary valve closure (P2), right ventricular S4, long harsh murmur with delayed peak are the features of severe valvular PS.

Pulmonary Stenosis with Ventricular Septal Defect (Fig. 7)

Classically, it is found in tetralogy of Fallot (TOF). ESM across right ventricular outflow tract (RVOT) in TOF shows a typical inverse relation between its length

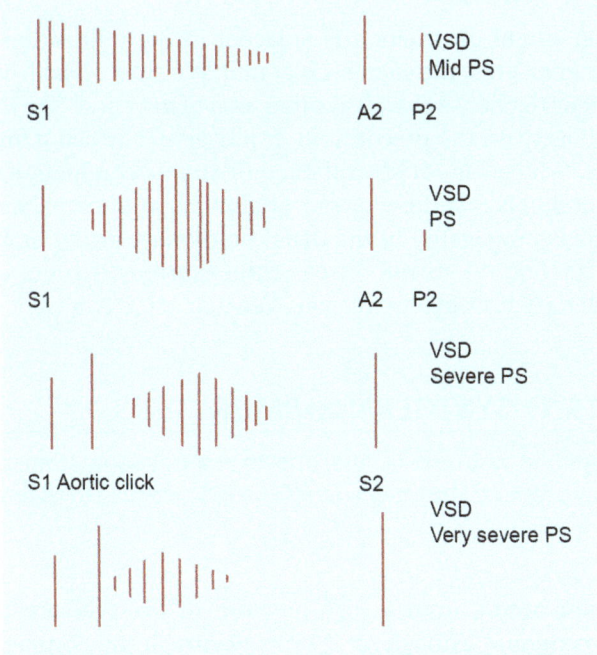

(A2: aortic component; P2: pulmonary component; S1: first heart sound; S2: second heart sound)

Fig. 7: Ventricular septal defect (VSD) with pulmonary stenosis (PS): When PS is mild, it will be a long decrescendo murmur of VSD, not of PS. In tetralogy physiology, murmur originates due to right ventricular outflow tract stenosis. Severe the stenosis, shorter will be the murmur. P2 and aortic click will behave accordingly.

and loudness versus severity of PS. Flow from right ventricle across RVOT is restricted in early ejection phase, when right ventricle contains most blood and develops peak pressure. Right ventricle decompresses through large ventricular septal defect (VSD) in aorta. Thus, more severe is the RVOT obstruction, right ventricular pressure becomes progressively more inadequate. Another mechanism is infundibular contraction in late systole, which retards late systolic flow and shortens murmur. More severe the stenosis is, more vigorous is the infundibular contraction. Both the ventricles eject most of their content into the aorta before the closure of aortic valve. Thus, the flow and murmur end before A2. In mild TOF, right ventricle can maintain the gradient in late systole. Thus, the flow and murmur across RVOT extends over A2.

Grade of the murmur may range from 1 to 5. In classical TOF, it may be grade 2–4. Flow across RVOT is against a significant gradient, which may impart a high-grade murmur and even thrill.

Shape of the murmur varies from diamond-shaped, reverse-kite shaped, and kite-shaped for very severe, severe and mild TOF, respectively. In contrast, murmur of only PS varies from diamond-shaped and kite-shaped for mild and severe stenosis, respectively.

Peripheral Pulmonary Artery Stenosis

Most common site of obstruction is adjacent to the bifurcation of the main pulmonary artery. Often, the stenosis is at multiple sites. Hence, best site of the murmur is left or right base as well as other area of the chest. The ESM is usually grade 3 in intensity on the precordium. It preserves the same intensity at the axillae or back, which cannot be explained by simple conduction of precordial sound. Explanation is that the murmur originating at the proximal pulmonary artery stenosis is propagated in the distal pulmonary artery branches, which may not be stenotic. S1 to the onset of the murmur is more delayed than that of valvular PS for obvious reason. Valvular click is absent and P2 may be loud.

REGURGITANT SYSTOLIC MURMUR

Regurgitant systolic murmur occurs due to regurgitation from high-pressure ventricle to low pressure atrium or shunt from left ventricle to right ventricle.

Physiology

As regurgitation occurs from a high-pressure to low-pressure chamber, the regurgitation continues throughout systole, mostly in same intensity. Classical pansystolic murmur starts after the atrioventricular pressure pulse crossover, in early part of isovolumetric contraction phase. Thus, it begins with S1. As the gradient between two chambers persists in isovolumetric relaxation phase and beyond, the systolic murmur may continue to and beyond S2. Audibility of S1 and S2 depends on the intensity of those sound and site of auscultation.

Characteristic

- As the flow is from high pressure to low pressure chamber, but the flow is part of total stroke output, regurgitant systolic murmur is high frequency murmur and blowing in nature. In severe regurgitation or shunt, the flow is also high and there may be low frequency component and the murmur may become harsh.
- Long R-R interval of postpremature beat or AF does not potentiate regurgitant systolic murmur. Though ventricle gets more blood during long R-R interval and during the following beat, it contracts more vigorously, regurgitant murmur intensity does not change much. Karliner and O'Rourke[10] proposed the hemodynamic explanation in their study—"*after a premature ventricular beat, reduced impedance to left ventricular ejection and augmented left ventricular contraction favour forward flow, and lead to volume equalization early during ejection when control and long cycles are compared. This mechanism explains the constancy of the murmur of mitral regurgitation in the beat after a premature ventricular contraction.*"

PANSYSTOLIC MURMUR

Most common pansystolic murmurs are MR, tricuspid regurgitation (TR), and VSD.

Mitral Regurgitation (Fig. 8)

In MR, left ventricular-left atrial pressure gradient persists more or less same throughout systole. For this reason, the regurgitation continues throughout systole mostly in same intensity, resulting in a holosystolic or pansystolic

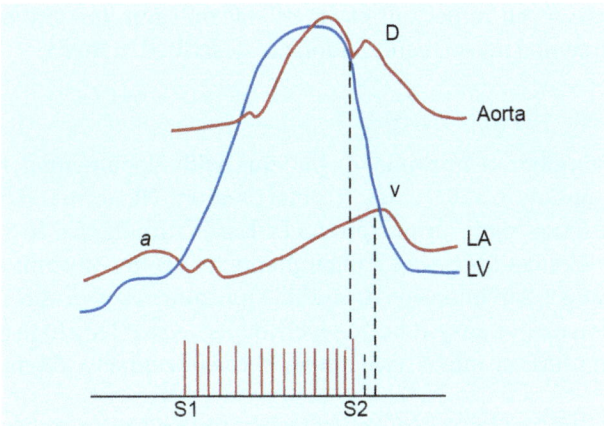

(LA: left atrium; LV: left ventricle; S1: first heart sound; S2: second heart sound)

Fig. 8: Physiology of mitral regurgitation (MR) murmur: It starts after the atrioventricular pressure pulse crossover, in early part of isovolumetric contraction phase. Thus, it begins with S1. Even after A2, left ventricular pressure remains high than left atrial pressure during early isovolumetric relaxation phase. Thus, pansystolic murmur continues beyond A2.

murmur. It starts after the atrioventricular pressure pulse crossover, in early part of isovolumetric contraction phase. Thus, it begins with first heart sound. Even after A2, left ventricular pressure remains high than left atrial pressure during early isovolumetric relaxation phase. Thus, pansystolic murmur of MR continues beyond A2. However, it may not be always appreciable. S1 and A2 may mask the initial and last part of murmur, simulating the murmur starting after S1 and ending at A2.

Mitral regurgitation murmur is usually plateau shaped. Mild MR may produce a murmur with late accentuation; smaller regurgitant volume is producing lesser intensity during early part of filling phase with enhanced late systolic flow, due to fanning out of sound vibration. Severe MR with enhanced flow during rapid filling phase may impart an impression of mid systolic murmur. Insignificant MR, acute MR, and chronic severe MR with noncompliant small left atrium with a large v wave may produce tapering murmur.

Thus, MR murmur is essentially pansystolic with variable configuration, namely plateau shape, tapering or early, mid and late systolic accentuation.

Mitral regurgitation murmur is best heard at the apex with the diaphragm of the stethoscope firmly pressed, preferably at left lateral decubitus position, which increases the intensity of the murmur. Its common radiation is to the axilla, back or at the base when posterior leaflet is involved.

There is an excellent correlation between intensity of murmur and severity of MR.[11] MR murmur more than grade 4 intensity indicates severe MR (regurgitant fraction >40%) in 91% cases, whereas less than grade 2 MR murmur indicates nonsevere MR in 88% cases. Grade 3 murmur does not have any correlation to severity of MR. This relation is weaker in functional MR or ischemic MR. Intensity of murmur may be reduced by associated conditions such as heart failure, large left atrium, and mitral stenosis. Heart failure, due to reduced force of contraction of left ventricle, is an important cause of soft murmur, in spite of severe MR. Causes of congenital mitral regurgitation are described in **Box 4**.

Tricuspid Regurgitation

Tricuspid regurgitation murmur, in patients with documented regurgitation, might not be audible in >20% cases. Normal pressure TR, normal right ventricular pressure or a large right atrium produces lesser turbulence. In consequence, murmur may be inaudible even if regurgitation is severe. Murmur is usually not more than grade 2, 3 in intensity. An audible murmur always indicates severe TR.

Murmur is usually pansystolic. In severe hypertensive TR, a high gradient, high flow situation murmur might have a high frequency quality. TR murmur is best

---

BOX 4 | **Congenital mitral regurgitation.**

- Cleft mitral valve
- Congenitally corrected transposition of the great arteries
- Parachute mitral valve
- Anomalous left coronary artery from pulmonary artery

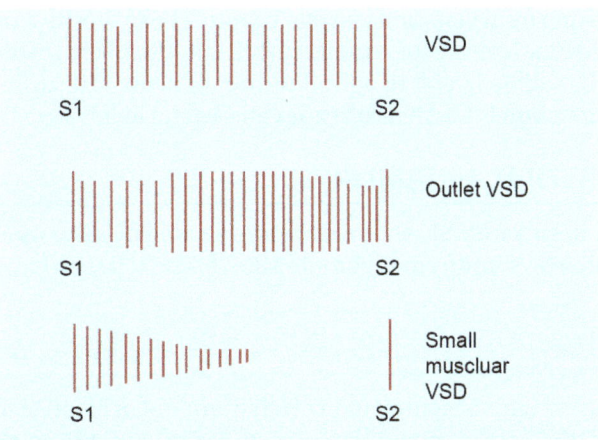

(S1: first heart sound; S2: second heart sound)

Fig. 9: Ventricular septal defect (VSD): Usually, the murmur is pansystolic and plateau shaped. Murmur of outlet (doubly committed) VSD may show an ejection systolic pattern. Murmur of small muscular VSD may show an early systolic pattern.

heard at left lower parasternal area, in 4th and 5th intercostal space. The murmur may radiate to right lower parasternal area, below the right costal margin and over the hepatic surface. When the dilated right ventricle forms the apex, TR murmur may radiate to the apex. However, the murmur never radiates to the axilla.

Inspiratory increase in the intensity of the murmur, known as Carvallo's sign, is a characteristic sign of TR murmur. The enhancement in the grade may be transient and detectable only in first one or two beats. Carvallo's sign may be absent in presence of severe right ventricular failure.

Hepatojugular reflux, by increasing venous return, increases TR murmur.

Maneuvers such as squatting, Müller's maneuver, and release phase of Valsalva increase the intensity of TR murmur by increasing right heart filling. On the other hand, maneuvers such as erect posture and strain phase of Valsalva decrease the intensity by reducing right heart filling.

In contrary to MR murmur, long-short cycle in AF affects TR murmur. Long cycle increases JVP as well as TR murmur.

Ventricular Septal Defect (Fig. 9)

Ventricular septal defect murmur is best heard at left parasternal area with radiation down to right parasternal area. Outlet VSD is best heard in upper parasternal area, muscular VSD in lower parasternal area, and perimembranous VSD in between. Murmur is not affected by respiration. Large VSD may be associated with third heart sound (S3), wide split S2, and diastolic flow murmur. P2 is usually normal or loud in VSD, whereas it is normal or down in PS. In nonrestrictive VSD or VSD with severe pulmonary arterial hypertension (PAH), murmur may be absent.

In VSD arising from ventricular septal rupture (VSR) due to acute myocardial infarction, murmur is always of lesser grade. This is best heard medial to apex and at apex. It is inaudible lateral to apex. Murmur of acute MR secondary to acute myocardial infarction is best heard at apex and lateral to it.

EARLY SYSTOLIC MURMUR

This murmur begins with S1, ends well before S2, and behaves as a decrescendo murmur. Acute MR, some form of chronic MR, TR, and VSD can have early systolic murmur.

Acute Mitral Regurgitation (Fig. 10)

Acute MR causes sudden regurgitation of large amount of blood in the left atrium, which is a smaller, less accommodative chamber in comparison to chronic MR. This results in sharp rise of left atrial pressure with a large v wave. In the later part of systole, this large v wave causes equilibrium of left atrial and ventricular

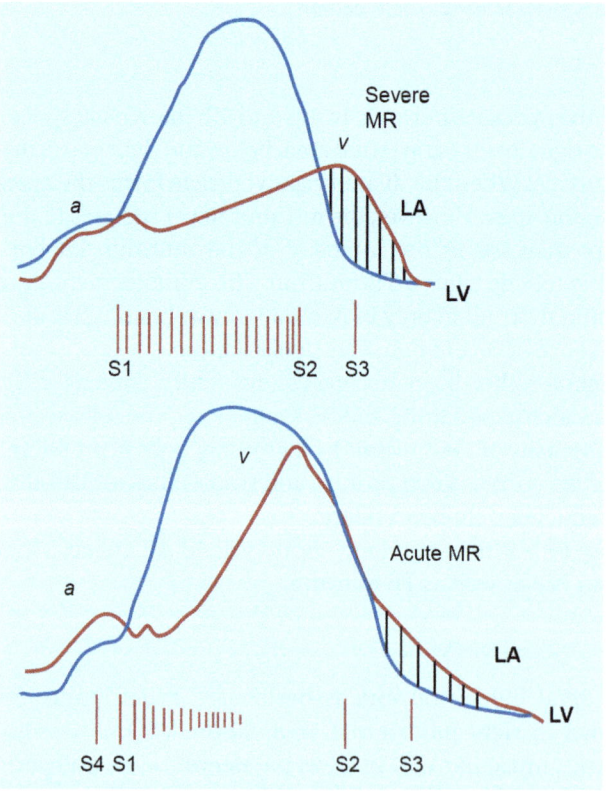

(S1: first heart sound; S2: second heart sound; S3: third heart sound; S4: fourth heart sound)

Fig. 10: Mitral regurgitation (MR): chronic severe MR—due to higher flow of the regurgitant blood from left atrium (LA) and rapid relaxation of left ventricle (LV), in diastole, S3 is found in severe MR; acute MR—it creates very large v wave with high mean LA pressure, reducing LV-LA gradient. Thus, the MR murmur will become early systolic.

> **BOX 5** **Causes of primary/low-pressure tricuspid regurgitation (TR).**
> - Ebstein anomaly
> - Right-sided infective endocarditis
> - Right ventricular infarction
> - Trauma
> - Rheumatic heart disease
> - Device-lead induced TR
> - Carcinoid disease

pressure and regurgitation flow is reduced. This results in early systolic murmur. Acute myocardial infarction, infective endocarditis, rheumatic carditis, and trauma are common causes of acute MR. S4, rather than S3, and loud P2 are common findings.

Primary Tricuspid Regurgitation (Box 5)

Primary or low pressure TR, in contrast to hypertensive TR, is often early systolic. Here, as gradient between right ventricle and right atrium is minimum, in later part of systole, right atrial pressure becomes equal to right ventricular pressure. This causes a low and medium frequency soft, early systolic murmur. Severity of TR can be assessed by RV S3, diastolic flow murmur, large v and y wave in jugular pressure pulse.

Other Causes

Mitral regurgitation secondary to left ventricular dilatation, mitral annular calcification, and small muscular VSD cause early systolic murmur.

LATE SYSTOLIC MURMUR

Mitral Valve Prolapse

Myxomatous degeneration of mitral valve is most common cause of mitral valve prolapse (MVP). It is associated with click and consistent changes on dynamic auscultation. MVP is sometimes associated with precordial whoop or honk, which is a loud, high-pitched musical murmur.

Ischemic/Functional Mitral Regurgitation

In ischemic/functional MR, regurgitation murmur may be pansystolic, late systolic or early systolic in timing. When MR is severe, murmur is usually pansystolic. As the mitral valve becomes incompetent only after the interaction of tethering and closing forces, murmur may begin well after the first sound and may behave as late systolic murmur. In presence of relatively good left ventricular systolic function, murmur may be early systolic. Tethering force is reduced during late-systolic ventricular contraction, when its volume becomes smaller, whereas closing force is enhanced. In consequence, late systolic regurgitation is curtailed, and murmur becomes decrescendo in nature. In severe MR with a large v wave, late systolic part may be absent, and murmur may have an ejection systolic pattern. Shape of the murmur may be variable in a single patient, depending on the hemodynamic variable. Unlike rheumatic MR murmur, secondary murmur may change with long-short cycle of AF or postectopic pause, which changes left ventricular filling and volume. Tethering force is variable and changes with the left ventricular volume and force of contraction.

DIASTOLIC MURMUR (BOX 6 AND FIG. 11)

Aortic Regurgitation

There is conceptual contradiction regarding intensity versus severity of aortic regurgitation murmur. More severe the aortic regurgitation, louder the intensity had been described in study.[12] Severe aortic regurgitation usually produces a grade 3 murmur. Severe aortic regurgitation with heart failure sometimes produces a short soft murmur. On the contrary, a mild aortic regurgitation may occasionally produce a loud murmur.

BOX 6	Diastolic murmur.
Early diastolic murmur:	**Mid diastolic murmur:**
• Aortic regurgitation	• Mitral stenosis
• Pulmonary regurgitation	• Tricuspid stenosis
• Dock murmur	• Carey Coombs murmur
• Chronic renal failure	• Austin Flint murmur
	• Rytand murmur
	• Other murmur

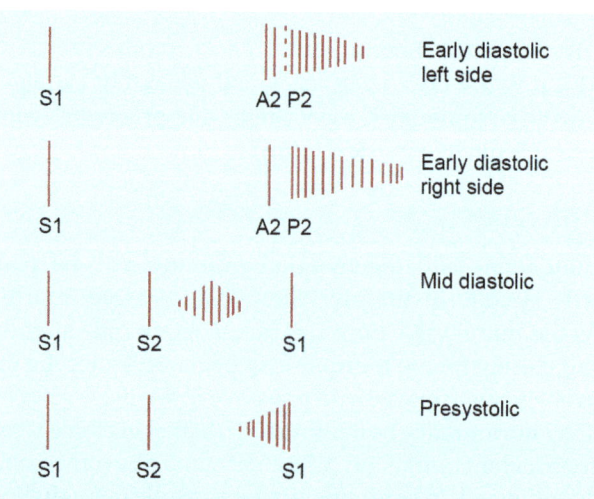

(A2: aortic component; P2: pulmonary component; S1: first heart sound; S2: second heart sound)

Fig. 11: Different diastolic murmur.

There is high aortic-left ventricular diastolic gradient with smaller flow in, aortic regurgitation producing high frequency murmur. The frequency is similar to respiratory sound. For this reason, murmur is often missed and needs special method to elicit. More severe the murmur more is the flow and murmur becomes a mixed frequency of high and medium frequency. In severe or free aortic regurgitation, a combination of very high flow and not that high gradient produces a murmur of medium and dominating low frequency murmur, which is harsh in quality. In severe aortic regurgitation, with very high flow, aortoventricular gradient and thus velocity of reflux may be reduced, leading to a pure low frequency murmur.

Aortic regurgitation murmur is classically described as decrescendo in shape. As reflux goes on, aortoventricular gradient falls due to reducing aortic diastolic pressure and increasing ventricular diastolic pressure. As a result, murmur is decrescendo in shape, tapering in late diastole.

Reflux begins after isovolumetric relaxation phase, when left ventricular pressure is minimum and aortic diastolic pressure is maximum. At this maximal aortoventricular gradient, murmur may behave as crescendo shape for a brief period.

Most important determinant regarding aortic regurgitation severity that can be gathered from aortic regurgitation murmur is the length of aortic regurgitation murmur. In mild aortic regurgitation, a brief murmur just after A2, high frequency and low amplitude, is often missed. Severe the aortic regurgitation, longer is the murmur, which may extend to S1. The length becomes pandiastolic, preserving the decrescendo nature. On the other hand, in severe aortic regurgitation and in aortic regurgitation with heart failure, when late aortoventricular gradient is reduced, murmur may not extend to late diastole.

Aortic regurgitation murmur, being high frequency, is soft blowing in nature. The murmur becomes harsh in quality, when it becomes low frequency.

Musical murmur, cooing-dove or seagull murmur is found in perforated or everted leaflet of infective endocarditis, ruptured sinus of Valsalva (RSOV), and trauma (luetic aorta is no more seen). The murmur is resonating in nature with pure frequency. Mid and late diastolic part of the murmur imparts a musical tone.

Aortic regurgitation murmur is best heard at left parasternal area, on second to fourth intercostal space. Severe aortic regurgitation murmur may be audible more downward and at apex. In elderly, murmur may be best audible at apex. This is the usual site, when aortic regurgitation is valvular in origin. Right parasternal area, third to fifth intercostal space, is the best site, when aortic regurgitation is aortic root in origin. Dilated aorta is displaced rightward and superiorly, leading to a selective radiation of murmur on right of sternum. Common causes are aortic aneurysm, RSOV, aortic dissection, and selective perforation or eversion of right coronary cusp. Audibility of aortic regurgitation murmur has been described even at axilla, known as Cole-Cecil murmur.

How to Assess Severity of Aortic Regurgitation?

More severe the aortic regurgitation is, longer is the murmur. It should envelope at least more than half of the diastole, in significant aortic regurgitation. Other features of severity are: Pulsus bisferiens and water-hammer pulse, Duroziez's murmur, positive Hill's sign, diastolic pressure below 60 mm Hg, down and outward–shifted apex, paradoxical split and diminished intensity of S2, functional AS murmur, and Austin Flint murmur (**Fig. 12**).

Acute Aortic Regurgitation

Basic hemodynamic in acute aortic regurgitation is the acute severe volume overload of the nondilated left ventricular, with sudden increase of left ventricular end-diastolic pressure (EDP). Due to high EDP, diastolic murmur is relatively short. Other features of high EDP are: Premature closure of mitral valve resulting in soft or absent S1, features of PAH, and absence of S4 (high EDP excludes effective left ventricular filling during left atrial systole).

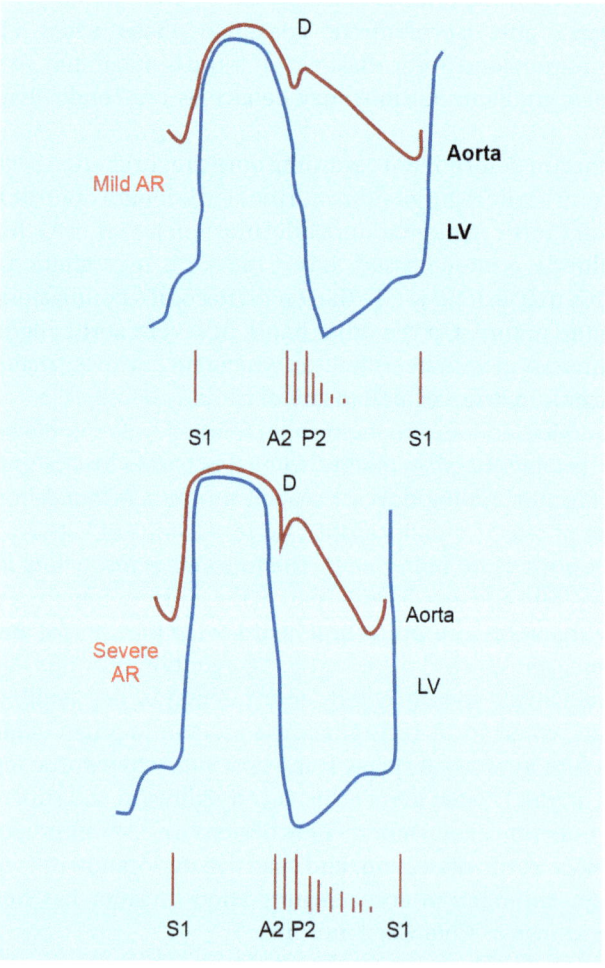

(A2: aortic component; LV: left ventricle; P2: pulmonary component; S1: first heart sound; S2: second heart sound)

Fig. 12: Murmur of aortic regurgitation (AR): More severe, longer will be its duration, and wider will be the pulse pressure.

Pulmonary Regurgitation (Fig. 13)

Hypertensive Pulmonary Regurgitation

The murmur of hypertensive pulmonary regurgitation (PR), popularly known as Graham Steell murmur, begins with loud P2. The high-pitched, decrescendo murmur is localized in left 2nd and 3rd sternal space. Inspiration does not increase its intensity appreciably, because the hypertrophied noncompliant right ventricle, associated with pulmonary hypertension, cannot accommodate any extra volume during inspiration. Length of the murmur varies. It may be

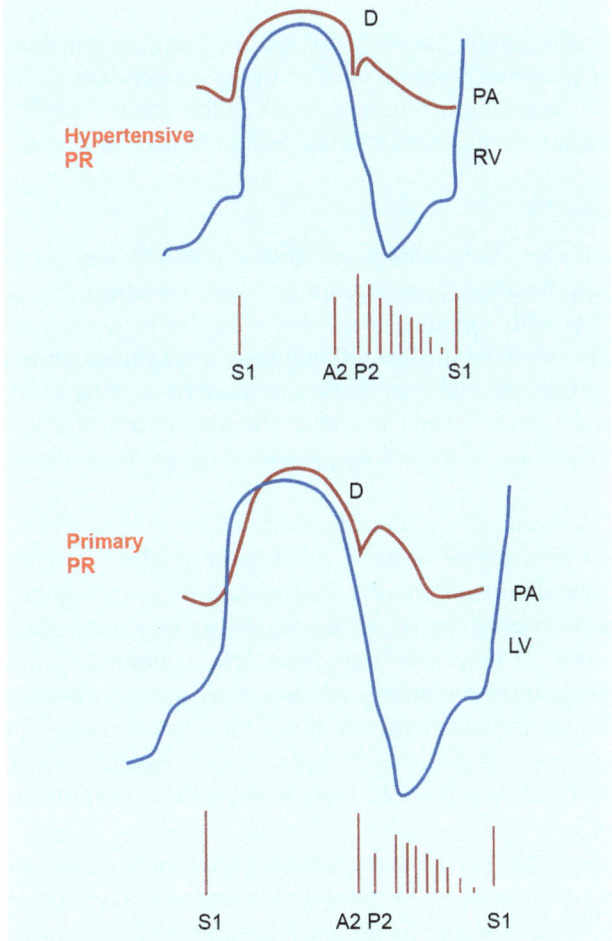

(A2: aortic component; LV: left ventricle; P2: pulmonary component; PA: pulmonary artery; RV: right ventricle; S1: first heart sound)

Fig. 13: Murmur of pulmonary regurgitation (PR): hypertensive PR—murmur starts with loud P2, decrescendo, long, near holodiastolic, occasionally short, high-pitched; primary PR—murmur starts well after soft P2, decrescendo, brief, low-pitched.

pandiastolic in pulmonary hypertension due to Eisenmenger syndrome, where right ventricular diastolic pressure may remain normal. Murmur may be brief in pulmonary hypertension due to postcapillary hypertension.

Normal Pressure Pulmonary Regurgitation

Unlike hypertensive PR, normal pressure PR is low-pitched rumbling murmur that starts well after P2. Important clinical clue is loudness of P2, which is not booming and even may be absent, as in congenital absent pulmonary valve. It is shorter in duration and increases appreciably with inspiration. Normal pressure PR is found in idiopathic dilatation of pulmonary artery, pulmonary valvotomy, right-sided endocarditis, and congenital absence of pulmonary valve syndrome.

Dock Murmur

In 1967, Dock described[13] an early diastolic murmur in a patient with critical stenosis in the proximal segment of left anterior descending artery. It is a short localized early diastolic murmur best heard in the left 2nd and 3rd parasternal space. The murmur disappeared after successful revascularization.

Mitral Stenosis

Mid-diastolic is very characteristic of significant mitral stenosis. Patient should be in left lateral position; apex should be localized where the bell should be placed. It starts with opening snap, denoting the beginning of rapid filling phase. Then it is reduced in slow filling phase. It reappears during active atrial contraction, producing the presystolic component, ending in S1. Essentially, it is a decrescendo-crescendo murmur. Presystolic murmur is described as accentuation, because of the waning phase of the murmur during slow filling phase.

From the duration of the diastolic murmur, severity of mitral stenosis can be decided. In mild mitral stenosis, as pressure gradient between left atrium and left ventricle dissipates shortly, the murmur does not extend much in late diastole. It may or may not reappear in presystolic with a silent phase in between. Sometimes, murmur may have only presystolic component without the mid diastolic phase. In moderate mitral stenosis, there are two distinct components, with a decrescendo phase in between. In severe mitral stenosis, with a persistent left atrial-left ventricular gradient throughout, mid-diastolic murmur extends in late diastole and ends as presystolic component at S1. Longer the murmur, severe is the stenosis.

Hemodynamically being a low gradient, high flow situation, mitral stenosis murmur is of low frequency in nature. As being low frequency murmur, it is very much localized. It is best heard in left lateral position, at apex only with the bell of stethoscope being pressed on chest wall very lightly. A few sits up make the murmur more prominent. In high output situation such as fever, infection murmur may become of mixed frequency, rougher and more audible over wider area.

Intensity of mid-diastolic murmur is not related to severity of mitral stenosis. Rather high flow across the stenosed valve may produce excess turbulence and high-grade murmur. However, flow remaining constant, severe the stenosis more will be the turbulence across the valve. Thus, intensity of murmur may have a thin relation to severity of mitral stenosis. In low flow situations, such as heart failure, severe pulmonary hypertension, and severe mitral stenosis itself, intensity of mid-diastolic murmur may be diminished. Concomitant severe aortic regurgitation or AS, by enhancing left ventricular diastolic pressure, may reduce intensity of the murmur. In Lutembacher's syndrome, as left atrium is decompressed through atrial septal defect (ASD), intensity of mid-diastolic murmur may be reduced. On the other hand, intensity of mid-diastolic murmur may be increased during tachycardia, post-short cycle length of AF, and associated MR.

Presystolic component can be heard in all cases of mitral stenosis, even when mitral stenosis is mild. A pressure gradient across mitral valve as low as 5 mm Hg can produce presystolic murmur. This may be present not only in sinus rhythm but also in AF, which denote mechanism other than late atrial contraction for this presystolic component. Initial concept was that the component is due to vibration of the anterior mitral leaflet or due to tricuspid valve closure. There is progressive narrowing of the mitral valve annulus in the last phase of ventricular diastole. In fact, the valve closure starts 60 ms before final closure and S1. In presence of significant gradient, flow continue through the closing valve, producing the presystolic component. At the same time, motion of the anterior mitral leaflet contributes to the murmur (**Fig. 14**).

Atrial contraction may have a role, when the rhythm is sinus. Atrial contraction reinforces the forward flow, as a result of which the impact of forward flow and closing leaflet is more pronounce and the presystolic component starts earlier. Thus, in mitral stenosis with AF, presystolic component does not have any contribution from atrial contraction and starts later than that in sinus rhythm. In presence of AF, presystolic component occurs after short cycle, as there is inadequate emptying and left atrial pressure remains high in compare to the long cycle.

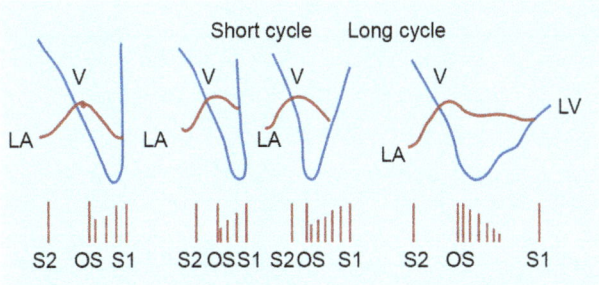

(LA: left atrium; LV: left ventricle; OS: opening snap; S1: first heart sound; S2: second heart sound)

Fig. 14: Mitral stenosis (MS) in atrial fibrillation (AF): Typically after short cycles, short diastolic murmurs are crescendo with presystolic components and after a long cycle, it is a decrescendo murmur without presystolic component.

How to Elicit?

Patient should be in left lateral position; apex should be localized where the bell should be placed.

How to Assess Severity?

Severe the stenosis, longer is the murmur. Severe the stenosis higher is the gradient and shorter will be the A2-OS interval. Associated PAH indicates severe mitral stenosis (**Fig. 15**).

Silent Mitral Stenosis

Severe stenosis may reduce the cardiac output with reduction of flow across the valve, which makes the murmur softer or even absent. Similarly, severe stenosis

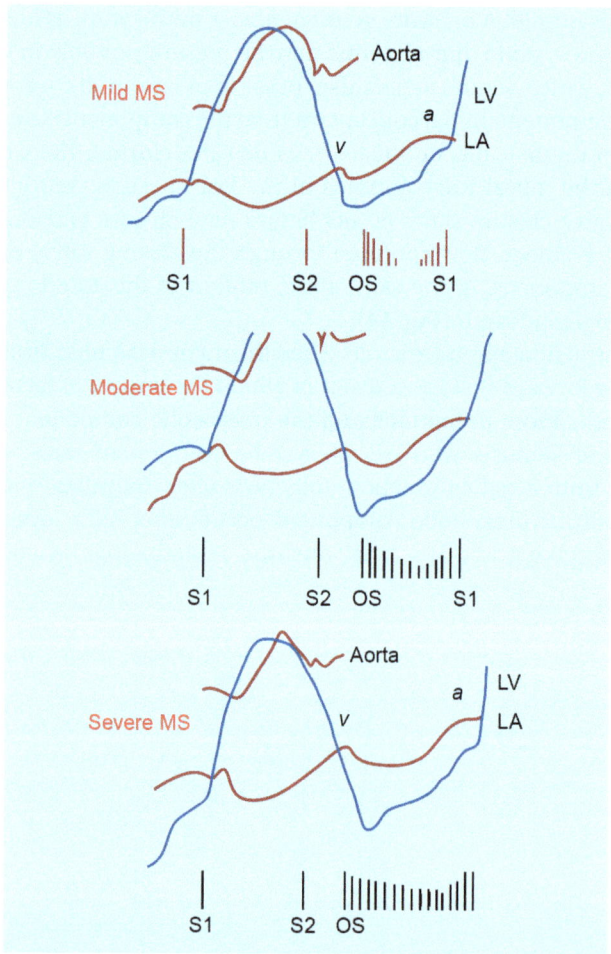

(LA: left atrium; LV: left ventricle; OS: opening snap; S1: first heart sound; S2: second heart sound)

Fig. 15: Severity of mitral stenosis (MS): In mild MS, it is a short mid-diastolic decrescendo murmur, followed by a presystolic crescendo murmur. In severe MS, it is a long diastolic murmur ending with the presystolic component.

leading to PAH causes right ventricular dominance, which occupies the apex, making the murmur inaudible. According to Levine and Love, mitral stenosis may be silent in 5–10% cases (**Box 7**).[14]

Tricuspid Stenosis

Tricuspid stenosis murmur has two components, such as mitral stenosis murmur, namely presystolic and mid-diastolic. Presystolic or atriosystolic murmur is the major component in presence of sinus rhythm, corresponding to maximum gradient produced during atrial systole. The presystolic murmur shows characteristic crescendo-decrescendo nature instead of crescendo character of mitral stenosis. Earlier explanation ascribed was prolonged PR interval, which accompanied tricuspid stenosis. More plausible explanation for the decrescendo nature of presystolic murmur is offered by the hemodynamic observation of earlier right atrial systolic summit than that of left atrium.[15]

In most of the cases, mid-diastolic component is present along with presystolic murmur, as because significant mid-diastolic gradient. The murmur has higher pitch than that of mitral stenosis murmur sometimes superficial with a scratchy or musical character.

Inspiration appreciably increases the intensity of diastolic murmur due to increased gradient across tricuspid valve. In presence of AF, murmur behaves like that of mitral stenosis. In short diastolic cycle, gradient remains constant and murmur is pandiastolic, whereas in long diastolic cycle, murmur behaves as a decrescendo and ends well before S2 (**Box 8**).

Austin Flint Murmur

Austin Flint, the American physician, first described this murmur in 1862. For him the eponym is Austin Flint murmur, which is mid-diastolic murmur with presystolic accentuation. It is a low frequency murmur, which begins with S3 and is localized to apex.

Initial theories for the Austin Flint murmur were:
- Diastolic MR—increased left ventricular EDP with a reverse ventriculoatrial gradient, flow occurs from left ventricle to left atrium.
- Increased velocity of antegrade flow across a closing mitral valve.

BOX 7	Common causes of left ventricular inflow obstruction.
• Mitral stenosis	• Ball-valve thrombus
• Left atrial myxoma	• Cor triatriatum

BOX 8	Common causes of right ventricular inflow obstruction.
• Isolated tricuspid stenosis	• Carcinoid disease
• In associated with rheumatic mitral stenosis	• Constrictive pericarditis
• Systemic lupus erythematosus	• Right atrial myxoma

- Oscillation of anterior mitral leaflet between two opposite antegrade and retrograde flow.
- A specific aortic cusp has to be involved with a direction of regurgitation jet directing to anterior mitral leaflet, which is deflected in the pathway of antegrade flow, producing the murmur.

Fortuin and Craige[16] use simultaneous phonocardiogram, apex cardiogram, and echocardiogram. They offered the following mechanism for Austin Flint murmur. The mitral valve remains open in diastole for a brief period of time. This is due to increasing left ventricular diastolic pressure, resulting in reverse ventriculoatrial gradient in major part of diastole. As antegrade filling period is shortened, velocity of antegrade flow is increased. At the same time, mitral valve is closing, leading to reduced orifice size. These two factors lead to turbulence, creating the mid-diastolic component of Austin Flint murmur. Atrial emptying is always incomplete. Distended atria contract forcefully. At the same time, left ventricular EDP is high, which prevents complete opening of valve at the end of presystole. These two factors, vigorous contraction of left atrium and incomplete valve opening, lead to presystolic accentuation of the murmur. They concluded—"Austin Flint murmur, which is commonly heard in patients with severe aortic regurgitation, is in essence a flow rumble produced by antegrade flow across the mitral valve".

In mild-to-moderate aortic regurgitation, mild alteration of left ventricular diastolic pressure occurs and Austin Flint murmur is absent. With moderate-to-severe aortic regurgitation, there is late diastolic rise of left ventricular pressure following atrial systole, leading to rapid valve closure following an opening movement. A crescendo presystolic Austin Flint murmur is present. With severe aortic regurgitation, diastolic pressure is elevated from mid-diastole onward and the murmur begins in mid-diastole and extends to presystolic. In very severe aortic regurgitation, mitral valve is opening only in mid-diastole. Thus, murmur is restricted in mid-diastole, losing its presystolic component.

A prominent *a* wave in apexcardiogram is common in aortic regurgitation, in presence of Austin Flint murmur. It represents the late diastolic left ventricular response to left atrium. This wave occurs simultaneously with left atrial *a* wave and S4. Distended left atrium contracts vigorously upon a noncompliant left ventricle, having EDP is already high, leading to tall *a* wave in apexcardiogram and S4. This wave is inconspicuous in case of mitral stenosis. Thus, in a patient with aortic regurgitation along with a mid-diastolic rumble, prominent *a* wave in apexcardiogram indicates isolated aortic regurgitation and diastolic rumble is due to Austin Flint murmur and not due to mitral stenosis.

The murmur can easily be differentiated from aortic regurgitation murmur. Later is usually high-pitched and decrescendo murmur, whereas Austin Flint murmur is low-pitched and crescendo murmur.

Isometric handgrip cannot differentiate Austin Flint murmur from mitral stenosis murmur. Handgrip results in increased peripheral resistance and reflux, which increases the grade of Austin Flint murmur. Increased reflux may increase left ventricular EDP so high, that mitral leaflet fails to open in presystolic, resulting in abolishing the presystolic component. Isometric handgrip does not have any immediate effect on diastolic murmur of mitral stenosis. Sometimes, increased heart rate and venous return may increase mitral stenosis murmur. However, presystolic component is not affected. Transient arterial occlusion of both arms is more objective maneuver, which increases aortic regurgitation murmur loudness by increasing afterload. As arterial pressure, heart rate, cardiac output, and both systemic and vascular resistance remain constant, mitral stenosis murmur is not affected. Amyl nitrite inhalation reduces peripheral resistance and reflux from aortic regurgitation, leading to decreased loudness of Austin Flint murmur, whereas shortened diastole and increased output augment diastolic murmur of mitral stenosis.

Carey Coombs Murmur

Carey Coombs, the British physician, described[17] the short mid-diastolic murmur in acute rheumatic fever with carditis. He is remembered eponymically for the description of that murmur. This short diastolic murmur, usually preceded by S3, is found in rheumatic mitral valvulitis. This is an acute inflammatory process that leads probably to valve edema, produces flow acceleration and the murmur. Usually found in children during active carditis and disappears after it gets resolved.

Chronic Renal Failure[18]

A diastolic murmur of aortic regurgitation may be found in 9% cases of end-stage renal disease (ESRD) and may disappear after replacement therapy. It is found in patients with volume overload, anemia, and hypertension. Origin is probably due to transient pulmonary hypertension and dilatation of pulmonary root leading to PR. Calcific AS along with aortic regurgitation, due to secondary hyperparathyroidism, is relatively common in ESRD.

Other Causes

- *Rytand murmur*: This is a mid-diastolic murmur found in some patients in complete heart block. Increased flow due to bradycardia may be the mechanism.
- Excessive flow across the mitral valve in severe MR, large VSD, and patent ductus arteriosus can lead to a mid-diastolic rumble at the apex.
- Similarly, excessive flow across the tricuspid valve in large ASD can lead to a mid-diastolic rumble at the parasternal area.

CONCLUSION

René Théophile Hyacinthe Laennec discovered stethoscope, which over 200 years, has become a symbol of medicine. He narrated his discovery as—*"In 1816, I was consulted by a young woman laboring under general symptoms of diseased heart, and in whose case percussion and the application of the hand were of little avail on* *account of the great degree of fatness. The other method just mentioned [immediate auscultation] being rendered inadmissible by the age and sex of the patient..........I rolled a quire of paper into a sort of cylinder and applied one end of it to the region of the heart and the other to my ear, and was not a little surprised and pleased, to find that I could perceive the action of the heart in a manner much more clear and distinct than I had ever been able to do by the immediate application of the ear...**"

For him only, we have so many murmur and for him only, clinical cardiovascular science is so much fascinating.

REFERENCES

1. Laennec R (Ed). De l'Auscultation Médiate. Paris, France: Brosson et Chaudé; 1819.
2. Levine SA. The systolic murmur: its clinical significance. JAMA. 1933;101:436-8.
3. McDonald DA (Ed). Blood Flow in Arteries. London: Edward Arnold Publishers Ltd; 1960.
4. Bruns D. A general theory of the causes of murmurs in the cardiovascular system. Am J Med. 1959;27:360-74.
5. Ranganathan N, Sivaciyan V, Saksena FB. The art and science of cardiac physical examination. Humana press: Springer; 2006. p. 219.
6. Pringle SD, Fitzsimmons S, Gudmundsdottir IJ, et al. Cardiovascular signs. In: The ESC Textbook of Cardiovascular Medicine. Oxford University Press; 2019. p. 11.
7. Robert WC, Perloff JK, Costantino T. Severe valvular aortic stenosis in patients over 65 years of age. Am J Cardiol. 1971;27:497.
8. Criley JM and Siegel RJ Has obstruction hindered our understanding of hypertrophic cardiomyopathy? Circulation. 1985;72:1148-54
9. Stewart BF, Siscovick D, Lind BK, et al. Clinical factors associated with calcific aortic valve disease. Cardiovascular Health Study. J Am Coll Cardiol. 1997;29:630-4.
10. Karliner JS, O'Rourke RA, Kearney DJ, et al. Haemodynamic explanation of why the murmur of mitral regurgitation in independent of cycle length. Br Heart J. 1973;35:397-401.
11. Desjardins V, Enriquez-Sarano M, Tazik M, et al. Intensity of murmurs correlates with severity of valvular regurgitation. Am J Med. 1996;100:149-56.
12. Paulus WJ. Chronic aortic regurgitation. In: Crawford MH, Dimarco JP, Paulus WJ (Eds). Cardiology, 3rd edition. Philadelphia: Elsevier Ltd.; 2010. pp. 1293-304.
13. Dock W, Zoneraich S. A diastolic murmur arising in a stenosed coronary artery. Am J Med. 1967;42:617.
14. Levines A, Love DE. Mitral stenosis without murmurs. Cardiologia. 1952;21:599.
15. Bousvaros G, Stubington D. Some auscultatory and phonocardiographic features of tricuspid stenosis. Circulation. 1964;29:26.
16. Fortuin NJ, Craige E. On the mechanism of Austin Flint murmur. Circulation. 1972;45:558.
17. Coombs CF. Rheumatic Heart Disease. Bristol, England: John Wright & Sons Ltd.; 1924; (a) 8; (b) 9; (c) 27; (d) 65; (e) 233; (0325; (9) 330.
18. Alexander WD, Polak A. Early diastolic murmur in end stage-renal failure. Br Heart J. 1977;39:900-2.

---

* Forbes J. A Treatise on the Diseases of the Chest. Underwood, London; 1821.

CHAPTER 21

Continuous Murmur

INTRODUCTION

Continuous murmur starts in systole, enveloping S2, spills over diastole. There is difference in opinion on gradation of continuous murmur. In most of the continuous murmurs, the systolic component dominates. Thus, it is graded in usual way of any systolic murmur. Continuous murmur can be classified in different ways. One way of classification is according to hemodynamics (**Box 1**).[1]

Another way of classification is according to the site of drainage, i.e., receiving chamber and best site to pick up the murmur (**Table 1**) (**Figs. 1A and B**).[2]

PATENT DUCTUS ARTERIOSUS

Classical murmur in uncomplicated, moderately restrictive patent ductus arteriosus (PDA) is continuous with systolic reinforcement, peaking around

---

BOX 1 | Hemodynamic classification of continuous murmur.

- Communication between high-pressure and low-pressure chamber:
  - Patent ductus arteriosus
  - Aortopulmonary window
  - Ruptured sinus of Valsalva (RSOV)
  - Lutembacher's syndrome
- Excessive flow through tortuous vessel:
  - Arteriovenous fistula (pulmonary, coronary, any other vessels)
  - Major aortopulmonary collateral arteries:
    - Collaterals in coarctation of aorta
- Partial obstruction of vessel:
  - Peripheral pulmonary artery (PA) stenosis
  - Coarctation of aorta
- Excessive venous flow:
  - Venous hum
  - Mammary shuffle
  - Total anomalous pulmonary venous connection

TABLE 1: Classification of continuous murmur: Receiving chamber.

Draining chamber	Anomaly
Right atrium	• Coronary cameral fistula • Sinus of Valsalva • Total anomalous pulmonary venous connection
Right ventricle	• Coronary cameral fistula • Sinus of Valsalva
Proximal pulmonary artery	• Patent ductus arteriosus • Aortopulmonary window • Anomalous origin of left coronary artery from pulmonary artery • Coronary cameral fistula
Distal pulmonary artery	• Pulmonary artery stenosis • Pulmonary arteriovenous fistula
Left atrium	• Coronary cameral fistula
Left ventricle	• Sinus of Valsalva • Aortic-left ventricular tunnel

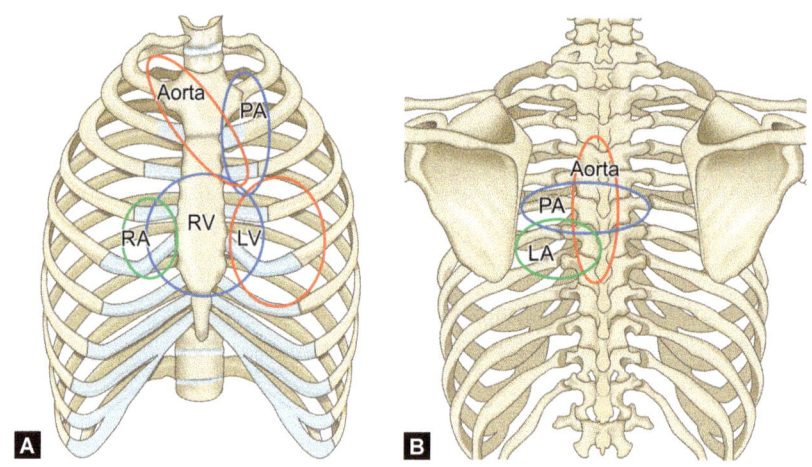

(LA: left atrium; LV: left ventricle; PA: pulmonary artery; RA: right atrium; RV: right ventricle)

Figs. 1A and B: (A) Drainage site on anterior chest wall; and (B) drainage site on posterior chest wall.[3]

second heart sound. Thus, it behaves as crescendo in systole and decrescendo in diastole. The murmur is described as machinery due to its roughness or Gibson murmur, which was described as, *"It persists through second sound and dies away gradually during the long pause. The murmur is rough and trembling. It begins softly and increases in intensity so as to reach its acme just about, or immediately after, the incidence of the second sound, and from that point gradually wanes until its termination."* In restrictive PDA, it is a soft and high-frequency murmur.

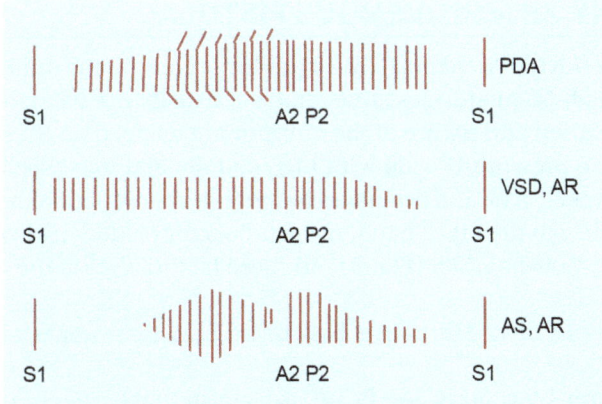

Fig. 2: Continuous murmur of patent ductus arteriosus (PDA): Peak around S2; to-and-fro murmur of ventricular septal defect (VSD) and aortic regurgitation (AR): Pansystolic, plateau murmur of VSD, ending in A2 and the decrescendo diastolic murmur starting with A2; to-and-fro murmur of aortic stenosis (AS) and AR: Diamond-shaped midsystolic murmur, late peaking before A2; decrescendo diastolic murmur, starting with A2.

This continuous murmur may occupy whole or part of systole and diastole, along with eddy sound in late systole and early diastole. Systolic enhancement is explained by the fact that pulmonary artery (PA) gets blood both from right ventricle (RV) and aorta in systole, whereas only from aorta in diastole. Eddy sound has been described due to head-on collision of two flows from RV and aorta. More reasonable explanation is an effect of torrential flow through a tubular structure, and not the effect of dual flow because it occurs also in diastole.

Murmur is best heard in left infraclavicular or 1st and 2nd intercostal space. Diastolic component may become less prominent down the precordium and at apex.

A large PDA can produce a mid-diastolic flow murmur at the apex, which may be masked by the diastolic component of PDA murmur. But it may be audible in PDA with hyperkinetic pulmonary hypertension, which makes the diastolic component unobvious, yet maintaining flow (**Fig. 2**).

A mitral diastolic flow murmur is also indicative of a large shunt. With progressive pulmonary hypertension, first the diastolic component, then the systolic component may disappear, making the ductus silent. Other causes of silent ductus are a tiny (Doppler) ductus and ductus with abnormally directed jet.

AORTOPULMONARY WINDOW

Continuous murmur is uncommon in aortopulmonary window (APW). When found in restrictive or moderately restrictive APW, its location is 3rd, 4th, and 2nd left intercostal space, i.e., lower down than PDA murmur. Diastolic component is brief. Eddy sounds are present. Location and brief diastolic component may be mistaken as ventricular septal defect (VSD) murmur. However, bounding pulse and eddy sound favor APW.

CORONARY ARTERIOVENOUS FISTULA

Coronary arteriovenous fistula (CAVF) produces continuous murmur, which is medium to high frequency, less than grade 4, usually not harsh and relatively localized. Location and nature of the murmur are decided on its' drainage site. As aortic pulse pressure is wide with high systolic and low diastolic pressure, gradient between CAVF and drainage chamber in systole should be higher than that in diastole. On the other hand, myocardial contraction during systole may retard systolic flow in CAVF (**Fig. 3**). All these factors decide the nature of the murmur.

- *Superior vena cava*: Murmur is best heard over right upper to mid sternal border.
- *Right atrium*: Murmur is best heard on right sternal border or over sternum. Continuous murmur shows systolic accentuation.
- *Right ventricle*: Murmur is best heard over mid to lower left sternal border. When it drains in outflow, it is best heard over upper left sternal border. Right ventricular contraction may retard systolic flow across the fistula, resulting in diastolic accentuation of the murmur.
- *Pulmonary artery*: Murmur shows systolic accentuation. Location is best at left upper sternal border. At this location, it may be confused with PDA murmur, which is characterized by eddy sound, notably absent in CAVF murmur.
- *Left atrium*: Murmur shows systolic accentuation. It is best heard at upper left sternal edge and may radiate to left anterior axillary line.
- *Left ventricle*: Murmur remains restricted only to early diastole, as left ventricular contraction obliterates systolic flow in systole. Location is variable, between apical and left parasternal area.

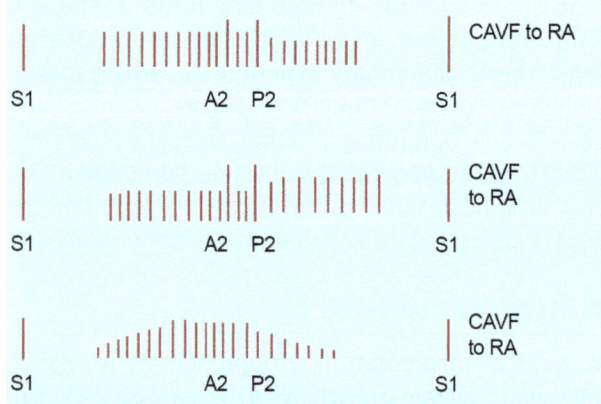

Fig. 3: Continuous murmur of coronary arteriovenous fistula (CAVF): CAVF to right atrium (RA)—systolic accentuation. CAVF to right ventricle (RV)—diastolic accentuation. CAVF to pulmonary artery (PA)—accentuation around S2.

RUPTURED SINUS OF VALSALVA

Site of the characteristic continuous murmur depends on the receiving chamber. When rupture is in right ventricular body, it is best heard in left parasternal area, at 3rd and 4th intercostal space; when in right ventricular outflow tract, it is best heard in 2nd and 3rd intercostal space. When rupture is in right atrium, it is best heard in right or left parasternal or lower sternal area. It is superficial harsh murmur, sawing in nature. Unlike PDA, continuous murmur of ruptured sinus of Valsalva (RSOV) is not accentuated around S2 with mostly systolic accentuation. When rupture is in either of the ventricle, its contraction during systole may reduce the systolic component with diastolic accentuation. Systolic component is best heard near the proximal chamber, aorta, i.e., at the base, whereas diastolic component in the receiving chamber, atrium or ventricle, i.e., at lower down position (**Fig. 4**).

PULMONARY ARTERIOVENOUS FISTULA

It is a soft low-grade murmur, best heard at the front or back of the chest, depending upon its location. It is commonly found in the lower lobes and right middle lobe. More often, it is systolic rather than continuous one. As the systolic gradient is significant and diastolic gradient is minimal, the murmur shows systolic accentuation with a brief, softer diastolic component. It is a late-onset late-crescendo murmur, as because the fistula is downstream from the RV requiring a time gap between right ventricular contraction and flow through the fistula. Another feature is its' inspiratory enhancement. Increased right ventricular flow and lowering of diaphragm with less compression of the lower lobe fistula during inspiration are the explanations. Posture affects the intensity of the murmur. Standing may enhance and lateral decubitus on the same side of the fistula may decrease the intensity.

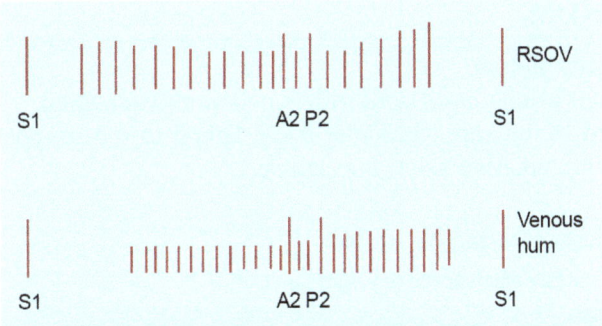

Fig. 4: Continuous murmur: ruptured sinus of Valsalva (RSOV)—may have systolic or diastolic accentuation; Venous hum—diastolic accentuation.

ANOMALOUS ORIGIN OF LEFT CORONARY ARTERY FROM PULMONARY ARTERY

Anomalous origin of left coronary artery from pulmonary artery (ALCAPA) occasionally can produce continuous murmur, though more commonly diastolic murmur, the source of which is the retrograde flow through intercoronary anastomoses connecting the right and the left coronary arteries. It is soft in systole and accentuated in diastole. Ventricular contraction during systole increases the transmural pressure, which decreases the flow, sometimes completely through these intercoronary channels during systole. The murmur is best heard on the left or right of the sternum, usually at the base.

SYSTOLO-DIASTOLIC MURMUR (TO-AND-FRO MURMUR)

Systolo-diastolic murmur also known as to-and-fro murmur mimics continuous murmur.[4] This murmur is a combination of systolic and diastolic murmur. It comprises a low-pitched crescendo-decrescendo systolic component and a decrescendo diastolic component with a short pause between the two, best heard at the mid-left parasternal border. Here, the systolic murmur does not spill over S2. Another important differentiating point from continuous murmur is that the frequency and character of the systolic and diastolic components are different (**Box 2**).

CONTINUOUS MURMUR IN CONGENITAL CYANOTIC HEART DISEASE

Continuous murmur is not uncommon in congenital cyanotic heart disease. In a large series, it was reported in 4% of 670 children with cyanotic heart disease.[5] Tetralogy of Fallot (TOF) with pulmonary atresia is the most common cause, where the source of continuous murmur is PDA or major aortopulmonary collaterals (**Box 3**).

VENOUS HUM

- Common in children.
- In adult, it is usually associated with hyperkinetic circulation.
- Best heard in the supraclavicular fossa, lateral to the sternocleidomastoid muscle, with radiation below the clavicle.

BOX 2   Causes of to-and-fro murmur.

- Ventricular septal defect, aortic regurgitation (AR)
- Aortic stenosis, AR
- Aortic-left ventricular tunnel
- Absent pulmonary valve syndrome
- Truncus arteriosus with incompetent truncal valve

> **BOX 3** **Causes of continuous murmur in cyanotic congenital heart disease (CCHD).**
> - Tetralogy of Fallot (TOF), pulmonary atresia
> - Truncus arteriosus
> - TOF
> - CCHD with surgical shunt
> - Pulmonary arteriovenous fistula
> - Total anomalous pulmonary venous connection

- Child should be in sitting position with the head rotated toward opposite direction to make the neck taut and stretched. Murmur is enhanced by inspiration.
- Compressing the internal jugular vein, relaxing the stretch, Valsalva maneuver, and lying posture reduces murmur.
- Accentuated in diastole.
- Internal jugular vein is deformed at the level of atlas during head rotation and its' laminar flow changes to turbulent flow and the murmur.

MAMMARY SOUFFLÉ

- Found in late pregnancy and early lactation period.
- A continuous musical murmur with systolic accentuation.
- Onset is delayed well after S1.
- Best heard in lying down position.
- Sitting posture and compression attenuate the intensity.
- Valsalva does not affect the intensity.
- Delayed onset, systolic accentuation, and no effect on Valsalva—all points toward an arterial origin of murmur.

CONCLUSION

George Alexander Gibson described the continuous murmur as—*"when the ductus arteriosus is permanently patent, a very distinct thrill is to be felt—a thrill which distinctly follows the systole of the heart and persists until the diastolic phase has existed for some time. The reason for this is obvious, in as much as the blood stream flows from the higher pressure of the aorta to the lower pressure of the pulmonary artery. It must, therefore, generally occur after the aortic pressure has reached a certain level and will persist until it has fallen, at least to some extent. In some of these cases the thrill is to be felt persisting throughout almost the entire cardiac cycle*".*

The description was so astute, so genuine; and to remind you the timing when he described in 1898! We should always describe the PDA murmur in the eponym of Gibson murmur.

---
*Boyer NH. Patent ductus arteriosus: some historical highlights. Ann Thorac Surg. 1967;4:570-3.

REFERENCES

1. Myers JD. The mechanisms and significances of continuous murmurs. Am Heart Association Monograph. 1975;46:201-8.
2. Huffman T, Leighton RF, Goodwin RS, et al. Continuous murmurs associated with shunts in the acyanotic adult. An anatomic classification. Am J Med. 1970;49:160-9.
3. Shah PM, Slodki SJ, Luisada AA. Revision of the 'classic' area of auscultation of heart. A physiologic approach. Amer J Med. 1964;36:160-9.
4. Gazit AZ, Singh GK. To-and-fro murmur in the young due to major congenital cardiac defects: is cardiac auscultation obsolete? Cardiol Young. 2010;20:707-8.
5. Campbell M, Deucher DC. Continuous murmur in cyanotic congenital heart disease. Br Heart J. 1961;23:173-93.

CHAPTER 22

Innocent Murmur and Sound

INTRODUCTION

Laennec thrilled by his own invention observed[1] in 1835: *"The bellows sound of the heart although frequently accompanying an organic affection of this organ, may exist without this."* It is a common clinical problem that a young boy or girl is being referred to cardiologist for evaluation of an incidentally detected murmur by the pediatrician. A murmur without structural heart disease is quite common in a growing child. It has been named as functional murmur, flow murmur, normal murmur or innocent murmur. The last one, i.e., innocent murmur, is the most appropriate one, as it conveys most strongly to the parents that nothing is serious.

PREVALENCE[2]

Prevalence of innocent murmur in infancy is around 60%. Its prevalence in school-going children is quite high and is around 75–90%. Prevalence of congenital heart disease at birth is around 6.1 per 1,000 and at school-going age is around 3.8 per 1,000. These data suggest that in majority of the children with a murmur will be an innocent murmur. Common causes of innocent murmur and sound are described in **Box 1**.

HOW TO ESTABLISH THE INNOCENCE

A thorough history and clinical examination establish the innocence in most of the cases. The triad in favor of innocence is (**Box 2**):
- No suspicious history suggestive of organic heart disease.
- Characteristic innocent murmur.
- No additional clinical findings in favor of organic heart disease.

STILL'S MURMUR

It is the most common innocent murmur. It is best heard in between apex and left lower sternal border. The murmur is low-pitched, musical, and vibratory in nature

BOX 1	Innocent murmur and sound.
Murmur:	**Sound:**
• Still's murmur	• Split S1
• Functional murmur in adult	• S3
• Innocent pulmonary murmur	• S4
• Pulmonary branch murmur	
• Supraclavicular murmur	
• Diastolic murmur	
• Venous hum	
• Mammary soufflé	

BOX 2	Features of innocent murmur.
• Should not be more than grade 3	• Mostly systolic
• Never louder at apex	• Never associated with click
• Never radiates to neck	• No clinical evidence of any chamber enlargement

without radiation, best heard with bell of the stethoscope. It is brief (100 ms), crescendo-decrescendo, grade 1 to 3/6 in intensity. Murmur is increased in intensity on recumbency, fever or exercise and decreased on Valsalva or standing. Most common age range is between 4 and 17 years and disappears at puberty onward. Murmur originates in left ventricle (LV) and is most likely due to periodic vibration of aortic valve or a LV "false tendon".

FUNCTIONAL MURMUR IN ADULT[3]

A grade 2, 3 midsystolic murmur is occasionally found in adult, typically in 2nd intercostal space, parasternal or downward. Echo Doppler study reveals increased intraventricular gradient (IVG) ranged from 0.7 to 5.2 m/s. In these patients with IVG, hypertension or renal insufficiency is more common. They have a higher LV mass index and a higher LV ejection fraction. Thus, patients with IVG have more vigorous systolic function and more severe concentric remodeling than patients without IVGs.

INNOCENT PULMONARY MURMUR

It is the second common innocent murmur, best heard at left upper parasternal area. It is a blowing, medium pitch, crescendo-decrescendo murmur, with transmission to axilla and back. Its intensity is increased by leg-raising, recumbency, and fever. Important issue is that it is heard better in expiration rather than inspiration. It is consistently present in straight-back syndrome. Murmur originates in right side of the heart and is caused by turbulent flow across the main pulmonary artery.

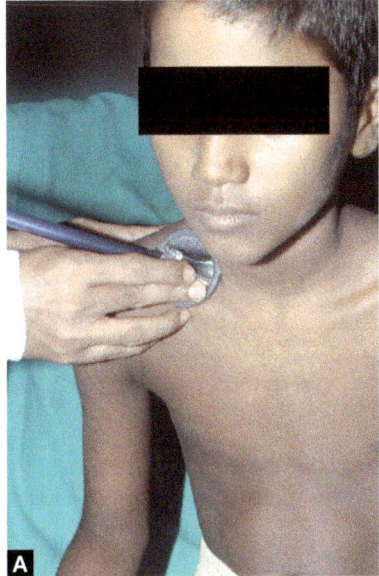 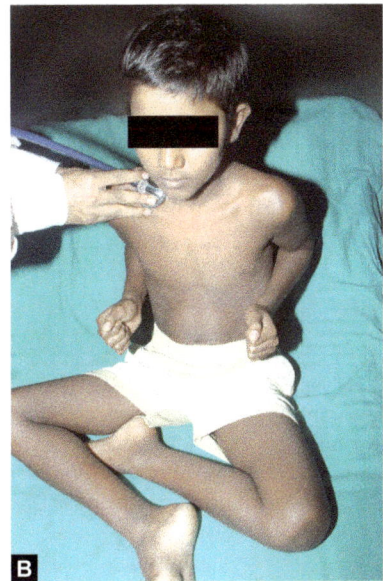

Figs. 1A and B: (A) Supraclavicular murmur: Best heard at supraclavicular fossa; and (B) murmur decreases or disappears on throwing back the patient's shoulder.

SUPRACLAVICULAR MURMUR/BRUIT

The bruit, rather murmur, is best heard in right supraclavicular fossa (**Figs. 1A and B**). It is early-systolic, harsh, high frequency in nature with a grade of 1 to 3/6. A light pressure on subclavian artery increases it, whereas it disappears on firm pressure. It disappears on raising the child's chin or throwing-back the shoulder. Its mechanism is the turbulence at the origin of the brachiocephalic artery.

PULMONARY BRANCH MURMUR

This murmur is best heard at left or right upper sternal border with radiation to back and axilla. It is brief, crescendo-decrescendo murmur with a grade of 1 to 3/6. The transient branch murmur is found in the newborn and is disappeared by 2 months of age. Mechanism is the turbulence produced at the relatively acute angle of bifurcation of the pulmonary artery or across the relatively hypoplastic pulmonary arteries of the newborn. As the infant grows along with pulmonary vasculature, angle of bifurcation becomes less acute and the murmur disappears.

DIASTOLIC MURMUR

Unless and otherwise proved, a diastolic murmur is always organic. Rarely, it may be innocent. One is transient solitary diastolic murmur of newborn. Mechanism is probably a closing duct. Another is found in school-going age. Best site is at the apex and LV in origin. Mechanism is like that of physiological S3 and simulates a "long" S3.

Concluding remark should be from a pioneer of auscultatory art, PM Latham:[4] *"Men are as often deceived by their ears as by their eyes, and they may hear ghosts as well as see them."*

CONCLUSION

The rule of thumb is all murmurs are not pathological and all apparently innocent murmurs are not always innocent.

REFERENCES

1. Laennec RTC. A treatise on disease of the chest and mediate auscultation. Philadelphia: DeSilver, Thomas; 1835.
2. Biancaniello T. Innocent murmur. Circulation. 2005;111:e20-e22.
3. Spooner PH, Perry MP, Brandenberg RO, et al. Increased intraventricular velocities. An unrecognized cause of systolic murmur in adults. J Am Coll Cardiol. 1998;32:1589.
4. Martin R (ed). The collected works of Dr P.M. Latham. London: New Sydenham Society; 1876.

CHAPTER 23

Dynamic Auscultation

INTRODUCTION

What really is the role of dynamic auscultation in present day cardiology practice? Amyl nitrite is not available at bedside for a long time. Even then a full chapter is on dynamic auscultation! This is just for the reason that the hemodynamic of a cardiac lesion is better understood by knowing the effect of various maneuver on heart sound and murmur.

PROMPT SQUATTING

Hemodynamics

Squatting is conventionally known to increase systemic vascular resistance. May be this is an overstatement. Schafer[1] in his experimental study described the effect of squatting on circulation. Mean pressure was increased immediately after squatting and *"thereafter mean pressure fell and eventually stabilized at a level which was higher than the standing or sitting level"*. He found two factors to explain the effect of increased mean pressure. The most important effect was due to *"increase in stroke output due to an increase in cardiac filing pressure due in turn to squeezing blood out of the veins of the legs"*. Second factor was increase in peripheral arterial resistance due to hydrostatic effect of postural change and kinking of the femoral arteries. Subsequent fall was due to increased mean pressure, leading to reflex baroreceptor-induced peripheral vasodilatation. The overall effects are:

- Momentarily increasing venous return and stroke volume.
- Increased peripheral resistance due to acute compression of the arteries in the leg.
- Increased mean arterial pressure due to the above two factors.
- Overall effect is increase in preload as well as afterload.
- Reflex bradycardia, due to rise of blood pressure.

Effect on Aortic Regurgitation

The rise in diastolic pressure and impairment of arterial run off result in an increase in the intensity of the diastolic murmur of aortic regurgitation (AR). Squatting is a simplest mean of amplifying AR murmur.

Effect on Hypertrophic Obstructed Cardiomyopathy

The systolic murmur of hypertrophic obstructed cardiomyopathy (HOCM) decreases with prompt squatting as a result of greater left ventricular filling, a large end-diastolic volume, and reduced obstruction.

Effect on Aortic Stenosis and Pulmonary Stenosis

The ejection murmur of aortic stenosis (AS) and pulmonary stenosis (PS) become louder during the first few beats after squatting as a result of increased venous return and stroke volume.

Effect on Mitral Regurgitation and Ventricular Septal Defect

The systolic murmur of mitral regurgitation (MR) and ventricular septal defect (VSD) increases because the greater impedance in the aorta leads to a rise in the left ventricular systolic pressure.

Procedure (Figs. 1A and B)

The examiner should be seated on a chair with stethoscope in place while the patient is still standing so that he can be prepared to assess any change occurring within the first few beats after the squatting posture is achieved. Squatting equivalent: In patients unable to perform squatting the same circulatory changes can be produced by bending the patient's knees on his abdomen while he is in supine position.

STANDING

Hemodynamic

The assumption of the erect posture results in the shifting of blood from the central venous reservoir to the lower part of the body, a decreased pressure in the right atrium and probably a decreased rate of ventricular filing.[2] Overall effects are:
- Venous pooling in the legs and splanchnic vessels with a reduction in venous return results in decreased preload.
- This results in a momentary decrease in heart size, stroke volume, and mean arterial pressure.
- Followed by a reflex increase in heart rate and systemic resistance.

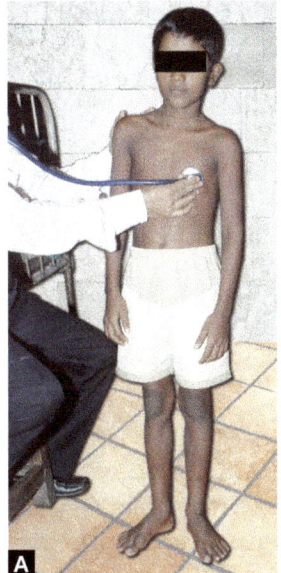 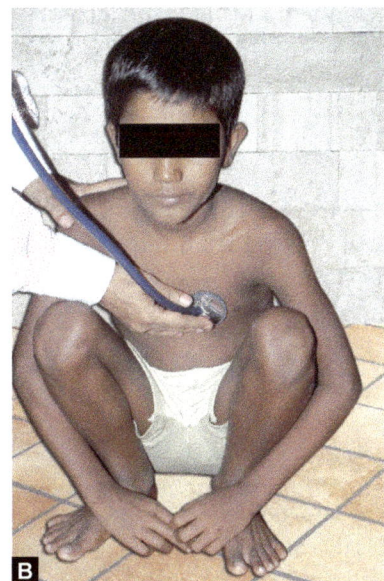

Figs. 1A and B: Initially, patient should be on standing position; examiner should sit beside with stethoscope in position. Then, patient should be asked to take a squatting position. Changes in the first few beats, thus, will be not missed.

Effect on Hypertrophic Obstructed Cardiomyopathy

The decrease in left ventricular volume results in an increase in the murmur of the HOCM.

Effect on AR, PS, MR, and Tricuspid Regurgitation

Standing results in decrease of all these murmurs.

Effect on S4-S1 versus S1-Ejection Sound

The fourth heart sound (S4) moves closure to first heart sound (S1) and may disappear altogether on standing. Standing has no effect on ejection sound. Thus, it helps to differentiate between S4-S1 combinations from the S1-ejection sound combination.

Effect on Physiological S3 versus Pathological S3

Physiological third heart sound (S3) disappears on standing, but the pathological S3 does not.

Effect on Mitral Valve Prolapse

Standing reduces left ventricular end-diastolic volume and results in early onset of click and the murmur since the mitral leaflet is closure to the position where prolapse begins. The click moves toward S1 and may merge with it. The murmur becomes longer and may occupy the whole systole.

Effect on Continuous Murmur of Patent Ductus arteriosus versus Venous Hum

The continuous murmur of patent ductus arteriosus may decrease in duration where that of venous hum becomes louder on standing position.

Procedure

Auscultation must be carried out immediately before and after standing since the effects may be transient, persisting for only 10–15 beats.

VALSALVA

In 1704, Valsalva described the maneuver to expel pus from the ear. Centuries passes, Valsalva maneuver remains as one of the most important maneuvers in clinical cardiology.

Hemodynamic

Phase 1: Sharp rise of blood pressure resulting from the direct transmission of the increased intrathoracic pressure on the large arteries.

Phase 2: Persistent straining impairs venous return, resulting in decrease in heart size, stroke volume, mean arterial pressure, and pulse pressure with reflex increase in heart rate.

Phase 3: With release of straining effect there is a further drop in arterial pressure in accordance with the fall in intrathoracic pressure.

Phase 4: Following this, there is a surge of venous return leading to an increase in stroke volume, cardiac output, and blood pressure (**Fig. 2**).

Overshoot phase occurs as a continuation of the preceding phase with further increase of arterial pressure, resulting in a brief phase of reflex bradycardia.

Effect (Fig. 3)

- Most of the changes occur in phase 2 and phase 4. Basic effect is decreased preload in phase 2 and increased preload in phase 4.
- *Phase 2*: Due to reduction of stroke volume, two common lesions with mid-systolic murmur, PS and AS, show decreased intensity. Most consistence effect is on HOCM. Due to reduction in heart size, murmur increases appreciably. It has similar effect on mitral valve prolapse (MVP). Due to reduction in heart size, click shifts toward S1 and systolic murmur lengthens. A2 and P2 become fused during this phase, excepting in atrial septal defect, where the split is maintained. Filling sound may disappear in this phase.

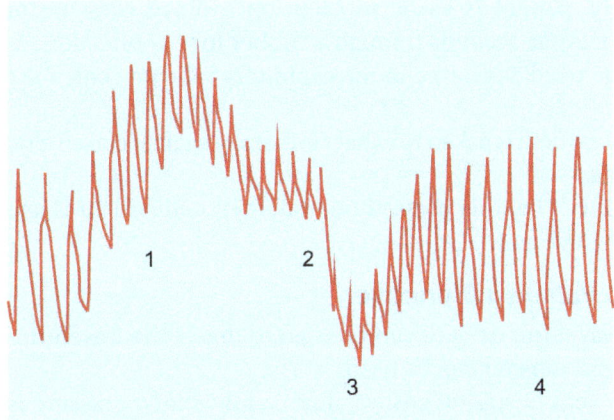

Fig. 2: Central aortic pressure tracing during Valsalva. Phase 1: Transient rise of aortic pressure; phase 2: Fall of aortic pressure; phase 3: Further decline of aortic pressure; and phase 4: increase in aortic pressure.

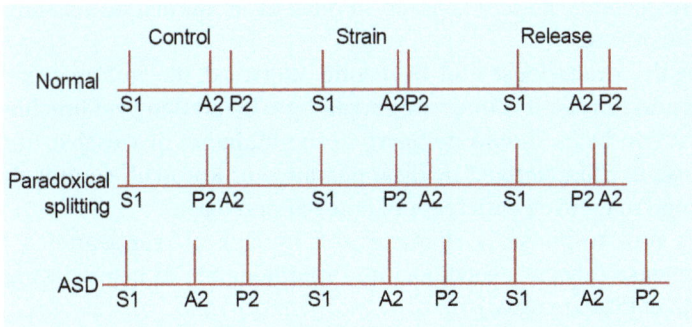

Fig. 3: Effect of Valsalva on S2. Physiological S2: During strain phase, A2-P2 gap narrow down; during release phase, it widens. Paradoxical split: During strain phase, P2-A2 gap widens; during release phase, it narrow down. Atrial septal defect (ASD): As hang-out interval has already been used maximally, Valsalva phases do not affect the A2-P2 split any further.

- *Phase 4*: Increased venous return during this phase causes augmentation of right-sided murmur in first few beats (1–2 beats). During those initial beats, left-sided murmurs do not get augmented. They are augmented after 5–6 beats. A2–P2 widens significantly and filling sounds are enhanced.
- Overshoot phase does not occur in patient with heart failure.

Valsalva Maneuver
- Ideal method is to perform the maneuver, with nose-clip maintaining for 15 second and standardized at 40 cm of water with a manometer connected to a mouthpiece.[3]

- Alternately, patient is asked to blow up a blood pressure manometer to 40 mm Hg for 30 seconds through a rubber tube connection. A small leak or a 20-gauge needle inserted in the expiratory tube prevents the closure of the glottis.[4]
- Or simply, patient is asked to exhale forcefully against closed glottis for around 15 seconds.
- Or, examiner's hand is pressed on abdomen and patient is asked to push it away with abdomen.

Steps to do Valsalva Maneuver

1. Arterial waveform devices can be used to detect the waveforms. At bedside, sphygmomanometer can be used.
2. Patient is kept in supine posture and systolic blood pressure is obtained by auscultatory sphygmomanometer at quietly breathing.
3. The cuff pressure is then raised 15 mm Hg above the systolic pressure and patient is asked to do the Valsalva maneuver at the end of normal inspiratory effort. Effective maneuver is evidenced by florid face, distended neck veins, and increased abdominal wall muscle tone.
4. After 10 seconds, patient is asked to relax his abdomen and resume normal quiet breathing.
5. During the strain phase and 15 second afterward, the cuff pressure is maintained and Korotkoff sounds are sought by auscultation over brachial artery.
6. At least two beats should be heard at the initiation of Valsalva. The normal response is characterized by disappearance of Korotkoff sounds during the sustained maneuver, with reappearance after release.
7. Square root response is characterized by lack of reappearance of sound after release (absent overshoot) and maintenance of beats throughout the maneuver (Square wave).
8. Effect of Valsalva is most pronounced on HOCM (**Fig. 4**) and mitral valve prolapse (**Fig. 5**).

MULLER MANEUVER

This maneuver is basically reverse Valsalva where patient is asked to inhale forcefully against closed glottis. Preload is increased. In effect, all right-sided murmurs are increased and second heart sound (S2) split becomes wider.

ISOMETRIC HANDGRIP

The effect of sustained hand grip to induce an effect of isometric exercise was first shown by Donald[5] in 1967. The normal response to isometric exercise is tachycardia, increase in cardiac output, and rise of both systolic as well as diastolic pressure. Tachycardia is due to release of vagal tone, pressor response is due to tachycardia, increase in cardiac output, and increase in peripheral vascular resistance mediated by the sympathetic nervous system.

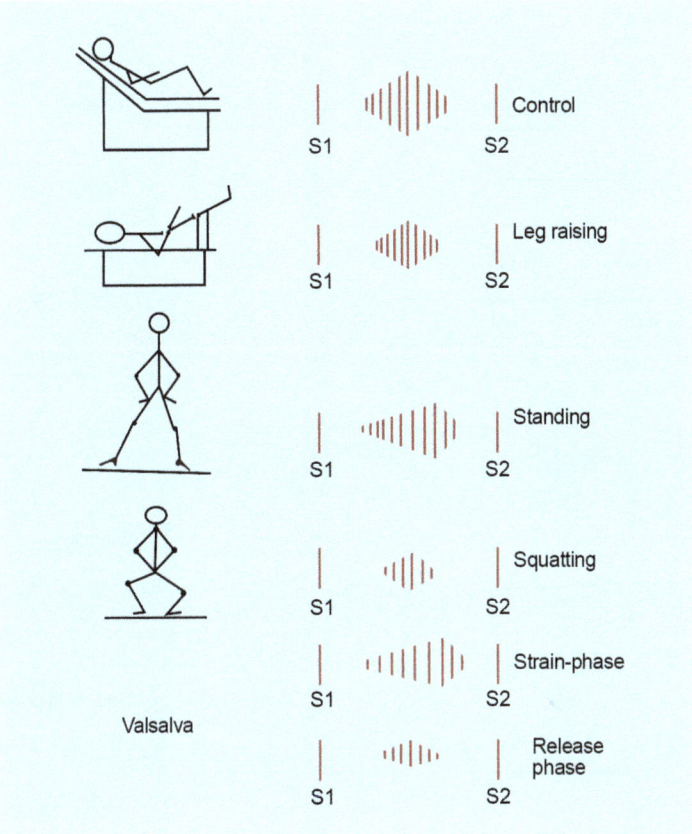

Fig. 4: Effect of maneuvers on murmur of hypertrophic obstructed cardiomyopathy.

Hemodynamic
- It effectively causes voluntary muscle contraction necessitating increased sympathetic tone and withdrawal of vagal tone.
- Thus, venous return, stroke volume, heart rate, and both arterial pressure are increased. Overall effect is increased afterload.

Effect
- Increased afterload augments the diastolic murmur of AR, and, sometimes, VSD and MR.
- Increased transmitral flow and shorter diastolic filling period due to tachycardia augment diastolic rumble of mitral stenosis (MS).
- Murmur of AS and, probably HOCM decrease in intensity due to increase in systemic resistance, which reduces the gradient.

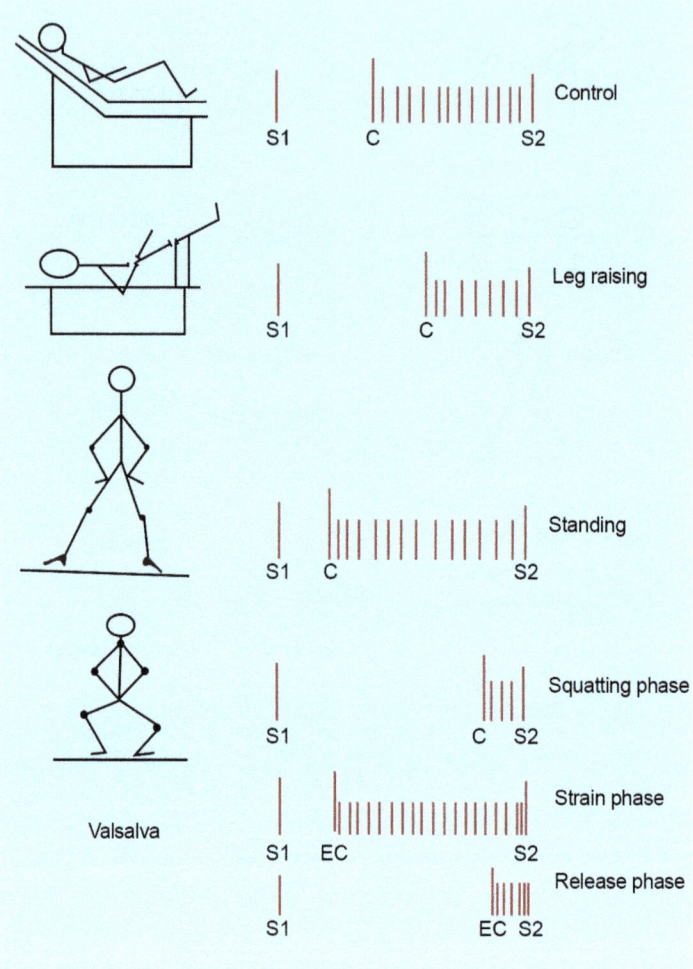

Fig. 5: Effect of maneuvers on the click (C) and murmur in mitral valve prolapse.

Procedure

By squeezing a towel, simply by clenching the fist or, if available, handgrip dynamometer (**Fig. 6**).

TRANSIENT ARTERIAL OCCLUSION[6]

Hemodynamic

- Transient arterial occlusion of a major peripheral artery produces an increase in afterload by decreasing compliance (increasing stiffness) of the arterial vessels proximal to the cuff occlusion.

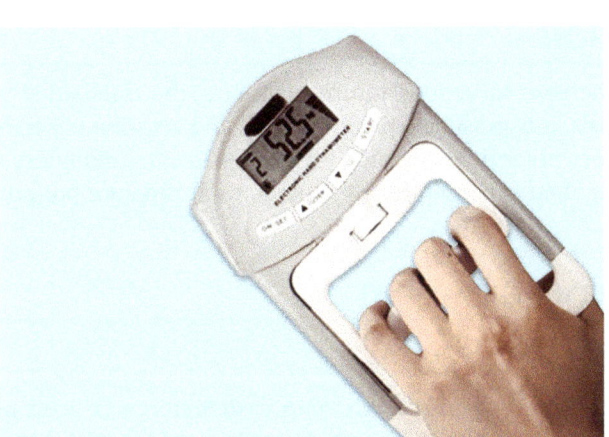

Fig. 6: Handgrip dynamometer.

- Arterial pressure, heart rate, cardiac output systemic, and vascular resistance remain constant.

Effect

The maneuver increases the left-sided regurgitation murmur, which includes AR, MR, and VSD. As the hemodynamic is simple, unlike handgrip and squatting, it can be used as useful maneuver to assess AR.

Procedure

- Sphygmomanometer is placed around each upper arm of the patient.
- Both cuffs are simultaneously inflated to 20–40 mm Hg above the patient's previously recorded systolic blood pressure.
- Twenty seconds after cuff inflation, the change in murmur intensity is compared with baseline.

PASSIVE LEG RAISING

As this maneuver increases the venous return, right-sided murmurs are increased in the first few beats. Carvallo sign [augmentation of tricuspid regurgitation (TR) murmur] is positive by this method, even in presence of congestive heart failure.

PREMATURE BEAT

Postectopic beat augments the murmur of AS, but that of MR does not change appreciably. Click moves toward S2 and murmur shortens in MVP.

RESPIRATION

Inspiratory increase in venous return augments the right-sided murmur, like TR and stenosis. It is most conspicuous in TR and was first observed by Rivero-Carvallo. It does not influence much the high-pressure pulmonary regurgitation murmur (described earlier) but augments normal-pressure pulmonary regurgitation murmur.

PHARMACOLOGIC AGENT

Vasodilator

- *Hemodynamic*: Amyl nitrite, a strong vasodilator, was used previously. In practice, it is no more used. Isosorbide can be used as a vasodilatory molecule.
- Amyl nitrite causes sharp decline of arterial pressure with reflex tachycardia and increased velocity of ejection. Venous return, hence preload may be increased. Overall effect is decreased afterload.
- Fall in afterload reduces diastolic murmur of AR, whereas shortened diastole and increased output augment diastolic murmur of MS.
- Fall in afterload and increased velocity of ventricular ejection augment ejection systolic murmur. In contrast, MR murmur diminishes due to fall in afterload.
- *VSD*: Vasodilator reduces systemic vascular resistance more than pulmonary vascular resistance. This explains why the small VSD murmur becomes softer. In a large VSD with hyperkinetic pulmonary hypertension, reduction in pulmonary vascular resistance is more pronounced. Here the murmur may actually augment, indicating the reversibility of pulmonary arterial hypertension.
- In VSD with PS, reduction in afterload enhances right to left shunt and reduces the flow across the right ventricular outflow tract. This makes the PS murmur softer in contrast to isolated PS murmur, which is augmented by vasodilator. It can be used as an important clue in pink tetralogy of Fallot.
- *How to use amyl nitrite*: Its vial is wrapped in towel, squeezed. Patient is asked to take around five normal inhalations. Peak effect is within 30 seconds. Alternately, isosorbide dinitrate can be used sublingually.

Vasoconstrictor

As parenteral vasoconstrictor is needed for using vasoconstrictor, its role in bedside cardiology is no more relevant.

CONCLUSION

We can conclude by narrating the concluding remarks by the masters of clinical cardiology, Grewe, Crawford, and O'Rourke in their review article on dynamic auscultation—"*The techniques described in this monograph will aid in the accurate identification of the origin of a cardiac murmur or abnormal heart sound. They do not necessarily reveal the presence or severity of cardiac disease. No maneuver is 100% accurate in elucidation of cardiac abnormalities, and a given maneuver's effectiveness varies in its application**".

REFERENCES

1. Sharpey-Shafer EP. Effect of squatting on the normal and failing circulation Brit Med J. 1956;1:1072.
2. Kjellberg SR, Lonroth H, Rudhe U, et al. Acta Physiol Scand. 1950;20:293.
3. Little WC, Barr WK, Crawford MH. Altered effect of Valsalva maneuver in left ventricular volume in patients with cardiomyopathy. Circulation. 1985;71:227-33.
4. Braunwald E, Oldham N, Ross J, et al. The circulatory response of patients with idiopathic hypertrophic subaortic stenosis to nitroglycerine and to the Valsalva maneuver. Circulation. 1964;29:422-31.
5. Donald KW, Lind AR, McNicol GW, et al. Cardiovascular responses to sustained (static) contractions. Circulation Research. 1967;20 Suppl I:15-32.
6. Lembo NJ, Dell'Italia LJ, Crawford MH. Diagnosis of left-sided regurgitant murmurs by transient arterial occlusion: A new maneuver using blood pressure cuffs. Ann Intern Med. 1986;105:368.

---

*Grewe K, Crawford MH, O'Rourke RA. Differentiation of cardiac murmurs by dynamic auscultation. Curr Probl Cardiol. 1988;13:669-721.

CHAPTER 24

Clinical Assessment: Congestion and Perfusion

INTRODUCTION

In a simplistic form, heart failure is associated with two hemodynamic abnormalities, namely reduced perfusion and increased ventricular filling pressure. The later is responsible for the congestive syndrome. Commoner presentation is due to congestion, rather than low cardiac output. Increased ventricular filling pressure has been described as *hemodynamic congestion*,[1] which may or may not be associated with clinical congestion. Decongestant medications and some adaptive mechanisms, namely increased lymphatic drainage, thickening of the alveolar-capillary barrier, and development of pulmonary arterial hypertension may prevent the clinical congestion to be manifested, even in presence of significant hemodynamic congestion. Clinical features of heart failure are described in **Box 1**.

WET OR DRY AND COLD OR WARM

As Stevenson chalked out the management of heart failure in 2006,[2] depending on the feature of congestion (wet or dry) and perfusion (cold or warm). When pulmonary capillary wedge pressure (PCWP) is ≥22 mm Hg, patient is wet and when PCWP is ≤22 mm Hg, patient is dry. Similarly, when cardiac index (CI) is ≤2.2 L/min/m², patient is cold and when CI is ≥2.2 L/min/m², patient is warm.

BOX 1 — Clinical features of heart failure.

Reduced perfusion:
- Weakness
- Fatigue
- Tachycardia
- Increased pulse pressure and decreased proportional pulse pressure

Increased ventricular filling pressure:
- S3
- Pulmonary congestion
- Systemic congestion

Pulmonary congestion:
- Dyspnea on exertion
- Paroxysmal nocturnal dyspnea
- Orthopnea
- Pulmonary rales/wheeze

Systemic congestion:
- Increased jugular venous pressure
- Edema in dependent part
- Hepatomegaly
- Weight gain

WET OR DRY/VENTRICULAR FILLING PRESSURE/CONGESTION (TABLE 1)

Congestion is the clinical expression of wet state or increased ventricular filling pressure. Congestion leads to following history and physical examination or H&P, which was used in ESCAPE (Evaluation Study of Congestive Heart Failure and Pulmonary Artery Catheterization Effectiveness) study **(Table 2)**.

Dyspnea on Exertion

Pulmonary congestion or pulmonary venous hypertension in the form of interstitial edema leads to reduced lung compliance and dyspnea on exertion.

Orthopnea

Orthopnea is more specific symptom of congestion and when present indicating PCWP is in the range of ≥28 mm Hg, ≥30 mm Hg, and ≥32 mm Hg, as described in ESCAPE trial.[4] Orthopnea requiring ≥2 pillows is more specific for elevated PCWP.

TABLE 1: Traditional view: Diagnostic value of symptoms/signs of heart failure.[3]

	Sensitivity	Specificity	Positive predictive value
Symptoms			
Dyspnea	66%	52%	45%
Orthopnea	66%	47%	61%
Signs			
Edema	46%	73%	46%
Raised JVP	70%	79%	85%
S3	73%	42%	66%

TABLE 2: Diagnostic value of H&P in heart failure: ESCAPE study.

H&P	Sensitivity	Specificity	PPV	NPV
Orthopnea ≥2 pillows	86	25	66	51
Crepts	15	89	69	38
Edema	41	66	67	40
JVP ≥12 mm Hg	65	64	75	52
+ Hepatojugular reflux	83	27	65	49

(ESCAPE: Evaluation Study of Congestive Heart Failure and Pulmonary Artery Catheterization Effectiveness; H&P: history and physical examination; JVP: jugular venous pressure; NPV: negative predictive value; PPV: positive predictive value)

Bendopnea

As discussed earlier, bendopnea is also a specific symptom of congestion. However, this symptom was not included in any major heart failure trial.

Edema

Edema responds quickly to decongestant medications. Besides, in a patient, who is on rest, fluid may be collected in the dependent part, i.e., in the sacral region and may be missed. Rapid improvement of edema without weight loss indicates redistribution of fluid. Edema does not always indicate increased ventricular filling pressure. It may be simply due to extravasations of fluid due to high vascular permeability and lower plasma oncotic pressure. When edema is associated with raised jugular venous pressure (JVP), it indicates high filling pressure.

Orthodema

Orthodema is a unique congestion score, described in DOSE-AHF (Diuretic Optimization Strategy Evaluation in Acute Decompensated Heart Failure) and CARRESS-HF (Cardiorenal Rescue Study in Acute Decompensated Heart Failure) trial.[4] Orthodema score is based on the symptom of orthopnoea (≥2 pillows = 2 points and <2 pillows = 0 point) and peripheral edema (trace = 0 point, moderate = 1 point, and severe = 2 points) (**Table 3**).

Increased JVP

Increased JVP is the most important physical sign of increased filling pressure. In ESCAPE study,[5] increased JVP was the one of only two physical signs (other is orthopnea), which correlated best with increased PCWP. JVP has a good correlation also to right atrial pressure (RAP) and can guide therapy.

Hepatojugular Reflux

Positive hepatojugular reflux in a patient with heart failure indicates PCWP >15 mm Hg.[6] JVP and hepatojugular reflux bear important prognostic factors. Those patients, who show positive reflux during discharge have a 6-month mortality of 16.7%, whereas those who show both positive reflux and increased JVP have a 6-month mortality of 33%.[7]

TABLE 3: **Orthodema score.**

Grade	Score
Absent	0
Low grade	1–2
High grade	3–4

(Orthopnea score: 2 pillows = 2 points and <2 pillows = 0 point. Edema score: trace = 0 point, moderate = 1 point, and severe = 2 points)

Pulmonary Rales/Wheeze

An acute elevation of left ventricular filling pressure can lead to extravasations of fluid in alveoli and one can get rales on auscultation. Chronic elevation, even up to 35-40 mm Hg, leads to increased lymphatic drainage and alveoli may remain relatively dry. Rales may be absent on auscultation. Patient should be asked to cough before listening rales.

COLD OR WARM/CARDIAC INDEX/PERFUSION

Perfusion is the clinical expression of cold or warm state or CI. Poor perfusion or cold state or low CI has the following H&P.

Fatigue

Fatigue is due to inadequate tissue oxygen delivery, due to reduced cardiac output. Patient may describe this as dyspnea on exertion.

Bendopnea

Bendopnea is a physical sign of both congestion as well as low perfusion.[8]

Cold Extremity

Cold extremity, specifically legs, is a physical sign of poor perfusion. The sign has a sensitivity of around 20% only.[8]

CLINICAL AIDS

Beyond H&P, simple blood pressure instrument can aid to identify at bedside, both congestion and poor perfusion status.

Orthostasis[9]

Normal response from sitting to standing is a fall of systolic blood pressure around 4-5 mm Hg. In patients with high ventricular filling pressure, standing reduces preload and improves filling pressure, subendocardial ischemia, and mitral regurgitation. These altogether improve hemodynamics and cardiac output with increase in systolic blood pressure. This paradoxical postural rise of blood pressure, orthostasis, is an indicator of increased filling pressure.

Proportional Pulse Pressure[10]

Proportional pulse pressure [(systolic pressure–diastolic pressure)/systolic pressure] is a simple measurement of low perfusion and its value <25% in heart failure patient may identify 90% of patient with CI <2.2 L/min/m². This has an 88% predictive accuracy of low cardiac output. However, it has a poor sensitivity.

Valsalva Maneuver

Valsalva maneuver is a simple bedside technique to assess filling pressure. A normal response[11] with the maneuver, i.e., sine wave, is replaced by a square wave response in heart failure. In mild heart failure, phase 1 to 3 responses are normal, whereas a phase 4 response is absent. In severe heart failure, the elevation in blood pressure is maintained up to phase 3 and returns to baseline in phase 4. Arterial waveform devices can be used to detect the waveforms. At bedside, sphygmomanometer can be used.

Even looking at pulse during doing Valsalva by patient can help to decide, whether filling pressure is high or not. Patients with normal filling pressure responds to low preload at phase 2, by baroreceptor induced sinus tachycardia and phase 4, by sinus bradycardia. In those patients with high filling pressure, change in preload in phase 2 or phase 4 does not alter filling pressure significantly and does not induce either sinus tachycardia or bradycardia. Thus, in any patient, response to phase 2 Valsalva by sinus tachycardia indicates normal filling pressure (**Fig. 1**).[12]

"Considering the cost and time involved with currently available methods to objectively demonstrate the presence or absence of 'congestive heart failure (CHF)' (e.g. exercise testing, natriuretic peptide and norepinephrine blood levels, radionuclide ventriculography, and echocardiography, etc.), one must ask whether or not it is time to incorporate the simple 30 seconds bedside Valsalva maneuver into the routine office examination. The arterial pressure response (which correlates with functional capacity, level of neurohormones, and cardiac hemodynamics) that occurs during the Valsalva maneuver (which is

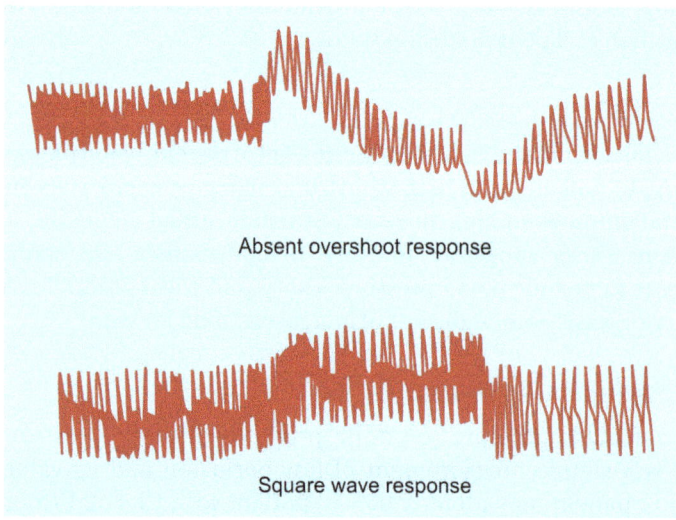

Fig. 1: Valsalva maneuver in heart failure patients with increased filling pressure. Absent overshoot arterial pressure response and square wave arterial pressure response.

totally noninvasive, does not expose the patient to ionizing radiation, and can be completed in <30 seconds) would appear to be a far more useful screening tool than either the chest radiograph or resting ECG."[13]

CONGESTION: RIGHT OR LEFT

Right atrial pressure is usually coupled to PCWP in heart failure. This is the basis of why increased JVP reflecting left ventricular filling pressure. However, these two sides are not always concordant. In around 30% of cases, it is feature of one side only. In these discordant cases, increased JVP only reflects increased RAP and right ventricular filling pressure. When there is disproportionate rise of right ventricular filling pressure over left ventricular filling pressure, manifested as RAP/PCWP ≥0.67, there is increased in-hospital mortality from heart failure and cardiorenal syndrome and 6-month mortality. Aggressive diuresis for management of congestion can lead to deterioration of renal function.[14] This RAP > PCWP concept renews the old concept of "right-sided heart failure." This is beyond "systemic venous congestion from backward-failure" concept. The higher RAP/PCWP ratio indicates an inadequacy of venous and pulmonary circulation to provide adequate preload for left ventricle, which remains underfilled leading to worsening renal function. Increased right ventricular filling pressure, ventricular interdependence, and stiff constraining pericardium in combination may be responsible for underfilling left ventricle (**Flowchart 1**).

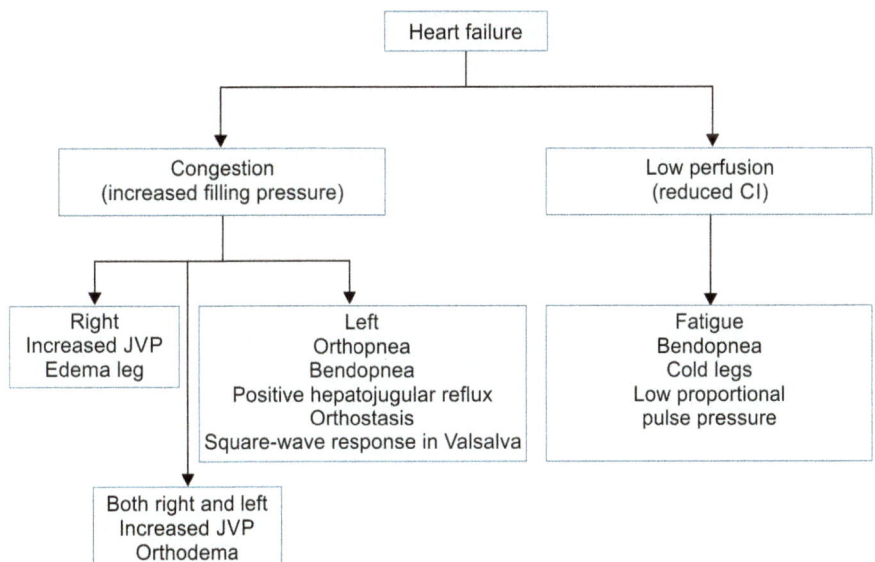

(CI: cardiac index; JVP: jugular venous pressure)
Flowchart 1: History and physical examination in heart failure patient to diagnose congestion and perfusion at bedside.

DIFFERENT CRITERIA FOR HEART FAILURE

Framingham Criteria for Heart Failure[15] (Box 2)

The Framingham Heart Study criteria are 100% sensitive and 78% specific for identifying persons with definite CHF.

Diagnosis of CHF requires the simultaneous presence of at least two major criteria or one major criterion in conjunction with two minor criteria.

Boston Criteria for Heart Failure (Table 4)

This criterion has been validated against PCWP and left ventricular ejection fraction measurements.[16]

No >4 points were allowed from each of three categories, and hence the composite score, the sum of the subtotal from each category, had a maximum possible of 12 points. The diagnosis of heart failure is classified definite for a score of 8-12 points, possible for a score of 5-7 points, and unlikely for a score of 4 points or less.

Ross Criteria of Heart Failure[17] (Table 5)

It was proposed to assess heart failure in infancy and early childhood and has been used in most of the heart failure studies.

BOX 2 | **Framingham criteria of heart failure.**

Major criteria:
- Bilateral moist rales
- Paroxysmal nocturnal dyspnea and/or orthopnea
- Neck vein distention in the semirecumbent position
- Peripheral venous pressure >16 cm H_2O
- Pulmonary edema by radiography
- S3 gallop
- Enlarging heart by radiography
- Hepatojugular reflux
- Weight loss of 4.5 kg in 5 days with treatment

Minor criteria:
- Bilateral ankle edema
- Nocturnal cough
- Dyspnea on ordinary exertion
- Hepatomegaly
- Pleural effusion
- Decrease in vital capacity by one third from maximum recorded
- Tachycardia (heart rate >120 beats/min)

TABLE 4: Boston criteria of heart failure.

Criteria	Point value
Category 1: History	
• Rest dyspnea:	4
○ Orthopnea	4
○ Paroxysmal nocturnal dyspnea	3
○ Dyspnea on walking on level	2
○ Dyspnea on climbing	1
Category 2: Physical examination	
• Heart rate abnormality (if 91–110 beats/min, 1 point if >110 beats/min, 2 points)	1–2
• Jugular venous pressure elevation (if >6 cm, 2 points, if >6 cm, plus hepatomegaly or leg edema, 3 points)	2–3
• Lung rales (if basilar, 1 point; if more than basilar, 2 points)	1–2
• Wheezing	3
• S3	3
Category 3: X-ray of chest	
• Alveolar pulmonary edema	4
• Interstitial pulmonary edema	3
• Bilateral pleural effusion	3
• Cardiothoracic ratio >0.50	3
• Upper zone flow redistribution	2

TABLE 5: Ross criteria of heart failure.

Ross criteria	
Grade of heart failure	Symptoms
Class 1	No limitations or symptoms
Class 2	Mild tachypnea or diaphoresis with feedings in infants, dyspnea on exertion in older children, and no growth failure
Class 3	Marked tachypnea or diaphoresis with feedings or exertion, and prolonged feeding times with growth failure
Class 4	Symptoms at rest with tachypnea, retractions, grunting, or diaphoresis

New York University Pediatric Heart Failure Index (PHFI) (Table 6)

In the proposed scoring system,[18] 0 is defined as no CHF and 30 as severe CHF.

TABLE 6: Pediatric Heart Failure Index.

Scoring system	
Features	**Score**
Failure to thrive	2
Prolonged feeding time	1
Retractions	2
Severe tachypnea	2
Resting sinus tachycardia	2
Hepatomegaly 3 cm below the costal margin	1
Marked cardiomegaly	1
High doses of diuretics	2
Digoxin	1
Angiotensin-converting enzyme inhibitor	1
Anticoagulants	2
Antiarrhythmic agents	2
Abnormal function by echocardiography	2
Single ventricle physiology	2

CONCLUSION

Heart failure is a syndrome, which is diagnosed at bedside. Its staging is also decided at bedside. So many decisions, including indication of device in heart failure, are decided at bedside with an addition of simple imaging like echocardiogram.

REFERENCES

1. Gheorghiade M, Filippatos G, De Luca L, et al. Congestion in acute heart failure syndromes: An essential target of evaluation and treatment. Am J Med. 2006;119(12 Suppl. 1): S3.
2. Nohria A, Tsang SW, Fang JC, et al. Clinical assessment identifies hemodynamic profiles that predict outcomes in patients admitted with heart failure. J Am Coll Cardiol. 2003;41:1797-804.
3. Chakko S, Woska D, Martinez H, et al. Clinical, radiographic, and hemodynamic correlations in chronic congestive heart failure: conflicting results may lead to inappropriate care. Am J Med. 1991;90:353.
4. Drazner MH, Hellkamp AS, Leier CV, et al. Value of clinician assessment of hemodynamics in advanced heart failure: the ESCAPE trial. Circ Heart Fail. 2008;1:170-7.
5. Lala A, McNulty SE, Mentz RJ, et al. Relief and recurrence of congestion during and after hospitalization for acute heart failure: insights from Diuretic Optimization Strategy Evaluation in Acute Decompensated Heart Failure (DOSE-AHF) and Cardiorenal Rescue Study in Acute Decompensated Heart Failure (CARESS-HF). Circ Heart Fail. 2015;8:741-8.
6. Ewy GA. The abdominojugular test: technique and hemodynamic correlates. Ann Intern Med. 1988;109:456-60.
7. Omar HR, Guglin M. Clinical and prognostic significance of positive hepatojugular reflux on discharge in acute heart failure: insights from the ESCAPE trial. Biomed Res Int. 2017;2017:5734749.

8. Thibodeau JT, Turer AT, Gualano SK, et al. Characterization of a novel symptom of advanced heart failure: bendopnea. J Am Coll Cardiol HF. 2014;2:24-31.
9. Tewart DJ, Cernacek P, Costello KB, et al. Elevated endothelin-1 in heart failure and loss of normal response to postural change. Circulation. 1992;85:510.
10. Stevenson LW, Perloff JK. The Limited Reliability of Physical Signs for Estimating Hemodynamics in Chronic Heart Failure. JAMA. 1989;261(6)884.
11. Zema MJ, Restivo B, Sos T, et al. Left ventricular dysfunction—bedside Valsalva manoeuvre. Br Heart J. 1980;44:560.
12. Nishimura RA, Tajik AJ. The Valsalva maneuver and response revisited. Mayo Clin Proc. 1986;61:211-7.
13. Zema MJ. Diagnosing Heart Failure by the Valsalva maneuver. Isn't it Finally Time? Chest. 1999;116:851.
14. Grodin JL, Drazner MH, Dupont M, et al. A disproportionate elevation in right ventricular filling pressure, in relation to left ventricular filling pressure, is associated with renal impairment and increased mortality in advanced decompensated heart failure. Am Heart J. 2015;169:806-12.
15. McKee PA, Castelli WP, McNamara PM, et al. The natural history of congestive heart failure: the Framingham study. N Engl J Med. 1971;285(26):1441.
16. Carlson KJ, Lee DC-S, Goroll AH, et al. An analysis of physicians' reasons for prescribing long-term digitalis therapy in outpatients. J Chron Dis. 1985;38:733.
17. Ross RD, Daniels SR, Schwartz DC, et al. Plasma norepinephrine levels in infants and children with congestive heart failure. Am J Cardiol. 1987;59:911.
18. Connolly D, Rutkowski M, Auslender M, et al. The New York University Pediatric Heart Failure Index: a new method of quantifying chronic heart failure severity in children. J Pediatr. 2001;138:644.

CHAPTER 25

Clinical Assessment: Pulmonary Hypertension

INTRODUCTION

David Dresdale, a trainee under the great teacher Cournand first described *"Primary Pulmonary Hypertension"* in 1951. The gate to pulmonary circulation was then opened. Then came Paul Wood, Heath, Edwards, and the Wagenvoorts and eventually in 1973 World Health Organization proposed the first classification of pulmonary hypertension.

DEFINITION

Definition of pulmonary hypertension (PH) is a level of pulmonary artery pressure, which is, measured hemodynamically, by cardiac catheterization. It is defined as mean pulmonary arterial pressure (mPAP) ≥25 mm Hg at rest.[1]

CLINICAL CLASSIFICATION OF PULMONARY HYPERTENSION

First clinical classification of PH was proposed in 1973. It was modified, then in 1998 at the Evian conference (**Box 1**).[2] Further modifications were done at Venice conference[3] in 2003 and in 2008 at Dana Point.[4] European Society of Cardiology/European Respiratory Society (ESC/ERS) guideline made a modified clinical classification suggested by Simonneau (**Boxes 2 to 5**).[3]

BOX 1 | Clinical classification of pulmonary hypertension.

Group 1: Pulmonary arterial hypertension
Group 2: Pulmonary hypertension due to left heart disease
Group 3: Pulmonary hypertension due to lung disease or hypoxia
Group 4: Chronic thromboembolic Pulmonary hypertension
Group 5: Pulmonary hypertension due to unclear and/or multifactorial mechanism

> **BOX 2** **Pulmonary arterial hypertension.**
> - Idiopathic
> - Heritable
> - Congenital heart disease
> - Drugs and toxins
> - Connective tissue disease
> - HIV infection
> - Portal hypertension
> - Pulmonary veno-occlusive disease
> - Persistent pulmonary hypertension of the newborn

> **BOX 3** **Pulmonary hypertension due to left heart disease.**
> - Left ventricular dysfunction
> - Valvular disease
> - Left ventricular congenital inflow/outflow tract obstruction
> - Congenital cardiomyopathies
> - Congenital/acquired pulmonary veins stenosis

> **BOX 4** **Pulmonary hypertension due to lung disease or hypoxia.**
> - Chronic obstructive pulmonary disease
> - Interstitial lung disease
> - Obstructive sleep apnea

> **BOX 5** **Pulmonary hypertension due to unclear and/or multifactorial mechanism.**
> - Hematological disorders (hemolytic anemia, myeloproliferative disorder, and splenectomy)
> - Systemic disorders (sarcoidosis and neurofibromatosis)
> - Metabolic disorders (glycogen storage disease, Gaucher disease, and thyroid disorder)

HEMODYNAMIC CLASSIFICATION (TABLE 1)

Precapillary versus Postcapillary Pulmonary Hypertension

After the diagnosis of PH, the next hemodynamic issue is whether PH is precapillary or postcapillary, depending on left ventricular filling pressure (left ventricular end-diastolic pressure or pulmonary artery capillary wedge pressure). Postcapillary PH is PH with pulmonary capillary wedge pressure (PCWP) >15 mm Hg due to increased left ventricular end-diastolic pressure with a backward transmission, whereas precapillary PH is PH with PCWP <15 mm Hg. Precapillary PH includes above-mentioned group 1, group 3, group 4 and some group 5, whereas postcapillary PH includes group 2.

Pulmonary Arterial Hypertension

Pulmonary arterial hypertension (PAH) is a precapillary PH along with pulmonary vascular resistance (PVR) >3 Wood unit in absence of other cause of precapillary

TABLE 1: Hemodynamic versus clinical classification.

Pulmonary hypertension pattern	Criteria	Clinical classification
PH	mPAP ≥25 mm Hg	
Precapillary PH	mPAP ≥25 mm Hg PCWP ≤15 mm Hg	• PAH • Lung disease or hypoxia • CTEPH • Unclear and/or multifactorial mechanism
Postcapillary PH	mPAP ≥25 mm Hg PCWP >15 mm Hg	• Left heart disease • Unclear and/or multifactorial mechanism
Isolated postcapillary PH	DPG <7 mm Hg PVR ≤3 Wood unit	
Combined postcapillary and precapillary PH	DPG ≥7 mm Hg PVR >3 Wood unit	

(DPG: diastolic pressure gradient; mPAP: mean pulmonary arterial pressure; PAH: pulmonary arterial hypertension; PH: pulmonary hypertension; PCWP: pulmonary capillary wedge pressure; PVR: pulmonary vascular resistance; CTEPH: Chronic thromboembolic pulmonary hypertension)

PH. PAH has diverse etiologies as mentioned above, with same pathophysiology in which small muscular pulmonary arterioles show enhanced contractility, endothelial dysfunction, remodeling and proliferation of both endothelial and smooth muscle cells, and in situ thrombi.[5]

Postcapillary Pulmonary Hypertension

Postcapillary PH is mostly due to group 2 diseases, i.e., left heart diseases and some of the group 5 diseases. PH in left heart disease develops due to passive backward transmission of increased filling pressure and grade of PH is in proportionate to PCWP. This is traditionally known as passive PH. However, in some patients the backward transmitted passive pressure triggers vasoconstriction, increases endothelin expression, reduces nitric oxide availability, and sets remodeling of small-sized pulmonary arterioles. This remodeling leads to further increases in mean pulmonary artery pressure, much higher than PCWP and eventually pulmonary vascular disease. This is traditionally known as reactive PH.

Transpulmonary and Diastolic Pressure Gradient

Transpulmonary pressure gradient (TPG) was used to differentiate between passive and reactive PH. Passive PH was said to be present when TPG is <12 mm Hg and reactive PH when TPG is >12 mm Hg. TPG is the difference between mPAP and PCWP. TPG was later found a poor determinant of pulmonary vascular disease, because it is affected by several factors flow, resistance, and left heart filling pressure. However, diastolic pulmonary artery pressure and diastolic pressure gradient (DPG) is the difference between diastolic pulmonary artery pressure and PCWP are less influenced by the above factors and are better determinant of pulmonary vascular disease. Normally, DPG is 1–3 mm Hg. Isolated postcapillary PH (previously known as passive) is said to be present, when DPG is <7 mm Hg. Combined postcapillary and precapillary PH (previously known as reactive PH) is said to be present, when DPG is >7 mm Hg.

Borderline Pulmonary Hypertension

Normal mPAP is 14 ± 3 mm Hg and upper limit is 20 mm Hg (mean + 2 SD). By definition, mean PH is >25 mm Hg. Thus, a gray zone exists between 21 and 25 mm Hg. This is named as borderline PH. Patients with connective tissue disorder and heritable PH when present with this borderline PH, should be followed up closely, as many of them will develop PH.[6]

Exercise Pulmonary Hypertension

Exercise PH is defined as resting mean pulmonary artery pressure <25 mm Hg and exercising mean pulmonary artery pressure >30 mm Hg and PVR more the 3 Wood unit.

CLINICAL FEATURES

Dyspnea

Dyspnea on exertion is the most common symptom. 60% of patients present with dyspnea and 98% of patients suffer from dyspnea at the time of diagnosis. Mechanism of dyspnea on exertion is multifactorial.[7] Most important cause is right ventricle is unable to increase cardiac output due to its decreased contractile reserve and further increase in afterload during exercise. Normally, pulmonary artery pressure falls on exercise due to pulmonary vascular recruitment and distensibility of the resistive vessels. It does not happen in patients with PH. Low cardiac output results in chronically reduced blood supply to exercising muscle leading to skeletal myopathy. The combination of reduced cardiac output and skeletal myopathy results in impaired oxygen delivery and extraction along with early anaerobiosis. In consequence, there is increased production of carbon dioxide, which increases alveolar ventilation. Patents with PH show chronical hyperventilation, due to heart failure and increased chemosensitivity. Chronic hyperventilation reduces $PaCO_2$. This increases ventilatory demand in relation to carbon dioxide output, which is already increased. This is a state of ventilatory inefficiency. In PH due to chronic thromboembolic PH, increased physiological dead space is the major contributing factor for ventilatory insufficiency. Ventilation-perfusion mismatch also plays a role. Severe PH opens up the stretched patent foramen ovale with right-to-left shunt, which increases hypoxemia and hyperventilation further through stimulation of peripheral chemoreceptors (**Box 6**).

> **BOX 6** **Mechanism of exertional dyspnea in pulmonary hypertension (PH).**
> - Reduced cardiac output due to reduced right ventricular contractile reserve and further increase in PH during exertion
> - Skeletal muscle dysfunction
> - Early anaerobiosis
> - Increased CO_2 production
> - Hyperventilation leading to decreased $PaCO_2$
> - Increased physiological dead space
> - Above factors lead to ventilatory insufficiency
> - Right-to-left shunt through stretched patent foramen ovale

Fatigue

Fatigue is quite common and presenting symptom in 19% of patients and 73% at the time of diagnosis. Fatigue is due to reduced cardiac output and skeletal myopathy.

Syncope

Syncope may be a presenting symptom in 8% of patients and 36% of patients at the time of diagnosis. Syncope is common during effort and due to reduced cardiac output during exercise. Occasionally, it may be due to fatal arrhythmia.

Bendopnea

Bendopnea may be an associated symptom, due to reduced cardiac output. Bending may precipitate syncope due to reduced venous return.

Angina

Angina may be present in 47% of patients at the time of diagnosis. Angina is due to right ventricular ischemia for obvious mechanism. Rarely, it may be due to compression of left main coronary artery by dilated pulmonary artery.

Other Symptoms

Hoarseness is due to compression of recurrent laryngeal nerve by dilated pulmonary artery. Hemoptysis is due to rupture of hypertrophied bronchial arteries. Dry cough and exercise-induced nausea and vomiting are minor symptoms.

Jugular Venous Pulse

A prominent large *a* wave is the characteristic finding in jugular venous pulse. A large *v* wave may be present when there is associated tricuspid regurgitation (TR).

Palpation

Palpation reveals a parasternal impulse ranging from grade 1 to 3. Apical impulse is diffuse. P2 and pulmonary artery pulsation and occasional pulmonary click are palpable. Pulmonary regurgitation (PR) murmur may be associated with thrill in 10% cases.

Hallmark of PH is loud P2, which is most consistent and found in 93% cases. Others are not always consistent. Right-sided S3 and S4 are found in 23% and 38% cases. Murmurs of TR and PR are found in 40% and 13% cases, respectively (**Box 7**).

Pulmonary Ejection Click

Pulmonary ejection click is a sharp, high-pitched, clicking, early ejection sound, which is often palpated overlying the dilated pulmonary artery pulsation. It is best heard on second and third left intercostal space and can be heard at lower left sternal edge and even apex, when apex is formed by right ventricle.[8] Like pulmonary valvular click, vascular click is also described by Perloff—*"selective attenuation during inspiration and amplification during expiration."*[8] However, pulmonary vascular click has been described by others as less variable with respiration. Higher the PH, more specifically pulmonary artery diastolic pressure, the later the right ventricular ejection begins and more delayed the ejection click occurs (**Table 2**).

Pulmonary Ejection Murmur

Pulmonary ejection murmur is due to ejection of blood in dilated pulmonary artery. The murmur is grade 2 to 3, best heard at second left intercostal space. It starts after ejection click, superficial, symmetrical in shape with a crescendo-decrescendo configuration.

Tricuspid Regurgitation Murmur

Pulmonary hypertension causes functional incompetence of tricuspid valve and produces high-pressure TR murmur. Unless there is dilatation of tricuspid annulus, TR murmur does not occur.

BOX 7 Auscultatory features of pulmonary hypertension.

- Pulmonary ejection click
- Pulmonary ejection murmur
- Tricuspid regurgitation murmur
- Graham Steell murmur
- Right ventricular S4, S3
- Mid-diastolic murmur
- Typical S2

TABLE 2: Pulmonary valvular versus vascular click.

Events	Pulmonary valvular click	Pulmonary vascular click
S1-click	Closer gap	Wider gap
Respiratory variation	Inconstant	Lesser variable
Audibility	More localized	Wider area

Graham Steell Murmur

Graham Steell narrated in 1888—*"There is occasionally heard over the pulmonary area… and below this region for the distance of an inch or two along the left border of the sternum, and rarely over the lowest part of the bone itself, a soft blowing diastolic murmur immediately following, or, more exactly, running off from the accentuated second sound, while the usual indications of aortic regurgitation afforded by the pulse, etc., are absent.…When the second sound is reduplicated, the murmur proceeds from its latter part. That such a murmur as I have described does exist, there can I think, be no doubt."*[9]

As the hypertensive PR murmur is high-pressure, low-flow murmur, it is high frequency, soft blowing murmur, best heard in left second and third intercostal space. But it may be heard in lower left sternal edge and even at aortic area.[8] As soon as pulmonary pressure pulse crosses right ventricular pressure pulse, i.e., at dicrotic notch, the murmur starts immediately after loud P2. As pulmonary artery to right ventricular diastolic gradient may persist throughout diastole, the murmur, usually decrescendo, may occasionally be pandiastolic.[8] The murmur of Eisenmenger syndrome is usually pandiastolic, whereas the murmur in postcapillary PH is early diastolic. The murmur may be associated with thrill in 10% of cases. As high-frequency and blowing, the murmur is often missed. Serotonin selectively increases pulmonary artery diastolic pressure and was used in the past to selectively increase Graham Steell murmur.[10]

Right-sided S4 and S3

Right-sided S4 is common. S3 occurs, when there is right ventricular failure secondary to PH.

Mid-diastolic Murmur

Mid-diastolic murmur has been occasionally reported in patients with severe PH. There had been various explanations regarding the origin of this murmur. The most interesting explanation was describing the murmur as right-sided Austin Flint murmur[11] occurring with pulmonary hypertensive regurgitation murmur.

Second Heart Sound

Expiratory splitting of second heart sound (S2) usually persists in PH. Inspiratory splitting depends on two opposing factors. PH causes prolonged right ventricular ejection with delayed P2. At the same time, it causes decreased pulmonary capacitance and hangout time resulting in narrow S2. Inspiratory splitting is usually preserved. Loud P2, however, may mask A2 in pulmonary area. In that case, split can better be assessed at the apex. In mitral stenosis (MS) with PH, split is physiological. In mitral regurgitation (MR) with PH, split is wide. In idiopathic PAH, expiratory splitting can be appreciated, and inspiratory splitting is narrower. Splitting in Eisenmenger syndrome has been described later.

P2 is equal to A2 in mild PH, louder than A2 in moderate PH, and it becomes audible all through the precordium in severe PH. In atrial septal defect (ASD), as apex is formed by right ventricle, P2 may be audible at the apex with normal pulmonary arterial pressure. Apical transmission of loud P2 in PH caused by MS and ventricular septal defect is somehow rare.[12] A very loud P2 can mask A2 in pulmonary area. Then the single component at pulmonary area can be compared with the counterpart in aortic area and if found louder, indicates that P2 is loud.

Why P2 is louder than A2 in PH? Pulmonary arterial diastolic pressure rarely crosses aortic diastolic pressure. Intensity of second heart sound closure depends on the amplitude of the second heart sound, related to the rate of change of the DPG. In patients with PH, the rate of change of this gradient across pulmonary valve is increased. Still, it did not equal the rate of change of the pressure gradient that developed across the aortic valve, implicating that there must be some other explanation, beyond hemodynamic explanation. As Stein et al.[13] pointed out in their study—*"pulmonary valve is larger in surface area, lighter, thinner and more distensible than the aortic valve. These findings suggest that the pulmonary valve would tend to deflect with a greater velocity than the aortic valve when caused to vibrate by a comparable driving force."*

CLINICAL GRADING OF PULMONARY HYPERTENSION

Pulmonary hypertension is expressed as mean pulmonary artery pressure. How to grade PH according to systolic artery pressure? Proposed upper limit of normal systolic pulmonary artery pressure is 30–35 mm Hg[14] and a pressure >35–40 mm Hg is taken as pulmonary arterial systolic hypertension.[15] Intensity of P2 correlates roughly with degree of PH. Leatham in his phonocardiographic versus cardiac catheterization study[16] showed that pulmonary systolic artery pressure must be >50 mm Hg to get louder P2. Apical transmission of P2 occurred only when pulmonary artery systolic pressure was in the range of 80 mm Hg (**Table 3**).

TABLE 3: Clinical grading of PH.

P2 Grading	Pulmonary artery pressure grading (mm Hg)
Normal: P2 < A2	Normal; mean PAP <20–25; systolic PAP <30–35
Grade 1: P2 = A2	Mild PH; mean PAP >25; systolic PAP >35–40
Grade 2: P2 > A2	Moderate PH; mean PAP >40; systolic PAP >50
Grade 3: P2 audible down to 3rd and 4th left ICS	
Grade 4: P2 audible at apex	Severe PH; mean PAP >50; systolic PAP >70–80
Grade 5: Very loud, booming P2	

(ICS: intercostal space; PH: pulmonary hypertension; PAP: pulmonary arterial pressure)

CONCLUSION

Most loudly audible sound in clinical cardiology is P2. Echocardiologist can miss PH due to inadequate tricuspid or pulmonary regurgitation jet. However, even a reluctant clinician cannot miss a loud P2—the hallmark of PH.

REFERENCES

1. Galiè N1, Hoeper MM, Humbert M, et al. Guidelines for the diagnosis and treatment of pulmonary hypertension: the Task Force for the Diagnosis and Treatment of Pulmonary Hypertension of the European Society of Cardiology (ESC) and the European Respiratory Society (ERS), endorsed by the International Society of Heart and Lung Transplantation (ISHLT). Eur Heart J. 2009;30(20):2493-537.
2. Rich S, Rubin LJ, Abenhail L, et al. Executive summary from the World Symposium on Primary Pulmonary Hypertension (Evian, France, September 6–10, 1998). Geneva, Switzerland: World Health Organization; 1998. pp. 1-27.
3. Simonneau G, Galiè N, Rubin LJ, et al. Clinical classification of pulmonary hypertension. J Am Coll Cardiol. 2004;43:S5.
4. Simonneau G, Robbins I, Beghetti M, et al. Updated clinical classification of pulmonary hypertension. J Am Coll Cardiol. 2009;54:S43.
5. Tuder RM, Archer SL, Dorfmüller P, et al. Relevant issues in the pathology and pathobiology of pulmonary hypertension. J Am Coll Cardiol. 2013;62(25 Suppl):D4-12.
6. Hoeper MM, Bogaard HJ, Condliffe R, et al. Definitions and diagnosis of pulmonary hypertension. J Am Coll Cardiol. 2013;62(25 Suppl):D42-50.
7. Dumitrescue D, Sitbon O, Weatherald J, et al. Exertional dyspnea in pulmonary arterial hypertension. Eur Respir Rev. 2017;26:170039.
8. Perloff JK. Auscultatory and phonocardiographic manifestations of pulmonary hypertension. Prog Cardiovasc Dis. 1967;9(4):303-40.
9. Steell G. The murmur of high pressure in the pulmonary artery. Med Chron. 1888;9:182.
10. Endrys J, Bartova A. Pharmacologic methods in the phonocardiographic diagnosis of regurgitant murmurs. Brit Heart J. 1962;24:213.
11. Wyckoff J, Bunim J. Observations on an apical diastolic murmur unassociated with valvular heart disease in cases of right ventricular hypertrophy. Tr Ass Amer Physicians. 1935;50:280.
12. Sutton G, Harris A, Leatham A. Second heart sound in pulmonary hypertension. Br Heart J. 1968;30:743.
13. Stein PD, Sabbah HN, Anbe DN, et al. Hemodynamic and anatomic determinants of relative differences in the amplitude of the aortic and pulmonary components of the second heart sound. Am J Cardiol. 1978;42:539.
14. Lam CS, Borlaug BA, Kane GC, et al. Age-associated increases in pulmonary artery systolic pressure in the general population. Circulation. 2009;119:2663-70.
15. McLaughlin VV, Archer SL, Badesch DB, et al. ACCF/AHA 2009 expert consensus document on pulmonary hypertension: a report of the American College of Cardiology Foundation Task Force on Expert Consensus Documents and the American Heart Association: developed in collaboration with the American College of Chest Physicians; American Thoracic Society, Inc; and the Pulmonary Hypertension Association. J Am Coll Cardiol. 2009;53:1573-619.
16. Leatham A, Gray I. Auscultation and phonocardiographic signs of atrial septal defect. Br Heart J. 1956;18:193-208.

CHAPTER 26

Segmental Approach in Congenital Heart Disease

INTRODUCTION

As Van Praagh described—*"Segmental approach is analysis of the heart in terms of its major developmental units or segments in a step-by-step fashion. The segments are the visceroatrial situs, the ventricular loop, and the conotruncus or more briefly, the atria, ventricles and great arteries."* Anderson used to name it as sequential segmental analysis. Heart is a three floor building, which include the atria as platform connected by atrioventricular (AV) junction to the ventricles which are first floor and connected by ventriculoarterial (VA) junction to great arteries which are the second floor (**Box 1**) (**Fig. 1**).[1]

BOX 1	Segmental approach.
• Cardiac position in chest	• Ventriculoarterial connection
• Situs	• Conus
• Atrioventricular connection	• Great artery spatial relations
• Atrioventricular alignment	• Associated cardiac anomalies
• Ventricular loop	

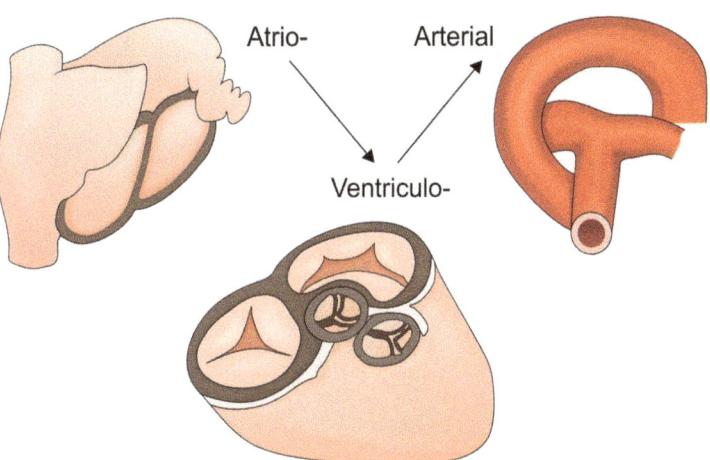

Fig. 1: Segmental building block approach.

CARDIAC POSITION

Cardiac position means whether the heart lies in the left or right hemithorax or in the midline. It also implies the apex which may point to left, to right or indeterminate. It has nothing to do with segmental connections, relations or associated intracardiac or visceral anomalies.

CARDIAC MALPOSITION

Cardiac malposition is used to describe both the location of the heart anywhere other than its usual position in the left hemithorax, or the location of the heart in the left hemithorax when other organs are in abnormal position such as situs inversus. They include dextrocardia, levocardia, and mesocardia. They indicate cardiac position only. Dextrocardia simply means a heart in right chest, levocardia a heart in left chest, and mesocardia a heart in midline.[2,3]

DEXTROCARDIA[4]

Dextrocardia was first reported by Fabricus in 1606. Dextrocardia is a cardiac positional anomaly in which the heart is located in the right hemithorax with its base-to-apex axis directed to the right and caudal (**Box 2**) (**Fig. 2**). It may be:

BOX 2	Simple classification of right-sided heart.
Primary	
• Situs solitus	
• Situs inversus	
• Situs ambiguous	
Secondary	

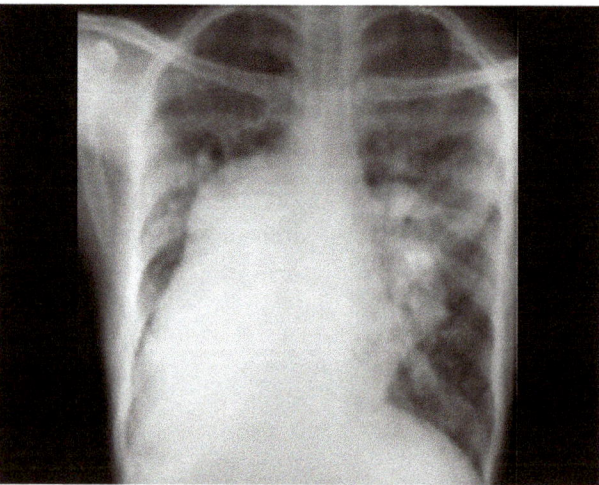

Fig. 2: Dextrocardia.

- Dextroversion/dextrorotation/pivotal dextrocardia means all right-sided hear with situs solitus. The heart appears as if the apex has been swung from left chest to the right.
- Isolated dextrocardia means the other organs are in the normal location with respect to the body and dextrocardia is an isolated finding.
- Dextroposition means the heart has been shifted rightward by external cause such as right lung hypoplasia, right pneumonectomy, or diaphragmatic hernia.
- Mixed dextrocardia means the dextrocardia with AV discordance.
- Mirror image dextrocardia means right-sided heart with situs inversus.

To avoid these jargons, one should describe all right-sided heart as dextrocardia along with mentioning other abnormalities.

The incidence of dextrocardia with situs inversus is between 1:2,500 and 1:20,000 living people, whereas dextrocardia with situs solitus is between 1:7,500 and 1:17,500. The incidence of congenital heart disease in primary dextrocardia is < 10% in situs inversus and > 90% in situs solitus (**Table 1**).

SITUS

The concept of situs refers to the configuration of asymmetric structures within an individual. They include abdominovisceral situs and thoracovisceral situs.

Abdominovisceral Situs

In situs solitus, liver, and inferior vena cava (IVC) are right sided, whereas stomach, spleen, and aorta are left sided. Reverse is found in situs inversus. Patients with heterotaxy syndrome show incomplete lateralization with a midline liver and stomach.

TABLE 1: Cardiac abnormalities in dextrocardia: Solitus versus inversus.

	Dextrocardia situs solitus	Dextrocardia situs inversus
Atrioventricular discordance	50%	25%
Single ventricle	25%	Uncommon
Ventricular septal defect	60%	60%
C-transposition of the great arteries (TGA)	50%	20%
TGA	10%	30%
Double outlet right ventricle	10%	30%
Normally related great arteries	40%	40%
Pulmonary stenosis/pulmonary artery	60%	50%
Right arch	5%	80%

Great Vessel Situs

Relationship is decided at the level of diaphragm. In situs solitus, aorta descends in front or slightly to the left of the spine, whereas IVC ascends to the right and anterior of the aorta. In polysplenia (double left sidedness), section of the IVC above the renal veins (right-sided structure) is absent. Here, venous drainage of the lower body is via an azygos or hemiazygos connection, ascends posterior to aorta in the paravertebral space, either right or left. There is separate entry of hepatic veins from the corner of the atrium. In asplenia (double right sidedness), aorta and IVC are on the same side of the spine. They may be side-by-side or IVC may be in front of aorta.

Thoracovisceral Situs

Lung lobation can also determine the situs. In situs solitus, the right lung is trilobed, and the left lung is bilobed. Reverse is found in situs inversus. In situs ambiguous, there is either bilateral trilobed lungs (polysplenia) or bilateral bilobed lungs (asplenia). Tracheobronchial tree can also determine the situs (**Fig. 3**). In situs solitus, the right main stem bronchus is short and eparterial (right upper lobe branch courses over the right pulmonary artery), more angulated with trachea (144°) and the left main stem bronchus is longer and hyparterial (courses below the left pulmonary artery) and less angulated (125°).

Atrial Situs

Atrial situs is usually consistent with visceral situs. However, in situs ambiguous with heterotaxy syndrome, abdominal situs is less consistent, whereas tracheobronchial anatomy is more predictable for atrial situs. Best way to differentiate right versus left atrium is their characteristic appendages and respective site of septum.[5] Fossa ovalis between thick superior and inferior limbus on right atrial site and flap valve of fossa ovalis on left atrial side are the other important clues (**Table 2**) (**Fig. 4**).

Situs Solitus, Dextrocardia

The systemic atrium is on the right with a right-sided trilobed lung, liver, gallbladder, and IVC. The pulmonary atrium is on the left with a left-sided bilobed

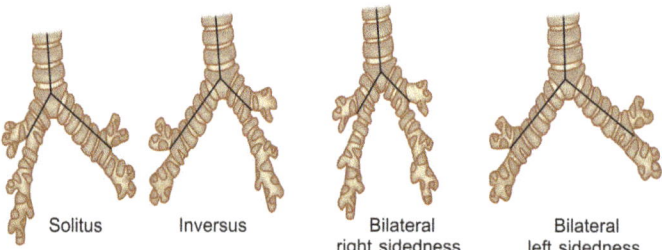

Fig. 3: Tracheobronchial situs.

TABLE 2: How to identify right and left atrium?

Right atrium	Left atrium
• It receives the superior vena cava, inferior vena cava, and the coronary sinus • Its musculature includes the crista terminalis and the tinea sagittalis • Its septal surface has superior and inferior bands of the fossa ovalis • Its appendage is broad-based, triangular, and anterior in location • Remnants of the embryonic venous valves, the Eustachian, and Thebesian valves guard the entrances to the inferior caval vein and the coronary sinus	• It receives the pulmonary veins • It has thin and few trabeculations • Its septal surface has the flap valve of the fossa ovalis • Its appendage is narrow-based, finger-like and posterior in location

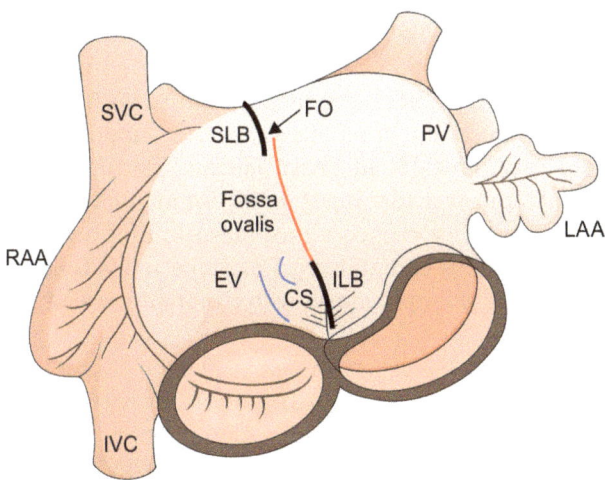

(CS: coronary sinus; IVC: inferior vena cava; LAA: left atrial appendage; RAA: right atrial appendage; SVC: superior vena cava; PV: pulmonary valve; EV: eustachian valve; SLB: superior limbus; ILB: inferior limbus)

Fig. 4: Morphology of right and left atrium.

lung, stomach, single spleen, and aorta. The incidence of congenital heart disease is very high, said to approach 100%. L-loop ventricle is very common, almost in 50% of cases. Single ventricle is found in 20% of cases. Isolated ventricular septal defect (VSD) is also common. VA discordance is the most common relation of great arteries. About half of these cases have also AV discordance. Normally, related great arteries are found in 40% of cases.

Situs Inversus

The systemic atrium is on the left with a left-sided trilobed lung, liver, gallbladder, and IVC. The pulmonary atrium is on the right with a right-sided bilobed lung, stomach, single spleen, and aorta. The cardiac apex is on the right. Situs inversus is seen in 0.01% of the population, and the incidence of congenital heart disease in patients with situs inversus is 3–5%. Transposition is more common. Double discordance is uncommon. Double outlet right ventricle (DORV) is relatively common. The most common abnormality is right-sided aortic arch, in around 80% of patients. Kartagener syndrome (which consists of situs inversus, nasal polyposis with chronic sinusitis, and bronchiectasis) is present in 20% of all patients with situs inversus. The bronchiectasis is caused by compromised mucociliary transport secondary to dynein protein structural and functional abnormalities (i.e., the immotile cilia syndrome). About 50% of patients with immotile cilia syndrome have situs solitus and 50% have situs inversus.

Sinus Ambiguous

Situs ambiguous tends toward symmetric morphology of normally asymmetric structure. To subclassify, it includes Asplenia syndrome, double right-sidedness, right isomerism, or Ivemark syndrome and Polysplenia syndrome, double left-sidedness, or left isomerism. The incidence of congenital heart disease in patients with heterotaxy is very high, ranging from 50% to nearly 100%. In asplenia (i.e., right isomerism or bilateral right-sidedness), both lungs have three lobes and eparterial bronchi. The main bronchus is located superior to the ipsilateral main pulmonary artery on each side. Associated cardiac malformations include common AV canal, univentricular heart, transposition of the great arteries, and total anomalous pulmonary venous return (seen in most cases). The complex cyanotic cardiac anomalies and abnormal immune status (because of absence of the spleen) result in a poor prognosis, with a mortality rate of up to 80% in the first year (**Fig. 5**).[6]

In polysplenia (i.e., left isomerism or bilateral left-sidedness), both lungs have two lobes and hyparterial bronchi. In this situation, the reverse is seen: The main bronchus passes inferior to the ipsilateral main pulmonary artery on each side. Cardiac anomalies are not as complex as in asplenic patients. The most common associated cardiovascular anomalies are azygos continuation of the IVC, partial anomalous pulmonary venous return, atrial septal defect, and endocardial

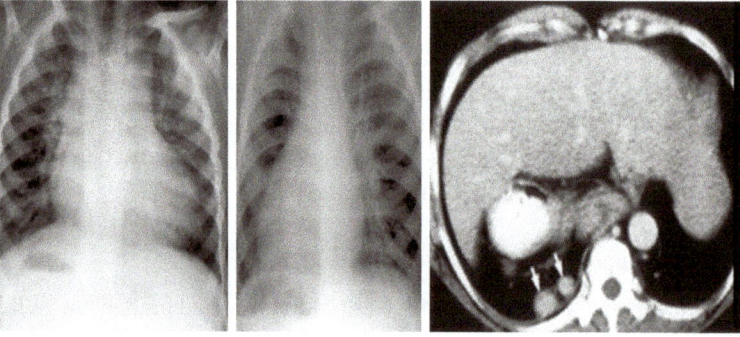

Fig. 5: Situs inversus (SI), levocardia; SI, dextrocardia, situs ambiguous (midline liver, stomach, two splenic nodules).

cushion defect. Up to 25% of patients have minor cardiac abnormalities, and the disorder may not be diagnosed until adulthood.

Heterotaxy

The critical structures to be evaluated with imaging in determining situs are:
- Position of the atria.
- Position of venous drainage below the diaphragm relative to midline.
- Position of the aorta relative to midline.
- Position of the stomach and presence of malrotation.
- Position of the liver and gallbladder.
- Position of the cardiac apex.
- Presence, appearance, and number of spleens.
- Presence of tri- or bilobed lungs, including presence or absence of bilateral minor fissures.

These anatomic structures may be evaluated with:
- Chest radiography
- Ultrasonography
- Computed tomography and magnetic resonance imaging
- Angiocardiography

Isolated Levocardia

Isolated levocardia, i.e., levocardia with situs inversus or ambiguous, is rare. The likelihood of associated intracardiac anomaly, such as corrected transposition, AV canal defect, total anomalous pulmonary venous connection, pulmonary stenosis or atresia is almost 100% and either asplenia or polysplenia is 80%.

Mesocardia

Mesocardia means the heart is on midline. Van Praagh found mesocardia a rare entity and only 0.2% in his autopsy series. He found higher incidence of situs abnormalities and malposition of great vessels. However, in many tall slender persons heart lies in midline, i.e., so called vertical heart which can be reported as mesocardia without any clinical significance.

Ectopia Cordis

Heart is partially or completely outside the thorax.

ATRIOVENTRICULAR CONNECTION

Atrioventricular connection is shown in **Box 3**:

BOX 3 — **Atrioventricular connection.**
- Double inlet ventricle
- Single inlet
- Common inlet

How to Define Ventricle?

A normal ventricle possesses an inlet, an apical trabecular component, and an outlet. This is the tripartite approach. However, the tripartite approach does not help to diagnose rudimentary abnormal ventricle. The most constant part of these three segments is apical trabecular segment. Thus, a good working definition of a ventricle is any chamber within the ventricular mass, which has an apical component.[7] When such ventricle also possesses inlet and outlet segment, it is normal ventricle, which may be left or right and which may be hypoplastic, more specifically the outlet portion, when there is severe stenosis or atresia in the outlet segment. One of the two ventricles of heart with univentricular AV connection is rudimentary and hypoplastic. Similarly, one of the ventricles in heart with AV valvar atresia is rudimentary and hypoplastic. However, most of these chambers are essentially tripartite, only they have been squeezed out of their ventricular cavity. When the heart possesses only one ventricle, which morphology is indeterminant from apical trabeculation, then only it's a true single ventricle of indeterminate morphology (**Table 3**) (**Fig. 6**).

TABLE 3: Morphological identification of ventricles.

Right ventricle	Left ventricle
• Right ventricle possesses an infundibulum and the tricuspid valve	• Left ventricle contains the bicuspid mitral valve with its paired papillary muscles
• Tricuspid valve consists of papillary muscle pattern of a single anterior muscle, multiple posterior muscles, and a conal muscle	• The mitral valve is in fibrous continuity with the aortic valve and there is no infundibulum
• The tricuspid valve is separated from the pulmonary valve by the crista supraventricularis	• Its trabeculations are fine
• A prominent trabecula septomarginalis is present on the septal surface	
• The trabeculations of the right ventricle are coarse	

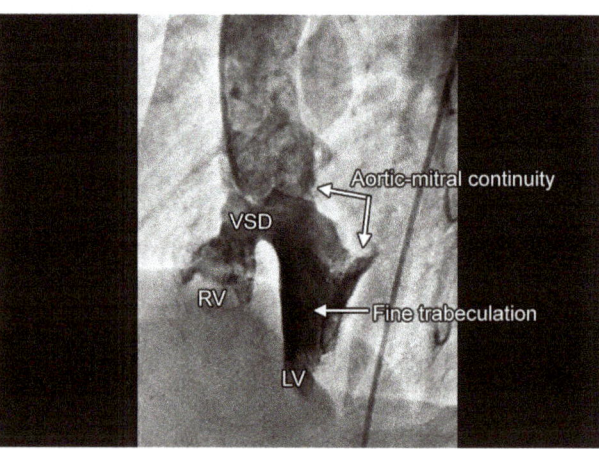

(LV: left ventricular; RV: right ventricular; VSD: ventricular septal defect)
Fig. 6: Right and left ventricular angiographic morphology.

Double-inlet Ventricle

Double-inlet ventricle is the typical univentricular (single or common ventricle)[8] connection where both the AV valves connect with the morphological left ventricle (LV) or right ventricle (RV). This connection has been described in various ways by Van Praagh (**Box 4**), Lev, Kirklin, Anderson, and others (**Fig. 7**).

Single Inlet

There is a single AV connection to one ventricular chamber. This form of univentricular connection results from absence or atresia of either right or left AV valve (**Figs. 8A and B** and **9A and B**).

Common Inlet Ventricle (Fig. 10)

- Both atria are communicating with one ventricle by a common AV valve.
- It is an association with AV septal defect with absence of the primum portion or whole of the atrial septum.
- It can be described as an extreme form of unbalanced AV septal defect. RV is the dominant ventricle with a hypoplastic RV.
- Situs is often ambiguous.

ATRIOVENTRICULAR ALIGNMENT

Atrioventricular alignment includes the following discussed here (**Box 5**).

BOX 4	Van Praagh classification double inlet ventricle.
• Double inlet left ventricle (DILV)	• Double inlet ventricle (mixed)
• Double inlet right ventricle (DIRV)	• Double inlet ventricle (indeterminate)

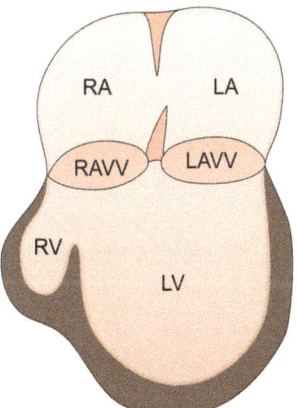

(LA: left atrium; LV: left ventricle; RA: right atrium; RV: right ventricle; LAVV: left atrioventricular valve; RAVV: right atrioventricular valve)

Fig. 7: Double inlet ventricle.

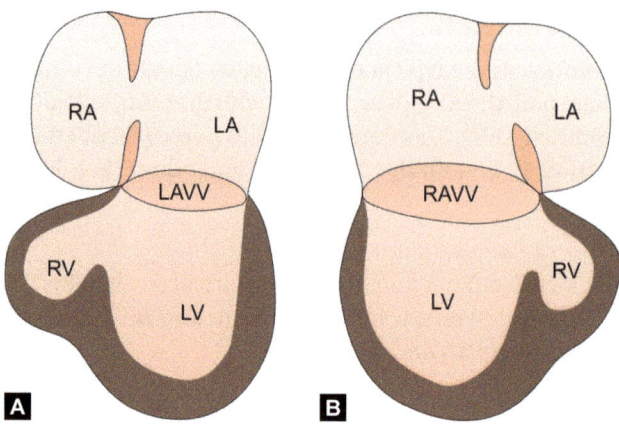

(LA: left atrium; LV: left ventricle; RA: right atrium; RV: right ventricle; LAVV: left atrioventricular valve; RAVV: right atrioventricular valve)

Figs. 8A and B: Single inlet ventricle: Absence of right and left atrioventricular connection.

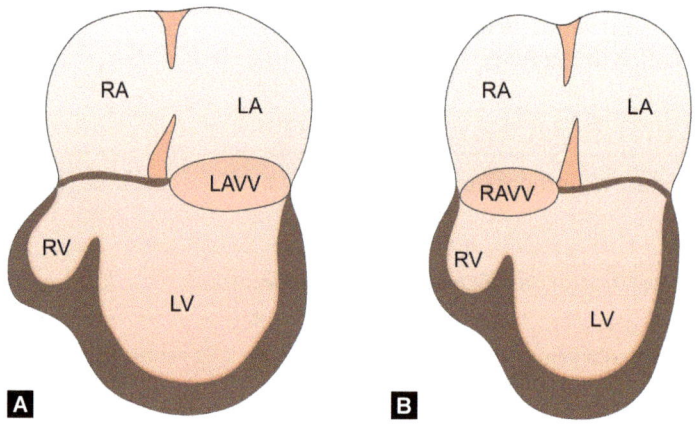

(LA: left atrium; LV: left ventricle; RA: right atrium; RV: right ventricle; LAVV: left atrioventricular valve; RAVV: right atrioventricular valve)

Figs. 9A and B: (A) Right atrioventricular (AV) valve atresia; and (B) Left AV valve atresia.

Atrioventricular Alignment: Concordance

Atrioventricular concordance is present when morphological right atrium connects with morphological RV, and morphological left atrium connects with morphological LV (**Fig. 11A**).

Atrioventricular Connection: Discordance

Atrioventricular discordance is present when morphological right atrium connects with morphological LV, and morphological left atrium connects with morphological RV (**Fig. 11B**).

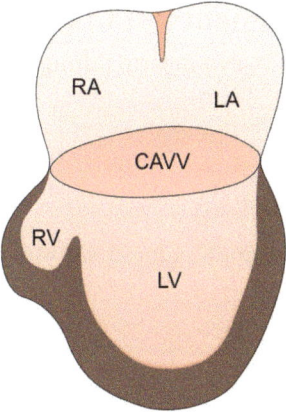

(LA: left atrium; LV: left ventricle; RA: right atrium; RV: right ventricle; CAVV: common atrioventricular valve)

Fig. 10: Common inlet ventricle.

BOX 5	Atrioventricular alignment.
• Concordant	• Ambiguous
• Discordant	• Straddling and overriding

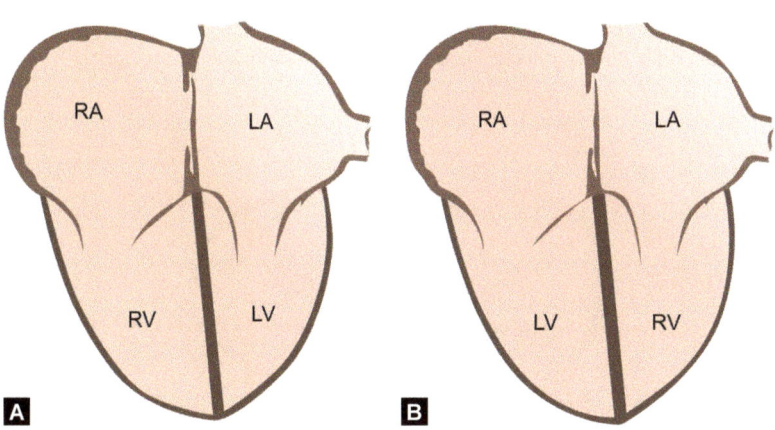

(LA: left atrium; LV: left ventricle; RA: right atrium; RV: right ventricle)

Figs. 11A and B: Atrioventricular alignment. (A) Concordant; and (B) Discordant.

Atrioventricular Alignment: Overriding

Overriding: Commitment of the AV valve annulus to the ventricular chamber. Malalignment between atrial and ventricular septum leads to overriding of the AV valve annulus (**Fig. 12A**).

Atrioventricular Alignment: Straddling

Tensor apparatus of one AV valve inserts through the VSD in the contralateral ventricle (**Fig. 12B**).

Atrioventricular Alignment: Both Overriding and Straddling

Rarely both overriding and straddling may be present in same patient (**Fig. 13**).

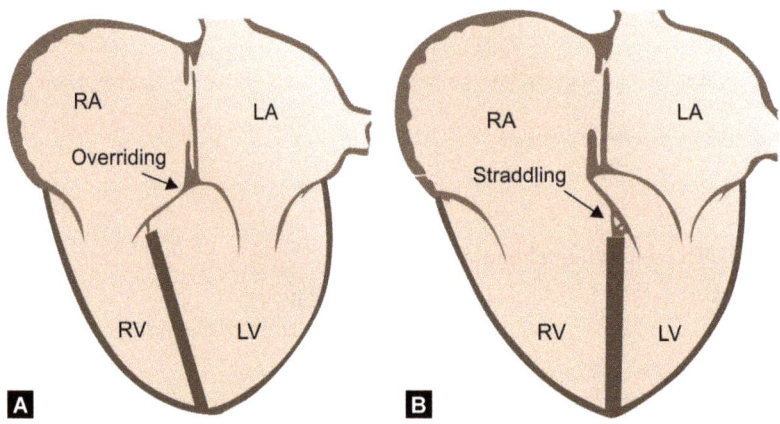

(LA: left atrium; LV: left ventricle; RA: right atrium; RV: right ventricle)

Figs. 12A and B: Atrioventricular alignment. (A) Overriding; and (B) Straddling.

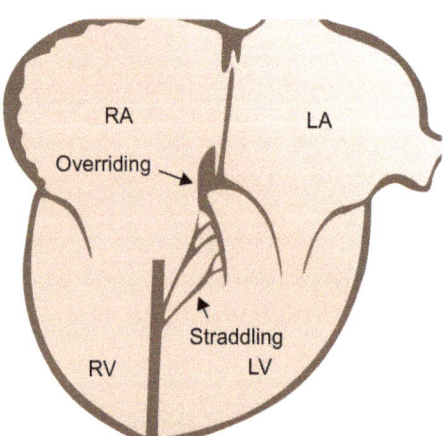

(LA: left atrium; LV: left ventricle; RA: right atrium; RV: right ventricle)

Fig. 13: Atrioventricular alignment: Both overriding and straddling in same heart.

LOOP

Loop refers to folding of the embryonic cardiac tube at about 23 days of gestation. The loop normally bends toward right (dextrally or D-loop). As a result, the portion of the primitive heart tube destined to become RV lies to the right of the anatomic LV. If it bends to the left (L-loop), RV lies to the left of LV. Thus, a D-loop is normal in situs solitus and an L-loop is normal in situs inversus (**Fig. 14**).

In situs solitus, L-loop ventricle and AV discordance are essentially synonymous. The morphologic RV develops from the bulbus cordis, and the morphologic LV develops from the ventricle of the bulboventricular loop. Thus, in D-loop, the morphologic RV is to the right of the morphologic LV and in L-loop, the morphologic RV is to the left of the morphologic LV. At the onset, with situs solitus and formation of a D-bulboventricular loop, the apex of the heart is in the right hemithorax.

At the end of the first month of fetal life, the apex of the heart migrates from the right thorax to the left. In situs inversus with formation of an L-loop, the apex of the heart swings from the left thorax to the right. In general, all D-bulboventricular loops should end development with the heart in the left hemithorax (levocardia), and all L-bulboventricular loops should become dextrocardia. Failure of this shift of the ventricular apex can result in dextrocardia with situs solitus (dextroversion) or levocardia with situs inversus (levoversion).

Dextrocardia can result from:
- D-bulboventricular loop that fails to undergo a shift into left hemithorax, or
- L-bulboventricular loop that completes its apical shift into the right hemithorax.
- Situs inversus, D-loop ventricles, and D-transposition of the great arteries (D-TGA) are a discordant AV connection and result in congenitally corrected D-TGA. This loop is uncommon, because discordant bulboventricular loop development is unusual even in situs inversus.
- Situs inversus, L-loop ventricle, and L-TGA are, on the converse, a concordant AV connection and result in L-TGA.

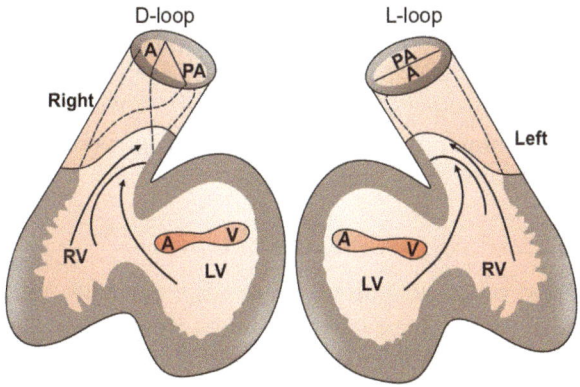

LV: left ventricle; RV: right ventricle; PA: pulmonary artery)

Fig. 14: Ventricular loop.

Loop: Congenitally Corrected TGA

Thus, L-loop in situs solitus is congenitally corrected L-TGA, while D-loop in situs inversus is congenitally corrected D-TGA. Both L-loop in solitus and D-loop in inversus result in AV discordance. It is unclear why discordant cardiac loops have such a strong association with TGA, resulting in congenitally corrected TGA. The discordant cardiac loop must somehow influence conotruncal development favoring VA discordance.

Interestingly, most cases of corrected TGA with situs solitus do not have dextrocardia, because the formation of the discordant cardiac loop appears to impede complete migration of the apex of an L-bulboventricular loop into the right hemithorax.

Loop: Transposition of the Great Arteries

D-loop in situs solitus with transposition is D-TGA, while L-loop in situs inversus with transposition is L-TGA. Both D-loop in solitus and L-loop in inversus result in AV concordance.

Bulboventricular Loop

- *L-loop with situs inversus, dextrocardia, and inverted great vessels*: Situs inversus totalis or the mirror-image dextrocardia.
- *D-loop with situs solitus, dextrocardia, and normally related great arteries*: Dextroversion
- *L-loop with situs solitus*: L-TGA (congenitally corrected TGA)
- *D-loop with situs inversus*: D-TGA (congenitally corrected TGA)
- *L-loop with situs inversus*: L-TGA
- *The classic type of corrected TGA is a discordant cardiac L-loop*: Situs solitus with L-loop ventricles and L-TGA (**Figs. 15** to **17**).

VENTRICULOARTERIAL CONNECTION

To ascertain VA connection, one will have to identify two ventricles, the septum and ventricular origin of both the arteries. This step does not need to identify spatial interrelations of the arteries or position of their coni (**Boxes 6** to **8**) (**Fig. 18**). That can be decided as a next step.

Van Praagh recommends that aberrations in conotruncal development be regarded as malpositions of the great arteries.

Normal Ventriculoarterial Connection

Usually, normally connected arteries are also normally related, with few exceptions. The aortic valve is posterior and on the opposite side of the LV in relation to the pulmonary valve. Thus, when the LV is on left side, a normally related aortic valve will be on the right side of the pulmonary valve and vice versa.

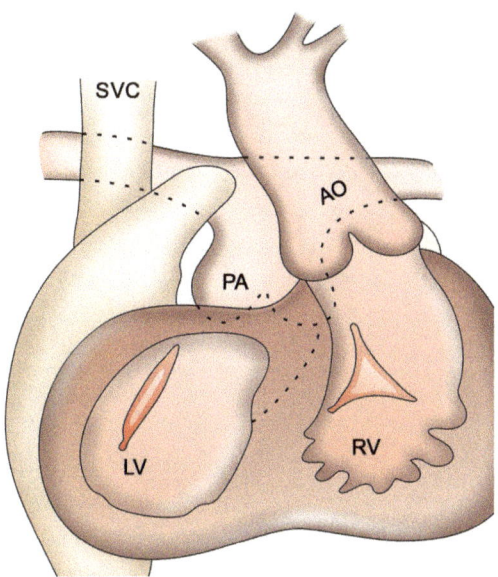

(AO: aorta; LV: left ventricle; RV: right ventricle; PA: pulmonary artery; SVC: superior vena cava)

Fig. 15: Classic congenitally corrected transposition of the great arteries (TGA): Situs solitus with L-loop ventricles and L-TGA.

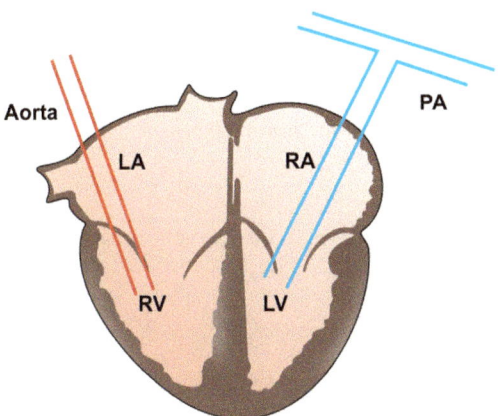

(LA: left atrium; LV: left ventricle; RA: right atrium; RV: right ventricle; PA: pulmonary artery)

Fig. 16: Situs inversus, atrioventricular discordance (D-loop), corrected transposition with D-malposition of aorta.

Transposition

Literally, the composite term "transposition" means "crossed position." Here, both great arteries are placed across the septum so as to arise from morphologically inappropriate ventricles. The term transposition describes the connection, whereas the terms d- or l- as applied to transposition are used to indicate the

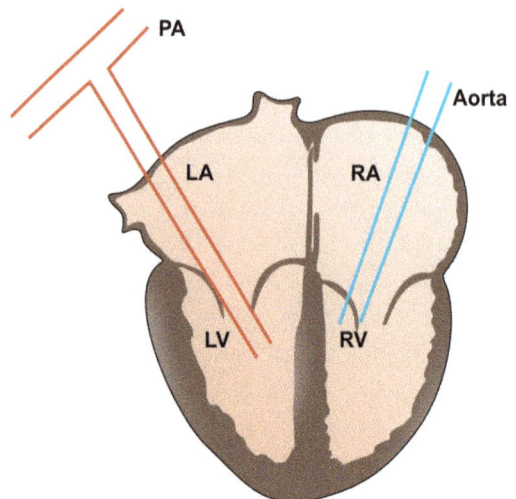

(LA: left atrium; LV: left ventricle; RA: right atrium; RV: right ventricle; PA: pulmonary artery)

Fig. 17: Situs inversus, atrioventricular concordance (L-loop), transposition with L-malposition of aorta.

BOX 6	Ventriculoarterial connection: Van Praagh.
• Transposition	• Double outlet left ventricle
• Double outlet right ventricle	• Anatomically corrected malposition

BOX 7	Ventriculoarterial connection: Tal Geva.

- Concordant
- Discordant:
  - Transposition of the great arteries (TGA) with ventricular D-loop
  - TGA with ventricular L-loop
- Double outlet right ventricle
- Double outlet left ventricle
- Atretic:
  - Pulmonary atresia
  - Aortic atresia
- Single outlet
- Ventriculoarterial connection

spatial relation of aortic to pulmonary valve, aortic valve to right or to left of the pulmonary valve and convey no information regarding VA connections. Even, rarely, aorta may be anterior (o-transposition) or behind (p-transposition) to pulmonary valve. Thus, it is best to think of TGA simply as formation of discordant VA connections rather than overemphasizing the anteroposterior relationship between the aorta and pulmonary artery.

> **BOX 8** **Ventriculoarterial connection: PS Rao.**
> - Type 1: NRGA
> - Type 2: D-TGA
> - Type 3: (great artery position abnormalities, other than D-transposition)
>   - Subtype 1: L-TGA
>   - Subtype 2: Double outlet right ventricle
>   - Subtype 3: Double outlet left ventricle
>   - Subtype 4: D-MPGA (anatomically corrected malposition)
>   - Subtype 5: L-MPGA (anatomically corrected malposition)
> - Type 4: Single outlet (truncus)
>
> *Anderson classification:*
> - Normal
> - Transposition
> - Double outlet
> - Single outlet
>
> (NRGA: normally related great arteries; TGA: transposition of the great arteries; MPGA: malposed great arteries)

Others are in opinion of two anatomic requirements:
1. Great arteries should reverse the interrelationships with the ventricles.
2. They should also reverse their mutual interrelationships.

Aberrant conotruncal development can lead to development of an infundibulum below the semilunar valve of the ascending aorta, moving it forward to form continuity with the morphologic RV, while the pulmonary artery forms a connection to the morphologic LV. In most of these cases, the main pulmonary artery is displaced posteriorly and oriented parallel to the aorta when viewed from the side, rather than spiraling around the ascending aorta. This disorder is termed "transposition of the great arteries."

When transposition occurs in the D-bulboventricular loop, the transposed aortic valve is usually located to the right of the transposed pulmonic valve. Hence, this is designated as D-TGA. When transposition occurs in the L-bulboventricular loop, the transposed aortic valve usually lies to the left of the transposed pulmonic valve. Therefore, this is designated as L-TGA.

Double Outlet

One and more than half of other arteries arising from the same ventricle. Bilateral conus is not a prerequisite. When >50% of aorta is from LV, it is Tetralogy of Fallot (TOF); >50% from RV, it is DORV; when >50% of pulmonary artery from LV, it is Taussig–Bing. Someone (including Kirklin) consider that aorticomitral discontinuity should be there to call it DORV, otherwise, it should be called as TOF even the overriding is >50%. Similarly, a subpulmonic conus must be present to call it Taussig–Bing, not the simple 50–50 rule. Interrelation of great arteries in DORV or double outlet left ventricle (DOLV) can be described as d- or l-malposition.

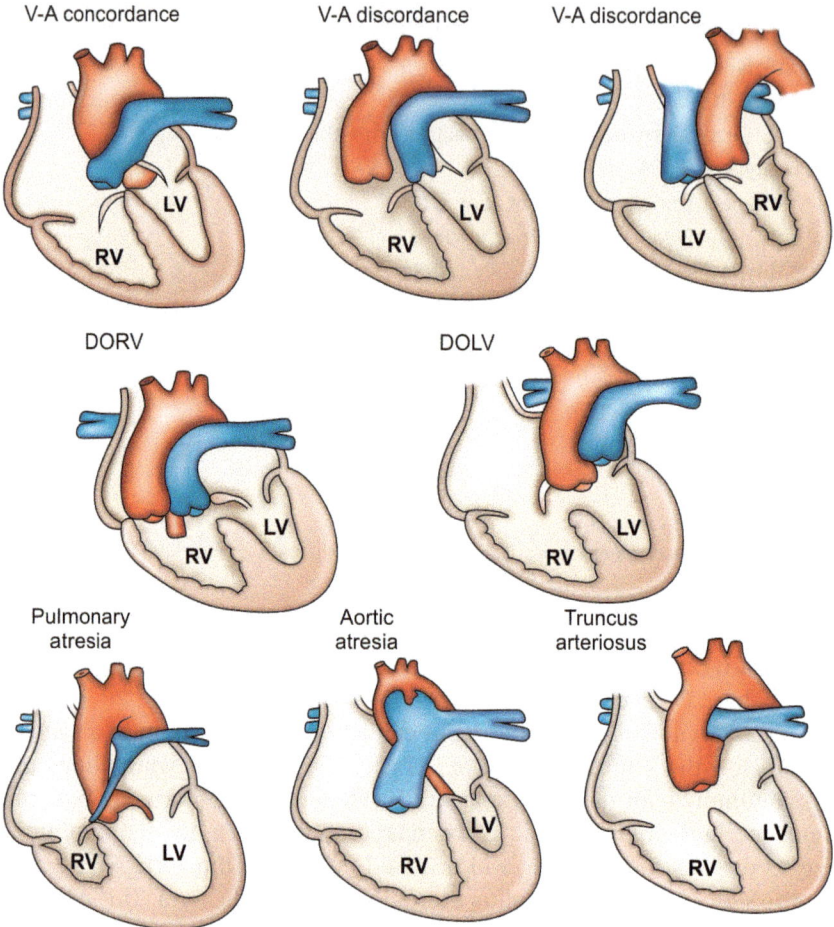

(DORV: double outlet right ventricle; DOLV: double outlet left ventricle; LV: left ventricle; RV: right ventricle

Fig. 18: Ventriculoarterial (VA) connection.

Single Arterial Trunk

Single trunk may be either common arterial trunk or solitary arterial trunk. When a single arterial trunk arises from ventricular mass through a common VA junction and gives origin of systemic, pulmonary, and coronary circulation, it is called common arterial trunk. When the origin of an atretic artery from ventricle cannot be ascertained and other artery arises from either of the two ventricles, or overriding the septum, it is called solitary trunk (aortic atresia or pulmonary atresia).

CONUS

The term "conus", applies to the muscular cardiac segment intervening between the semilunar and AV valves. Absorption reduces the length of the aortic conus from about 400 to 20 microns. Consequently, there is an aorticomitral fibrous continuity. The proximal half of the pulmonary conus is also absorbed, and its length is reduced from about 400 to 200 microns. As a result of the absorption of the proximal conus (underneath the aorta and the pulmonary artery) the distal conus with its septum acts as the conal septum of the subpulmonary portion of the ventricular septum (**Fig. 19**).

GREAT ARTERY SPATIAL RELATIONS

Great artery relation means interrelation of two great vessels in space (**Box 9**) (**Fig. 20**).

Spatial Relation: Anatomically Corrected Malposition (S, D, L)

Here, the great arteries are abnormally related to the ventricles and to each other but nonetheless arise above the anatomically correct ventricles. In the absence of associated malformations, anatomically corrected malposition is associated with

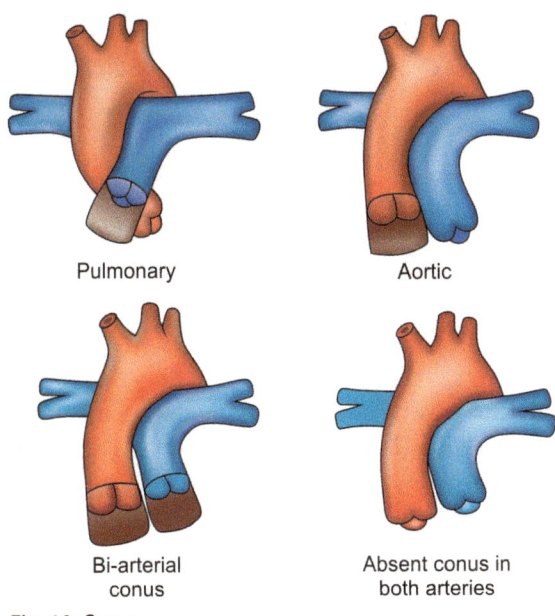

Pulmonary   Aortic

Bi-arterial conus   Absent conus in both arteries

Fig. 19: Conus.

BOX 9   **Great artery special relation.**

- Solitus
- Inversus
- D-malposition (aorta anterior and right)
- Anterior malposition (aorta anterior)
- L-malposition (aorta anterior and left)
- Posterior malposition (aorta posterior)

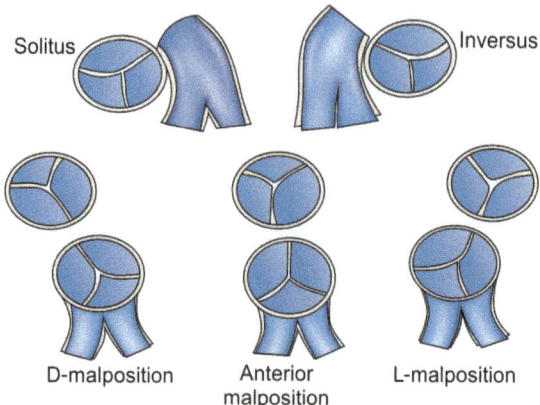

Fig. 20: Great artery spatial relation.

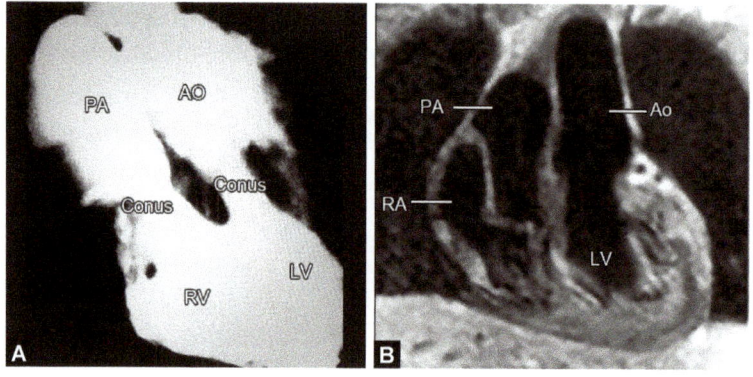

(AO: aorta; LV: left ventricle; PA: pulmonary artery; RA: right atrium; RV: right ventricle; RPA: right pulmonary artery)

Figs. 21A and B: Anatomically corrected malposition.

normal physiology and may be detected incidentally. Situs solitus of viscera and atria (S), ventricular D-loop (D), and L-malposition of great arteries (L). Aorta is superior, and leftward relative to the pulmonary valve and the great vessels are side-by-side. There is bilateral conus with aortic-mitral and pulmonary-tricuspid discontinuity (**Figs. 21A and B**).

Spatial Relation: Aorta in Congenitally Corrected TGA

Ascending aorta arises more anteriorly than the pulmonary trunk. Two great arteries run parallel to each other and never cross. Ascending aorta courses vertically upward or convex to the left. But it is never border forming on the right. Classical triad of ascending aorta on the right and aortic knuckle and pulmonary segment on the left heart border at the base of the heart is typically lost in congenitally corrected TGA. Most common relation is side-by-side with ascending aorta to the left of the medially placed pulmonary trunk, producing absent vascular shadow in the right base and unimpressive aortic shadow on left border. Sometimes, ascending aorta originates directly in front of the pulmonary trunk resulting in narrow stalk. Ascending aorta forms the base of the left border; depending upon the root size and spatial relation, aortic shadow might be absent, concave, straight, convex to strikingly convex (**Box 10**) (**Figs. 22A and B**).

Spatial Relation: Aorta

- *Levocardia, situs solitus*: Ascending aorta on the right, aortic knuckle on the left; descending aorta on the left vertebral border.
- *Dextrocardia, situs inversus*: Ascending aorta on the left, aortic knuckle on the right; descending aorta on the right vertebral border. Apex is formed by LV.
- *Dextrocardia, situs solitus, D-loop*: Ascending aorta on the right, aortic knuckle on the left; descending aorta on the left vertebral border. Apex is formed by RV.
- *Dextrocardia, situs solitus, L-loop*: Ascending aorta forms a prominent leftward sweep (L-loop/L-transposition), aortic knuckle on the right; descending aorta on the left vertebral border. Apex is formed by LV.
- *Levocardia, situs inversus*: Ascending aorta forms a prominent leftward sweep indicating D-transposition in situs inversus (congenitally corrected transposition), aortic knuckle on the right and descending aorta on the right vertebral border.

BOX 10	Spatial relation: Ascending aorta in left and anterior to pulmonary artery.
<ul><li>Congenitally corrected transposition of the great arteries (TGA)</li><li>TGA, situs inversus, L-loop: L-malposition of aorta</li><li>Anatomically corrected L-malposition of aorta</li></ul>	<ul><li>Aorta arising from inverted outflow chamber in univentricular connection</li><li>Double outlet ventricles</li><li>Cris-cross ventricles</li></ul>

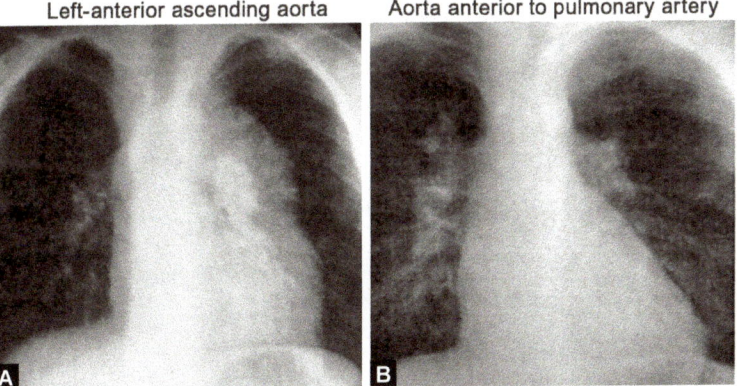

Figs. 22A and B: Spatial relation: Aorta in left anterior position and anterior position.

CONCLUSION

Segmental approach helps to formulate the complete diagnosis in congenital heart disease. A detailed clinical examination, ECG, and X-ray chest supported by echocardiogram build-up the multifloored building of segmental approach. Even a simple congenital heart disease like ASD or VSD should be evaluated by segmental approach, otherwise any associated lesion like partial anomalous venous drainage, or left-sided superior vena cava can be missed.

REFERENCES

1. Van Praagh R. The segmental approach to diagnosis in congenital heart disease. Birth Defects: Original Article Series. 1972;8:4.
2. Stanger P, Rudolph AM, Edwards JE. Cardiac malpositions: An over- view based on study of 65 necropsy specimens. Circulation. 1977;56:159.
3. Van Praagh R, Weinberg PM, Van Praagh S. Malposition of the heart. In: Moss AJ, Adams FH, Emmanouilides G (Eds). Heart Disease in Infants, Children and Adolescents, 2 edition. Baltimore, Williams & Wilkins Co., in press.
4. Van Praagh R, Viad P. Dextrocardia, mesocardia and levocardia. The segmental approach to diagnosis in congenital heart disease. In: Keith JD, Rowe RD, Vlad P (Eds). Heart Disease in Infancy and Childhood, 3 edition. New York, Macmillan Co.; 1978.
5. Melhuish BPP, Van Praagh R. Juxtaposition of the atrial appendages. Br Heart J. 1968;30:269.
6. Van Praagh R. How does the "segmental approach" help us understand complex lesions? In: Eldredge WJ, Lemole GM, Goldberg H (Eds). Current Problems in Congenital Heart Disease. New York, Spectrum Publications.
7. Lev M. Pathologic diagnosis of positional variations in cardiac chambers in congenital heart disease. Lab Invest. 1954;3:71.
8. Van Praagh R, Ongley PA, Swan HJC. Anatomic types of single or common ventricle in man. Am J Cardiol. 1964;13:367.

CHAPTER 27

Clinical Approach: Congenital Cyanotic Heart Disease

INTRODUCTION

The patient is having heart disease! He is having it since birth. Patient looks blue. So, a simple logic can establish that the patient is suffering from congenital cyanotic heart disease. Then, what is the final diagnosis? Let us do an echocardiogram and make the diagnosis! Otherwise, if we want to enjoy the charm of clinical approach, we should follow the following steps!

FIRST STEP

First step to approach common congenital cyanotic heart disease (CCHD) is to classify them into five major types, according to pathophysiology.

Pathophysiological Classification

- Tetralogy physiology
- Eisenmenger physiology (EP)
- Common mixing physiology
- Transposition physiology
- Mixed physiology

Tetralogy Physiology

Tetralogy physiology is obstruction at the outlet, which is supporting pulmonary circulation resulting in the supporting ventricular pressure at systemic level. This pulmonary ventricle decompresses through large septal defect, resulting in balanced or predominantly right to left shunt.

Transposition Physiology

Transposition physiology is a pattern, where systemic and pulmonary circulations are parallel. It includes D-transposition of the great arteries (TGA), double outlet right ventricle (DORV), and subpulmonic ventricular septal defect (VSD).

> **BOX 1 | Common mixing lesion.**
> - Tricuspid atresia, mitral atresia
> - Single ventricle
> - Truncus arteriosus
> - Total anomalous pulmonary venous connection
> - Common atrium
> - Double outlet right ventricle, double outlet left ventricle
> - Pulmonary atresia, aortic atresia

When transposition is associated with large VSD and pulmonary stenosis (PS), it behaves as tetralogy physiology. On the other hand, when transposition is associated with unobstructed pulmonary flow, it behaves as EP.

Eisenmenger Physiology
Eisenmenger physiology is pulmonary hypertension at systemic level with shunt reversal at the level of atrial septal defect (ASD), VSD, aortopulmonary window, and patent ductus arteriosus (PDA).

Common Mixing Physiology
A mixing chamber in which systemic and pulmonary venous return come together (**Box 1**).

Amongst the mixing lesions, when tricuspid atresia is associated with VSD, PS, and when univentricular connection is associated with PS, these two mixing lesions will behave as tetralogy physiology. On the other hand, when those two mixing lesions are associated with unobstructed pulmonary flow, they will behave as EP.

Mixed Physiology
Mixed physiology is found in complex cyanotic heart diseases, where effectively two physiologies act together:
- TGA, VSD, PS (transposition + Fallot's physiology)
- Tricuspid atresia, VSD, PS (mixing + Fallot's physiology)
- Univentricular connection, PS (mixing + Fallot's physiology)

SECOND STEP

History
A detailed history is utmost important, which includes day or week of presentation with cyanosis or heart failure or failure to thrive, evolution of symptoms, history of "cool down" of symptom, and history of spell (**Table 1**).

May be more important the usual age of presentation rather than specific cyanosis. This is because babies with cyanotic heart disease may present with other feature like heart failure, where cyanosis is trivial. There are several factors, which determine the age of presentation (**Tables 2 to 6**).

TABLE 1: Onset of cyanosis.

Earliest onset	Late onset
D-TGA	Eisenmenger physiology
PA, intact septum	TAPVC
PA, VSD	Ebstein's anomaly
Obstructed TAPVC	PS, stretched PFO
Tricuspid atresia	
Ebstein's anomaly	

(PFO: patent foramen ovale; PS: pulmonary stenosis; TGA: transposition of the great arteries; PA: pulmonary artery; VSD: ventricular septal defect; TAPVC: total anomalous pulmonary venous connection)

TABLE 2: Determinants of age of presentation with congenital heart disease.

Age	Physiological determinants	Change in physiology
0–3 days	Transitional circulation changing to neonatal circulation	Parallel nonmixing circulation and critically obstructed series circulation
4–14 days	• Ductus closing	• Obstructed pulmonary and descending aortic flow
	• Fall of neonatal pulmonary vascular resistance	• Pulmonary edema
2–18 weeks	Further remodeling of pulmonary circulation	Pulmonary edema
4–12 month	Growth, shifting of fetal hemoglobin, increasing activity	Appearance of cyanosis, growth retardation

TABLE 3: Congenital heart disease presenting from birth to 3 days of age.

Physiology	Disease
Parallel nonmixing circulation	Transposition of the great arteries
Critically obstructed series circulation	• Hypoplastic right heart syndrome
	• Severe Ebstein's anomaly
	• Hypoplastic left heart syndrome
	• Critical pulmonary stenosis
	• Obstructed total anomalous pulmonary venous connection

TABLE 4: Congenital heart disease presenting 4–14 days of age.

Physiology	Disease
Obstructed pulmonary flow	• Severe form of tetralogy of Fallot
	• Tricuspid atresia
	• TGA, VSD, pulmonary stenosis
	• Single ventricle, pulmonary stenosis
Obstructed descending aortic flow	Severe coarctation of aorta
Pulmonary edema	• Large PDA
	• Truncus arteriosus
	• Large arteriovenous malformation

(PDA: patent ductus arteriosus; TGA: transposition of the great arteries; VSD: ventricular septal defect)

TABLE 5: Congenital heart disease presenting 2–18 weeks of age.

Physiology	Disease
Heart failure	• Large VSD • AV canal defect • TAPVC • TGA, VSD • Single ventricle • ALCAPA

(ALCAPA: anomalous left coronary artery from the pulmonary artery; AV: atrioventricular; TAPVC: total anomalous pulmonary venous connection; TGA: transposition of the great arteries; VSD: ventricular septal defect)

TABLE 6: Congenital heart disease presenting 4–12 months of age.

Physiology	Disease
Appearance of cyanosis	Tetralogy physiology
Growth retardation or incidental detection of murmur	• VSD • PDA • ASD • Coarctation • Pulmonary stenosis • Aortic stenosis

(ASD: atrial septal defect; VSD: ventricular septal defect; PDA: patent ductus arteriosus)

BOX 2 | **Cyanosis with increased flow.**

- Transposition physiology
- TAPVC
- Common mixing lesions with unobstructed pulmonary flow
- PA, VSD with several MAPCAS

(MAPCAS: major aortopulmonary collateral arteries; PA: pulmonary artery; TAPVC: total anomalous pulmonary venous connection; VSD: ventricular septal defect)

History Suggestive of Increased Flow (Box 2)

Recurrent respiratory infection does not help much. More important is mother's description:
- Tachypneic kid with distressed breathing
- *Distress is more during feeding:* incomplete, interrupted, and prolonged feeding associated with sweating
- "Spoilt" kid, preferring mother's lap
- "Failure to thrive"
- Simple respiratory infection may become eventful
- Major pneumonia
- Beyond first year, those symptoms gradually cool down.

History: Gradual Cool Down of Symptoms of Increased Flow/Congestive Heart Failure
- Eisenmenger syndrome
- *Late onset PS:* Univentricular heart
- *VSD becomes restrictive:* Tricuspid atresia
- Acquired PS in large VSD (Gasul effect).

History of Spell
History of spell and a spontaneous folding of legs (knee-chest position) are suggestive of tetralogy physiology.

THIRD STEP

General Examination

Differential Cyanosis
Patent ductus arteriosus with pulmonary hypertension or PDA with aortic arch interruption or severe coarctation

Reverse Differential Cyanosis
Higher-lower-body SpO_2:
- Transposition complexes, PDA with or without aortic coarctation/interruption.
- Supracardiac total anomalous pulmonary venous connection (TAPVC) with patent ducts (rarely).

Pulse

Absent Lower Limb Pulsations
- Double outlet right ventricle, subpulmonic VSD
- Truncus arteriosus
- Univentricular heart.

Jugular Venous Pulse
- *Tetralogy of Fallot (TOF):* Jugular venous pulse (JVP) is usually inconspicuous. Ageing, systemic hypertension can produce prominent *a* wave. Heart failure due to different cause produces prominent *v* wave; postoperative: *a* and *v* waves.
- *Prominent a wave*: Tricuspid atresia, pulmonary atresia with intact septum, and PS with stretched patent foramen ovale (PFO).
- *Eisenmenger physiology*: Prominent *a* and *v* waves in ASD.
- *TAPVC*: Prominent *v* wave.
- *Ebstein's anomaly*: Prominent *a* and *v* waves are occasionally found due to hypokinetic tricuspid regurgitation and commodious right atrium.

Palpation
Thrill
- Exception, if cyanosis is very obvious
- PS, stretched PFO
- Double outlet right ventricle, restrictive VSD
- Tricuspid atresia, PS restrictive VSD
- Univentricular heart, across the bulboventricular communication
- TOF with absent pulmonary valve (APV).

Apical Impulse (Most Common is RV Type Apex)
- *Left ventricle (LV) type apex:*
  - Tricuspid atresia
  - Pulmonary atresia with intact septum
  - Univentricular (LV) heart
  - Ebstein's anomaly
  - Left superior vena cava to left atrial communication.
- *Absent RV activity*: Hypoplastic right heart syndrome.

Heart Sound
S1
- *Wide split with loud T1 component:* Ebstein's anomaly
- *Absent T1 component:* Tricuspid atresia.

S2
- *Fixed, wide:* TAPVC, ASD with shunt reversal
- *Normal/narrow/single:* PDA with shunt reversal
- *Single loud S2 (A2):* Any entity in tetralogy physiology with severe PS, CCHD with malposed great arteries
- *Single loud S2 (P2):* VSD with shunt reversal
- When cyanosis is mild and great arteries are normally related, P2, thought soft, may be preserved in tetralogy physiology
- A preserved P2, whatever may be the degree of cyanosis, excludes truncus arteriosus, pulmonary atresia, and TOF with APV.

S3/S4
- *Multiple heart sound:* Ebstein's anomaly
- *S4:* PS with stretched PFO, ASD EP
- *S4 (LV):* Corresponds the right atrial *a* wave and denoting a nonrestrictive ASD in tricuspid atresia.

Ejection Click
- *Pulmonary vascular click:* EP

- *Aortic click:* More severe the PS, more is the probability of getting it in tetralogy physiology.
- *Very prominent, high pitched:* Truncus arteriosus.

Murmur

Systolic Murmur
- Severe the cyanosis, lesser is the grade of the murmur
- Exception is the obligatory murmurs in DORV, VSD, PS, tricuspid atresia, VSD (more so when VSD is restrictive), and in univentricular heart (bulbo-ventricular flow).

Diastolic Murmur
- Truncal regurgitation
- TOF with APV
- TOF with aortic regurgitation
- Graham Steell murmur in EP

Continuous Murmur
- Major aortopulmonary collateral arteries/PDA
- Pulmonary arteriovenous fistula
- Post Blalock-Taussig shunt
- TAPVC
- Truncus arteriosus

Thus, from clinical examination, initial impression: CCHD with increased or decreased flow.

Increased flow:
- TGA
- TAPVC
- Truncus arteriosus
- L-R shunt leading to EP
- VSD, PA with several MAPCAs
- All other mixing physiology with unobstructed pulmonary circulation.

Decreased flow:
- Tetralogy physiology

FOURTH STEP: TO LOOK AT X-RAY CHEST FOR VASCULARITY

Fourth step is to look at X-ray chest for vascularity (**Figs. 1A and b**).

X-ray Chest with Increased Flow
- Equalization
- Pulmonary vessels can be traced in the lateral one-third of the lungs

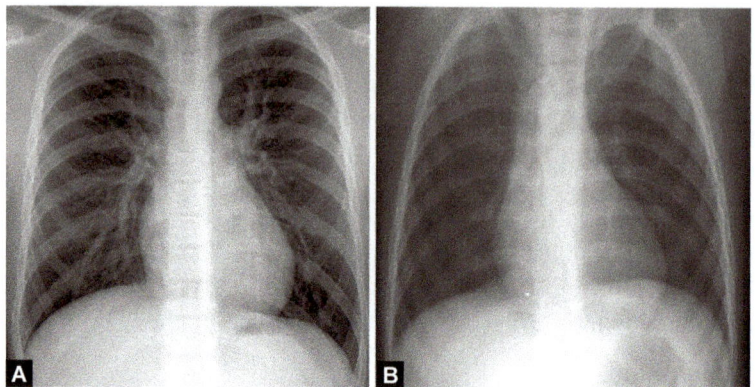

Figs. 1A and B: (A) Increased flow; (B) Reduced flow.

- Dense hilum with increased number of hilar pulmonary arteries, as evidenced by >3–5 end-on.
- Dilated right descending pulmonary artery, which can be traced below the diaphragm level.
- Diameter of the right descending pulmonary artery is larger than that of trachea. The diameter is measured at widest point distal to right middle lobe artery.[17]
- When it's diameter >16 mm.
- Artery-bronchial ratio (ABR) in upper lobe >1.
- The margins of the enlarged pulmonary vessels are sharp and clean.
- On left heart border, pulmonary artery segment may show more bulging.
- Cardiac size may be increased.

Increased Flow: TGA

Figure 2 shows increased flow: TGA.
Increased flow: TAPVC
Figure 3 shows increased flow: TAPVC.
Increased flow: Truncus arteriosus
Figure 4 shows increased flow: Truncus arteriosus.
ASD, Eisenmenger physiology
Figure 5 shows ASD, Eisenmenger physiology.

X-ray chest may identify the individual entities amongst the increased-flow group.
Increased flow—four common causes:
1. TGA
2. TAPVC
3. Truncus arteriosus
4. L-R shunt leading to EP (during the process; once developed, becomes reduced flow)

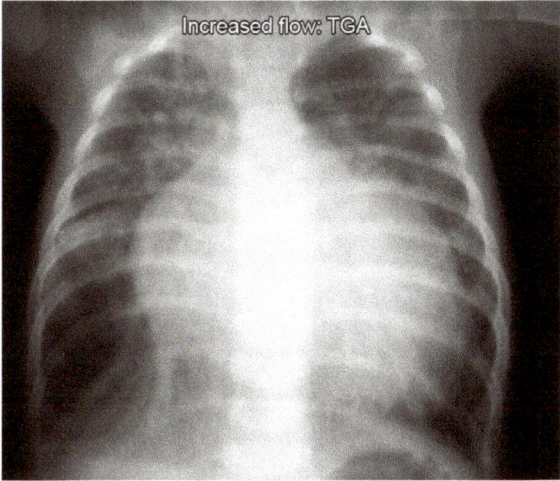

Fig. 2: Egg-on-side, narrow stalk, increased vascularity.

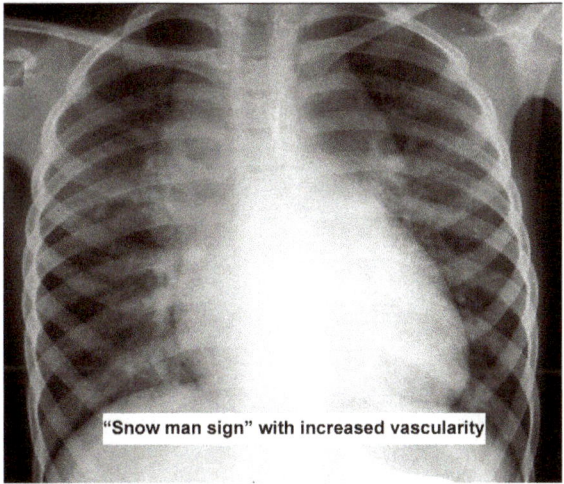

Fig. 3: Snowman sign of total anomalous pulmonary venous connection.

X-ray Chest with Decreased Flow

- Hilum appears less dense and smaller in size.
- All the linear shadows in normal lung fields are due to pulmonary vasculature. In consequence, when flow and therefore vessels sizes are reduced, lungs appear more radiolucent.
- Artery-bronchial ratio
- Normal bronchial artery supply to the lungs is usually so small as to be invisible on the plain X-ray. When there is oligemia due to PS or atresia, the bronchial arteries may dilate it such an extent as to be visible as a mottled appearance in the perihilar region.

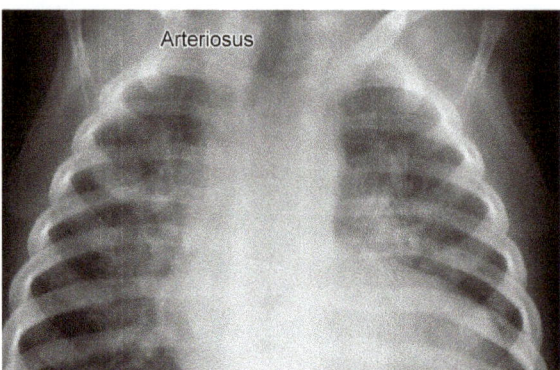

Fig. 4: Truncus arteriosus.

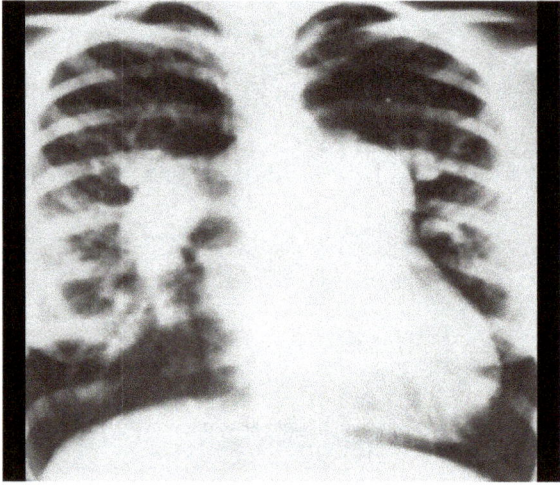

Fig. 5: Atrial septal defect Eisenmenger syndrome.

Then, probabilities are shortlisted to: Diseases under the umbrella of tetralogy physiology.

FIFTH STEP: TO LOOK AT ECG

Fifth step is to look at ECG (**Fig. 6**).

Now, probabilities are shortlisted:
- Tricuspid atresia
- Univentricular connection, noninverted outlet chamber.

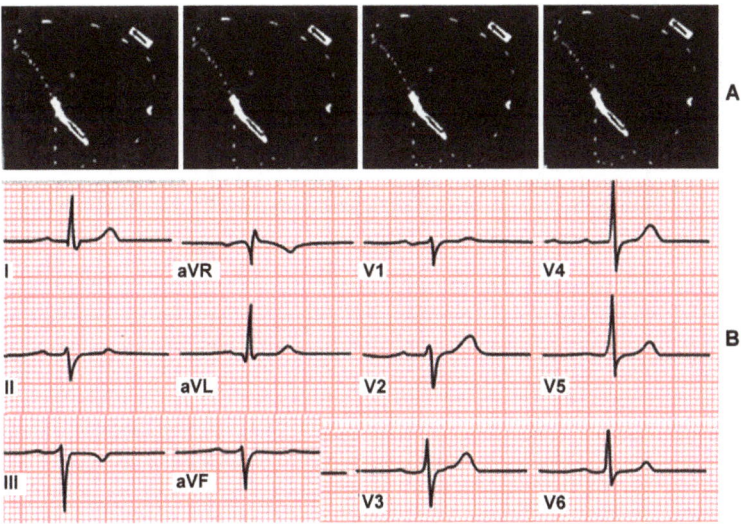

Fig. 6: Left axis, counterclockwise depolarization in frontal plane.

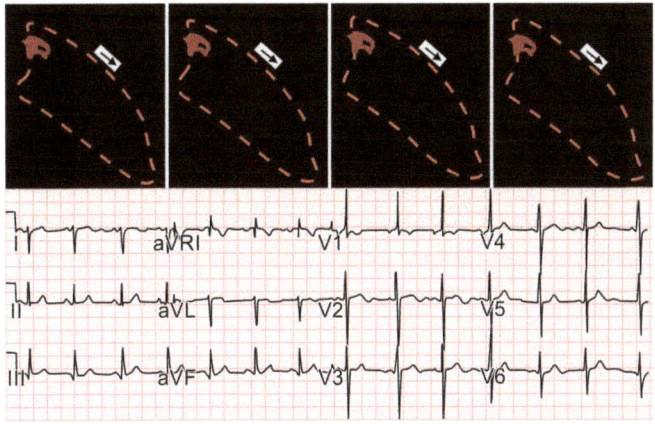

Fig. 7: Right, occasionally left axis, counterclockwise depolarization.

(From type of apex, ECG, and X-Ray chest, individual entity can be established).

Probability is shortlisted to: DORV and PS (**Fig. 7**).
*Then, probabilities are shortlisted to (**Fig. 8**):*
- TOF
- TGA, VSD, and PS
- Univentricular connection, PS, inverted outlet chamber.
(Individual entities described in tetralogy physiology).

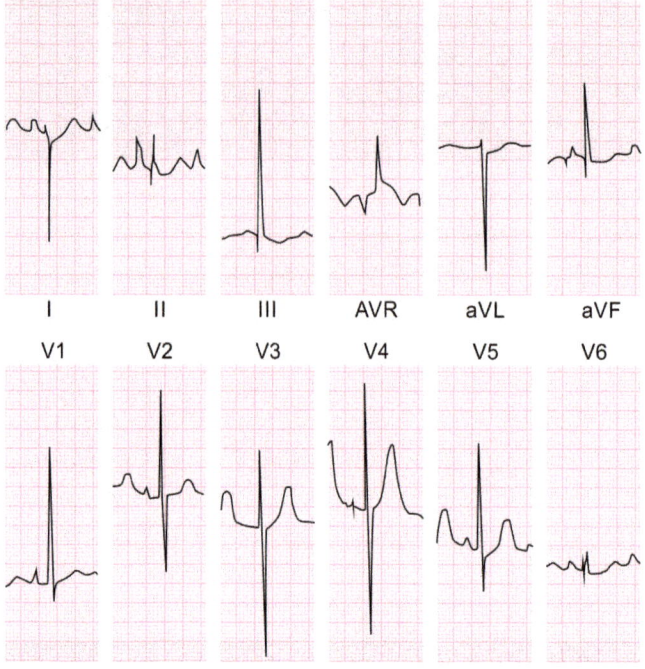

Fig. 8: Right axis, clockwise depolarization, right ventricular hypertrophy.

CONCLUSION

The simple clinical steps, ECG, and X-ray of chest can make a diagnosis in most of the congenital cyanotic heart disease. After this clinical exercise, we should proceed to proper and optimum imaging for final diagnosis.

CHAPTER 28

Clinical Approach: Tetralogy Physiology

INTRODUCTION

Tetralogy physiology is not a very defined entity. Amongst the congenital cyanotic heart diseases with low pulmonary flow, major lesions may be loosely grouped under this terminology. They are completely different in morphology but share a common hemodynamic.

Anatomically, they all share nonrestrictive ventricular septal defect (VSD) along with obstruction at outlet, which is supporting pulmonary circulation. As VSD is nonrestrictive, right and left ventricular (or a single ventricle) pressure and ejection forces are equal. Total pulmonary outflow resistance (TOR) versus systemic vascular resistance (SVR) decides the direction of shunt. Normally SVR is five times more than pulmonary vascular resistance (PVR). Downstream arteriolar beds determine these vascular resistances. SVR is normal, whereas PVR is normal or less than normal in tetralogy physiology. TOR is the combination of PVR and its supporting outlet obstruction at various level (infundibulum, annulus, valve, main, and branch pulmonary artery). TOR rather than only PVR is the actual hemodynamic factor.

When TOR > SVR, shunt is exclusively from pulmonary ventricle, across systemic ventricle toward systemic circulation. When TOR = SVR, shunt is balanced and bidirectional. May be occasionally, TOR < SVR and shunt is from systemic ventricle across pulmonary ventricle toward pulmonary circulation.

TETRALOGY PHYSIOLOGY: HEMODYNAMICS

- Septal defect is a nonrestrictive, large one, resulting in equalization of two ventricular pressure.
- Direction of the shunt will depend upon the resistance in the pulmonary and systemic circulation. It may be bidirectional with dominating right-left (R-L)/dominating left-right (L-R), or it may be exclusively R-L.
- As right ventricle, though working against systemic pressure, is decompressed through large septal defect, its' force of contraction will be not manifested in the jugular pulse pressure or precordium.

- As right ventricular blood is mostly shunted through VSD in systemic circulation, pulmonary flow and pressure will be inadequate to produce an audible P2. On the other hand, enhanced flow through aorta and its malposition may produce a loud A2 and aortic click.
- More severe will be the pulmonary stenosis (PS), more blood will pass in the aorta, resulting in shortening and softening of the murmur across the pulmonary outflow.
- In all the entities of tetralogy physiology, excepting tetralogy of Fallot (TOF), VSD pulmonary atresia and VSD, valvular PS, great arteries may be malposed.
- Commonly, aorta is right and anterior or left and anterior.
- This positional abnormality may alter the clinical finding. A2 may be more prominent, sometimes, palpable. Best audible position may be left or right base.
- Thus, the common hemodynamic feature in tetralogy physiology is equalization of two ventricular and aortic systolic pressure with a pressure gradient between pulmonary artery and the supporting ventricle.
- In TOF, the aortic saturation is higher than pulmonary circulation.
- When in mixing physiology situations, behaving as tetralogy physiology, mixing is adequate, saturation in both arteries should be same.
- In transposition physiology behaving as tetralogy physiology, saturation in pulmonary artery may be higher than the aorta.
- One should remember that the saturation in great arteries depends upon the mixing, streaming, and location of VSD in relation of the great arteries.

TETRALOGY PHYSIOLOGY: HOW TO GRADE SEVERITY?[1,2]

Severity is determined by the grade of PS. Accordingly, it is graded as mild, moderate, severe, and extremely severe.

Mild

- Usually acyanotic at rest; cyanosis is revealed on exercise.
- Aortic click is absent.
- A soft P2 may be audible with a wide split.
- Pulmonary ejection murmur is loud, grade 3 and 4, reaches at crescendo after midsystole and extends at A2, which is not obscured by the murmur.

Moderate

- Grade 2 cyanotic burden.
- Aortic ejection sound is absent.
- A2 is prominent; P2 is not audible.
- Pulmonary ejection murmur is grade 2-4 reaches peak at midsystole, and ends before A2.

Severe
- Grade 3 cyanotic burden.
- Aortic click may be found occasionally.
- A2 is louder.
- Pulmonary ejection murmur is grade 2 and 3, reaches at peak before midsystole and ends well before A2.

Extremely Severe
- Severe cyanotic burden.
- Aortic click is consistently present.
- A2 is louder.
- Pulmonary ejection murmur is soft, reaches early crescendo, ends long before A2.

UNDER UMBRELLA OF TETRALOGY PHYSIOLOGY

Group I (Pure)
- Tetralogy of Fallot.
- VSD, pulmonary atresia.
- VSD, pulmonary valvular stenosis.
- Double outlet right ventricle (DORV) and PS.
- Congenitally corrected transposition of the great arteries (CC-TGA), VSD, and PS.

Group II (Mixed Physiology)
- *Transposition + tetralogy physiology*:
  - TGA, VSD, and PS.
- *Mixing + tetralogy physiology*:
  - Tricuspid atresia, VSD, and PS.
  - Single ventricle (univentricular connection) and PS.

Tetralogy of Fallot
- Cyanosis typically appears between 6 weeks and 6 months of age. Hypoxic spell and squatting are classical symptoms.
- Jugular venous pulse (JVP) is found usually normal in uncomplicated classical TOF. Abnormal JVP may be found in conditions with increased right ventricular filling pressure. Prominent *a* wave (increased atrial support) is found when VSD has become restrictive or patient has developed systemic hypertension or aortic stenosis. Prominent *v/y* wave is found in progressive biventricular aortic regurgitation (AR), infective endocarditis of aortic valve, TOF with absent pulmonary valve with severe pulmonary regurgitation (PR), postoperative progressive PR, postoperative severe right ventricular diastolic dysfunction, and several major aortopulmonary collateral arteries (MAPCAs) leading to left ventricular failure.

- Pulse is usually normal in TOF. High volume collapsing pulse may be found in association with significant AR and aortopulmonary communication, namely large PDA or multiple large MAPCAs or surgically created aortopulmonary shunt. TOF, an increased aortic flow situation, is rarely, if ever, associated with coarctation or aortic arch interruption.
- A normal right ventricle occupies 2nd to 4th parasternal space, wider than normal left ventricular contact area on chest wall. But it does not produce any impulse, because right ventricle contracts less vigorously against low resistance pulmonary artery pressure, moves away and does not recoil back on chest wall in systole. Hypertrophied right ventricle contracts against systemic resistance in TOF. Thus, it should recoil back on chest wall and imparts a gentle impulse, like a normal left ventricle does. This may be described as a grade 1 parasternal impulse, which is a mild lift, easily compressible by counter pressure and sustained less than one-third of systole. As the obstruction is at infundibular level, impulse is best palpable in left 4th intercostal space and downward at subxiphoid area. A grossly hypertrophied right ventricle may displace left ventricle and occupies the normal apical area, imparting a diffuse apical impulse, continuous with the parasternal pulsation along with a lateral retraction.
- Second heart sound (A2) is louder, as aorta is dilated, dextroposed and pulmonary artery across it is relatively narrower. It may be even palpable. Ejection murmur, peaking well before aortic component contributes the clarity and makes it very clearly audible. Uncommonly, it is overshadowed by murmur. Pulmonary component is not appreciable in most of the cases on auscultation alone. Even phonocardiogram may not be able to record it. Reasons are obvious: Low pulmonary artery pressure distal to obstruction exerts a poor closing force, structurally abnormal pulmonary valve, commonly bicuspid, with restricted mobility results in slow closing movement. When audible or recordable, split is wider, may be around grade 3 (80–120 m/s).
- An ejection click in TOF is almost always an aortic click. This is called aortic vascular or aortic root click. More severe the grade of TOF more is the probability of getting the aortic vascular click. Click is best heard at right upper sternal border and may be appreciated at left upper sternal border and apex. Mechanism of aortic click is multifactorial: Aorta is dilated, which is dextroposed, pulmonary artery going across aorta is narrower than normal and more severe the right ventricular outflow tract (RVOT) obstruction more is the flow across aortic valve.
- Ejection systolic murmur across RVOT in TOF shows a typical inverse relation between its length and loudness versus severity of PS. Flow from right ventricle across RVOT is restricted in early ejection phase, when right ventricle contains most blood and develops peak pressure. Right ventricle decompresses through large VSD in aorta. Thus, more severe is the RVOT obstruction, right ventricular pressure becomes progressively more inadequate. Another mechanism is infundibular contraction in late systole, which retards late systolic flow and shortens murmur. More severe the stenosis is, more vigorous

is the infundibular contraction. Both the ventricles eject most of their content into the aorta before the closure of aortic valve. Thus, the flow and murmur end before A2. In mild TOF, right ventricle can maintain the gradient in late systole. Thus, the flow and murmur across RVOT extends over A2. Grade of the murmur may range from 1 to 5. In classical TOF, it may be grade 2-4. Flow across RVOT is against a significant gradient, which may impart a high-grade murmur and even thrill. Shape of the murmur varies from diamond-shaped, reverse kite-shaped, and kite-shaped for very severe, severe, and mild TOF, respectively. In contrast, murmur of only PS varies from diamond-shaped and kite-shaped for mild and severe stenosis, respectively.

- Regarding certain clinical findings,[3] is quotable: Dominant a wave, 3 cm above v wave in 20% of cases; moderate parasternal lift in 10% of cases; thrill in 75% of cases. Ejection systolic murmur is loud in 85%, moderate in 12%, and soft in 3% of cases.
- *ECG:* RVH is manifested as tall monophasic *r* wave in lead V1. From lead V2 onward, it changes to rS pattern. RVH and left ventricular hypoplasia causes right axis deviation, usually between 130° and 140°. QRS loop is clockwise, directed toward inferior, right, and anterior. Due to left ventricular hypoplasia and clockwise rotation, *r* wave is less than *s* wave in lead I, V5, and V6. In pink TOF or postcorrection TOF, left ventricle uses to get more blood. *r* wave becomes prominent, R/S ratio may be >1 and *q* wave may be prominent in V6. Inverted *t* wave in V1 as an indicator of RVH is present in 73% case. Inverted *t* wave beyond V1 is not usual in TOF (**Fig. 1**).
- *X-ray of chest:* Cardiac size is usually normal. Cardiomegaly may be found in situations leading to left ventricular dilatation. Left ventricular dilatation may be found when TOF is associated with significant AR, multiple MAPCAs (not very uncommon in classical TOF) or post Blalock–Taussig shunt. Boot-shaped heart or Cœur en sabot is the classical radiological feature of TOF. Cardiac apex forms the toe of the boot. Right ventricle forms the apex. Right ventricle enlarges

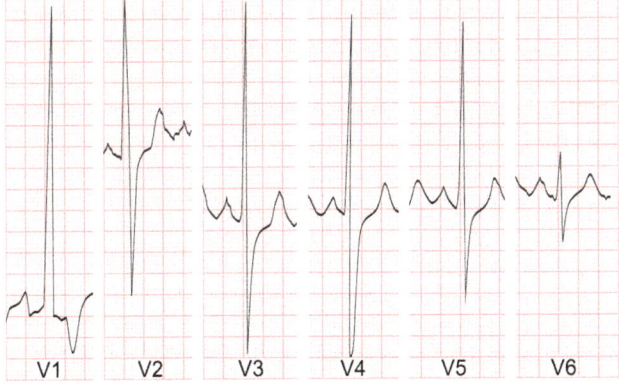

Fig. 1: ECG in typical tetralogy of Fallot; tall *r* in V1 with inverted *t*; transition from V2, where *t* wave is upright. In V6, R/S = 1 along with small q, indicating left ventricle is not underfilled.

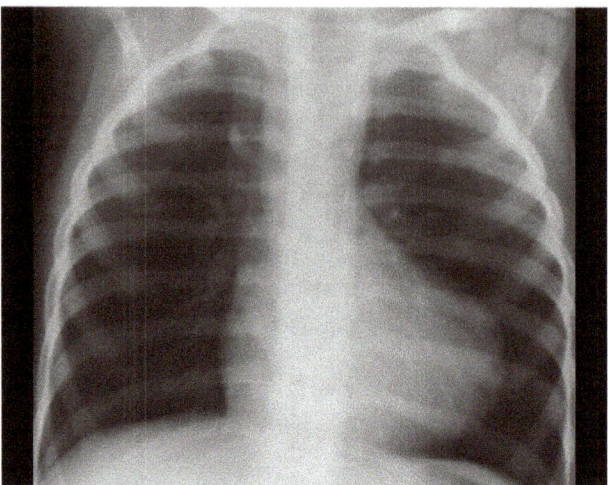

Fig. 2: X-ray in typical tetralogy of Fallot: Boot-shaped heart, reduced pulmonary vascularity, and right aortic arch.

superiorly, anteriorly, and toward left and not downward. Right ventricular hypertrophy (RVH) alone does not explain boot-shaped heart (**Fig. 2**). Severe PS leading to RVH or RVH due to acquired cause does not produce a tilted apex. Underfilled left ventricle and abnormal horizontal distribution of the interventricular septum may be the causative factors. The most characteristic feature of left heart border is concave pulmonary segment which is most consistent. Uncommonly, this segment may be full. When stenosis is at the os of the long tubular infundibulum, poststenotic infundibulum may impart an impression of fullness at pulmonary segment. When stenosis is predominantly valvular, poststenotic dilatation may make the segment full. However, classical poststenotic dilatation of isolated valvular PS is never seen. In TOF with mild-to-moderate stenosis without much rotation of right ventricular outflow, direction of pulmonary jet is toward left pulmonary artery, which may lead to poststenotic dilatation of left pulmonary artery. Bulging of this segment may be found in postcorrection TOF. Pulmonary vascularity is reduced, described as oligemic lung field in 47% cases, normal in 51% cases, and increased in 2% cases. Degree of oligemia depends upon the grade of pulmonary obstruction. In a neonate with mild obstruction, pulmonary vascularity may be even increased. In moderate obstruction, vascularity may be normal. In acquired TOF (Gasul phenomenon), vascularity may be even found enhanced in the initial phase.

Ventricular Septal Defect and Pulmonary Atresia

- Common presentation is sudden deterioration in early neonatal age, with deepening of cyanosis due to ductal closure, when pulmonary circulation is ductus dependent. More than 50% of children present with deep cyanosis at

birth. A delayed presentation of cyanosis occurs in those, who have MAPCAs as source of pulmonary circulation.
- History of spell or squatting is uncommon.
- Precordium is quiet. Apex is formed by right ventricle. However, when multiple MAPCAs are present, apex may be formed by left ventricle.
- S2 is always single.
- Aortic click, best heard at right upper sternal border and may be audible at left sternal edge and apex, i.e., it has wider range of audibility. The click does not vary with respiration. Its later onset in systole gives the impression of "wide splitting" of the first sound.
- Pulmonary ejection murmur is absent.
- A soft systolic murmur, due to flow into the aorta may be present.
- An early decrescendo diastolic murmur is audible due to AR, which occurs due to dilatated aortic route or infective endocarditis.
- Continuous murmur is the hallmark. It is present in 80% cases, best heard beneath the clavicle, back of the chest, right or left or both. Systolic portion may be prominent, and one may miss the diastolic part.
- *X-ray of chest*: Cardiac silhouette with tilted-up left heart border along with grossly concave pulmonary segment along with right-sided aortic arch is typical feature of TOF with pulmonary atresia. When intrapericardial pulmonary arteries are present, pulmonary vascularity is similar to classic TOF. In their absence, MAPCA-supported pulmonary circulation produces a typical pattern in pulmonary vascularity. The features include inappropriately large peripheral pulmonary vasculature compared with adjacent pulmonary vasculature, focal uneven distribution of pulmonary vasculature: When the pulmonary vascularity is increased or decreased in less than half lung field and asymmetrical to the opposite lung field (**Fig. 3**).

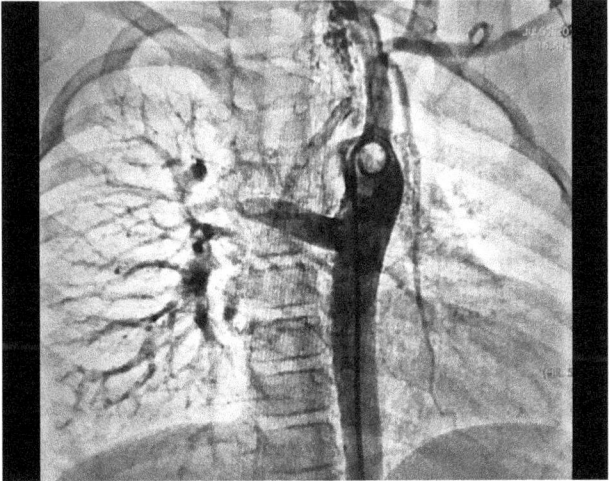

Fig. 3: Ventricular septal defect (VSD), pulmonary atresia: Major aortopulmonary collateral arteries.

Ventricular Septal Defect and Pulmonary Valvular Stenosis
- History of spell is uncommon.
- *Squatting*: In 20% of patients.
- Mostly pink at rest.
- Valvular ejection click is very closed to S1.
- Chance of getting a soft P2 is more probable.
- Ejection systolic murmur is prominent
- *ECG*: Left ventricular force may be present
- *X-ray*: Cardiomegaly; pulmonary segment is full.

Double Outlet Right Ventricle and Pulmonary Stenosis
- Clinically, it is indistinguishable from Fallot's tetralogy. This combination is found in 40% of cases of DORV. An underdeveloped subpulmonic conus or a bicuspid stenotic pulmonary valve constitutes PS. A restrictive VSD is another zone of obstruction.
- Cyanosis may be earlier and in 1st month of life in one series.
- Thrill is described in 40% of cases.
- In restrictive VSD and in presence of subaortic membrane, left ventricular impulse may be forceful.
- Systolic murmur across obstructed pulmonary outflow behaves as that of TOF. A long systolic murmur may be found in presence of restrictive VSD, due to obligatory flow from left ventricle. Perloff describes it as long decrescendo systolic murmur, whereas others described it as pansystolic murmur.[4]
- When great arteries are malposed and aorta is more anterior, A2 is relatively more prominent.
- *ECG*:[5,6] There is right axis deviation and RVH. Depolarization is counter-clockwise depolarization, with *q* waves in lead I and aVL. Deep and prolonged terminal forces like broad and slurred S in lead I, aVL, V5–6, and wide R in aVR are common. When PS is mild and occasionally when it is severe, axis may be left. Prominent left ventricular forces may be present. Right bundle branch block, AV delay with prolonged PR interval are various conduction defects (**Fig. 4**).
- X-ray of chest does not have any specific distinguishing feature.

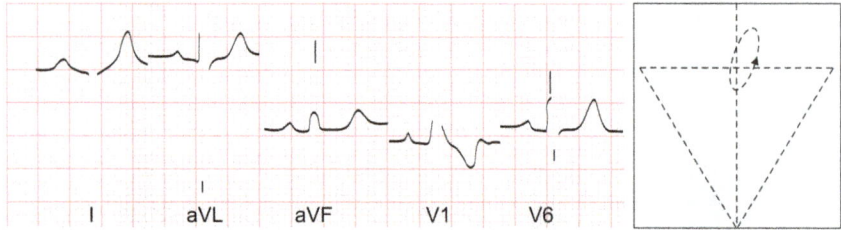

Fig. 4: ECG in double outlet right ventricle, ventricular septal defect, and pulmonary stenosis: Right axis deviation, counterclockwise depolarization, right ventricular hypertrophy, and preserved left ventricular force in V6.

Univentricular Heart and Pulmonary Stenosis

- In univentricular heart, presence of PS reduces streaming and increases mixing. Thus, cyanosis appears earlier.
- Hypoxic spell is uncommon. Squatting may be present. Spell is uncommon.
- Right atrioventricular (AV) valve atresia may lead to large *a* wave.
- Apex is formed by left ventricle.
- A visible and palpable systolic impulse in the 3rd left intercostal space is a result of the leftward and anterior position of an inverted outlet chamber. The second heart sound is palpable because the aorta is anterior whether the outlet chamber is inverted or noninverted. A systolic thrill at the mid left sternal border is evidence of subaortic stenosis caused by a restrictive outlet foramen.
- A2 may be louder because of anterior position of aorta. Aortic click may be present.
- Pulmonary stenotic murmur may be dampened because of the posterior position of pulmonary trunk. The murmur of subaortic stenosis caused by a restrictive outlet foramen is midsystolic and radiates from the mid left sternal border to the left or right base depending on whether the outlet chamber is inverted or noninverted
- *ECG*: High voltage is a characteristic feature. In fact, high voltage in ECG in cyanotic heart disease is suggestive of single ventricle. In a single morphologic left ventricle with a noninverted outlet chamber, the PR interval is usually normal. The QRS axis is directed away from the noninverted outlet chamber toward the main ventricular mass and is leftward and inferior or leftward and superior (left axis deviation). Initial depolarization forces are anterior and leftward, so small *q* waves occasionally appear in left precordial lead. Left ventricular hypertrophy is the prevailing pattern. Precordial QRS complexes may exhibit stereotyped patterns. When the outlet chamber is inverted, AV conduction is often abnormal and PR interval prolongation occasionally culminates in complete heart block. The *p* wave axis shifts to the left in the horizontal plane, so tall peaked right atrial *p* waves appear in mid and left precordial leads, a pattern that also occurs with noninversion of the outlet chamber. Ventricular depolarization is clockwise, so *q* waves appear in leads II, III, and aVF. Because initial forces of ventricular depolarization are posterior and leftward, *q* waves may be present in right precordial leads but do not appear in left precordial leads. Even though the univentricular heart is morphologically a left ventricle, precordial leads may show a dominant *r* wave in lead V1 and large equiphasic RS complexes in midprecordial leads (**Fig. 5**).
- *X-ray of chest*: The location of the outlet chamber is an important feature of the X-ray. An inverted outlet chamber forms a localized convexity at the left upper cardiac border and gives rise to an aorta that is convex to the left or that rises vertically as in CC-TGA. A noninverted outlet chamber and the aorta arising from it are not border forming. A transposed pulmonary outflow tract (i.e., inverted outlet chamber) lifts the right branch and produces a waterfall sign (**Fig. 6**).

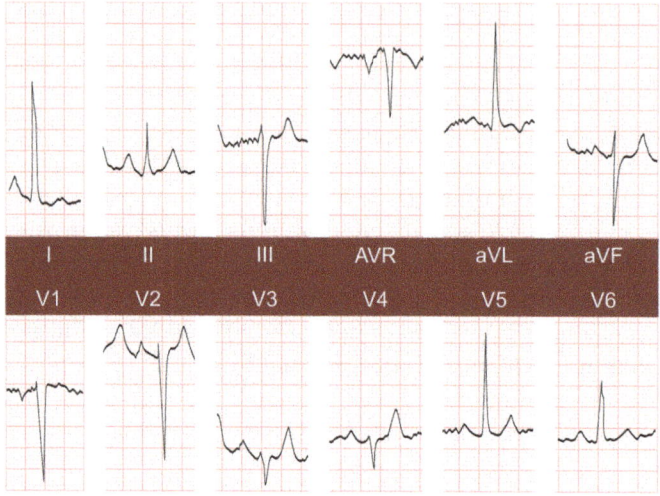

Fig. 5: ECG in single ventricle: Left axis, counterclockwise depolarization, and left ventricular dominance, high voltage.

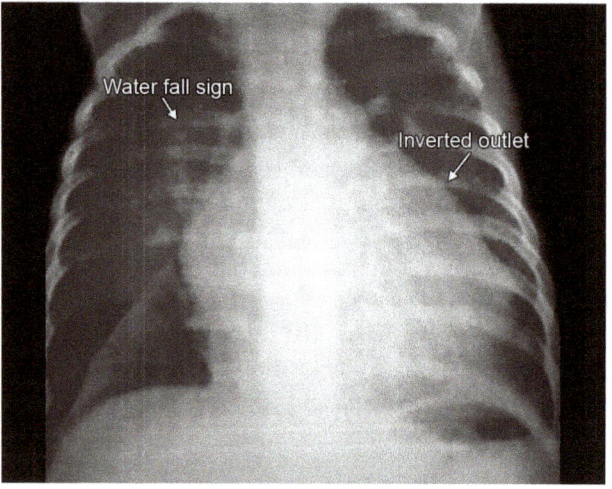

Fig. 6: X-ray of chest in single ventricle: Outlet chamber bulge in left heart border and waterfall sign.

Complete Transposition of Great Vessels (TGA), VSD, and PS (Left Ventricular Outflow Tract Obstruction)

- Incidence in male child significantly outnumbers female child.
- Without intervention, mortality in complete transposition is very high: 30% in 1st week; 50% in 1st month; and 90% in 1st year. Outcome is better in presence of VSD and PS.

- Pulmonary stenosis leading to left ventricular outflow tract (LVOT) obstruction is found in 15% of complete transposition cases. Isolated pulmonary valvular stenosis is rare. Subvalvular obstruction is either fixed or dynamic. In presence of VSD, malalignment and deviation of muscular septum into the left ventricle, producing subpulmonary outflow obstruction, is common. Other fixed obstructions are fibrous ridge leading to a tunnel-shaped LVOT, anomalous attachment of mitral valve chordae across LVOT, and septal aneurysm. Dynamic obstruction is due to bulging of ventricular septum.
- Cyanosis may be from day one. Cyanotic burden is always very high in these large babies. Heart failure is uncommon in presence of significant PS.
- Pulmonary stenosis leads to occasional spell, though unconsciousness is uncommon. Squatting is rare.
- Due to the large volume of highly unsaturated blood recirculating in the hyperkinetic low-resistance systemic vascular bed, pulse is bounding, scalp veins become varicosed and extremities are worm.
- As right ventricle is facing systemic circulation, its impulse is always palpable at left parasternal area. Left ventricular impulse is palpable in presence of significant LVOT obstruction. A2 may be palpable due to anterior placed aorta.
- Pulmonary ejection click is less audible due to posterior position of pulmonary artery. When audible, it is rather constant, as pulmonary valve is supported by left ventricle. S2 is single and louder due to anterior placed aorta.
- Ejection systolic murmur due to fixed obstruction at LVOT is audible from day one. Murmur due to dynamic obstruction appears weeks after birth. Murmur of fixed or dynamic PS murmur is best heard at left 3rd intercostal space with conduction to right base. Due to posterior position, the murmur is less audible.
- *ECG*: Peaked right atrial *p* waves appear in lead II and aVF and in lead V1. Pure RVH is reflected in marked right axis deviation, tall monophasic *r* waves in lead aVR and in V1, and deep *s* waves in left precordial leads. *t* waves are taller in right precordial leads than in left precordial leads.
- *X-ray of chest*: Classical picture of simple TGA is lost. Egg-on-side is not seen, as usually left heart chambers are small, occupied by right-sided chambers. There is decreased vascularity. Narrow pedicle is widened because of dilated ascending aorta (**Figs. 7A and B**).

Congenitally Corrected Transposition of the Great Arteries, VSD, and Pulmonary Stenosis

- *JVP*: Prolonged PR interval is manifested by increase in the interval between jugular *a* wave and carotid pulsation. Complete heart block is manifested as independent *a* waves and random cannon waves.
- *Pulse*: Bradycardia may be present.
- An inverted right ventricle occupies an anterior and leftward position with its medial border adjacent to the left sternal edge and its lateral border at the apex, an arrangement that accounts for the large topographic area generated by the right ventricular impulse.

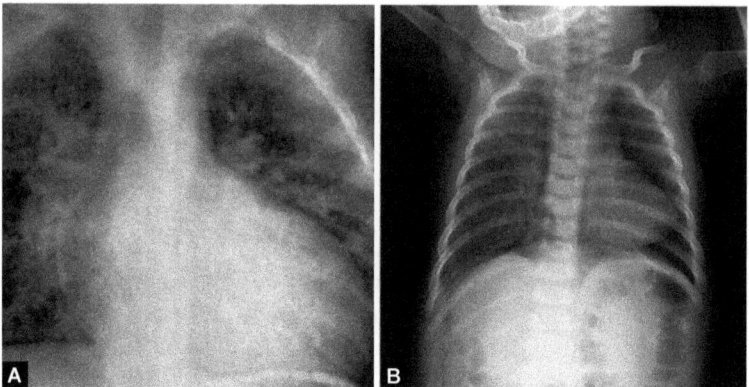

Figs. 7A and B: (A) Classical transposition of the great arteries (TGA); and (B) TGA, ventricular septal defect (VSD), and pulmonary stenosis (PS).

- There is no retraction medial to the interventricular sulcus because the sulcus lies too close to the left sternal border.
- The inverted left ventricle occupies a posterior and rightward position behind the sternum, where it cannot be felt even in the presence of PS.
- The ascending aorta is palpated when it is dilated and convex to the left, and the aortic component of the second heart sound is palpated because of the anterior position of the aortic root.
- The first heart sound is not loud, though Ebstein-like malformation of left AV valve is present, because the malformed anterior tricuspid leaflet is small and poorly mobile. First heart sound may further be soft due to prolonged PR interval.
- Second heart sound (A2) is significantly loud, because of anterior position of aorta.
- Aortic click may be heard.
- Pulmonary stenosis murmur is softer for a given degree of obstruction, because of the posterior position of pulmonary artery.
- Ejection systolic flow murmur across aorta may be heard.
- Left AV valve regurgitation generates systolic murmurs analogous to those of mitral regurgitation in hearts without ventricular inversion. Radiation tends to be toward the left sternal edge rather than into the axilla, because the malformed tricuspid leaflets direct the jet medially within the left atrium.
- *ECG*: Variable degree of heart block, starting from first degree to complete heart block is quite common. Complete heart block may be present in 30% of patients. Left axis deviation is common. When pulmonary ventricular (left) pressure is high due to PS, axis may be drifted toward right. As direction of septal depolarization is reversed, *q* wave is absent in left precordial leads, lead I and aVL and initial *r* wave may be absent in lead V1. *q* wave in lead III is deeper than that in aVF. Side-by-side ventricular positions are manifested by positive *t* waves in all the six precordial leads (**Fig. 8**).

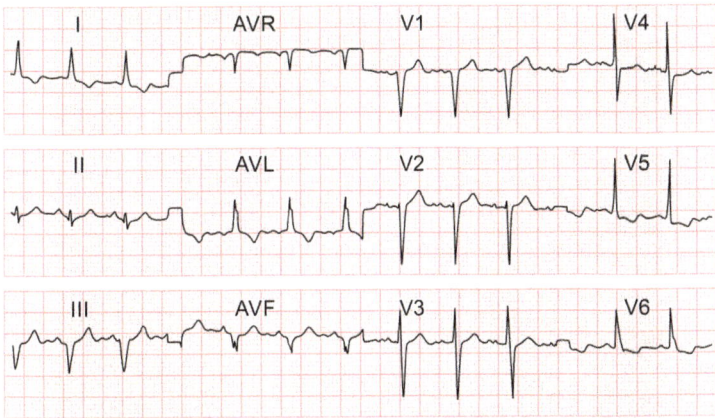

Fig. 8: ECG in congenitally corrected transposition of the great arteries (CC-TGA): left axis, absent *q* wave in V5, V6, I, and aVL; *q* wave in III is deeper than aVF; and positive *t* wave in all six chest leads.

- *X-ray of chest*: Ascending aorta is commonly forming the upper left heart border, producing a typical bulge. However, the left upper border will be less convex or even may not border forming, when aorta is exactly anterior to pulmonary artery. Pulmonary artery does not contribute in left heart border. Rather, it may push superior vena cava further right and forms a convex bulging in right upper cardiac border, simulating ascending aorta in normal heart. As right ventricle occupies left heart border, left atrial appendage does not come to left heart border. Rather, a prominent inverted infundibulum may form a hump-shaped appearance. Another feature is septal notch, which is an indentation on left heart border just above the left hemidiaphragm, indicating the apical position of interventricular groove (**Fig. 9**).

Tricuspid Atresia, VSD, and Pulmonary Stenosis
- Great arteries are nontransposed in 90% of cases with tricuspid atresia. Out of this, in 90% of cases, there is subpulmonic obstruction by the restrictive VSD. Obstruction due to bicuspid pulmonary valve is uncommon. When great arteries are transposed, subpulmonic obstruction is rare.
- Survival is best in nontransposed great arteries, when subpulmonic obstruction is optimum. VSD gets smaller and may be closed down within 1 year of age, giving rise to acquired pulmonary atresia with poor survival. In all forms of tricuspid atresia with unobstructed pulmonary circulation, survival is short.
- Hypoxic spell can occur due to closing down VSD. History of squatting may be present. Syncope has been described in baby by intermittent closure of interatrial communication by a large vena cava valve.
- A prominent *a* wave in the jugular pulse is characteristic feature of tricuspid atresia irrespective of other anatomical features.

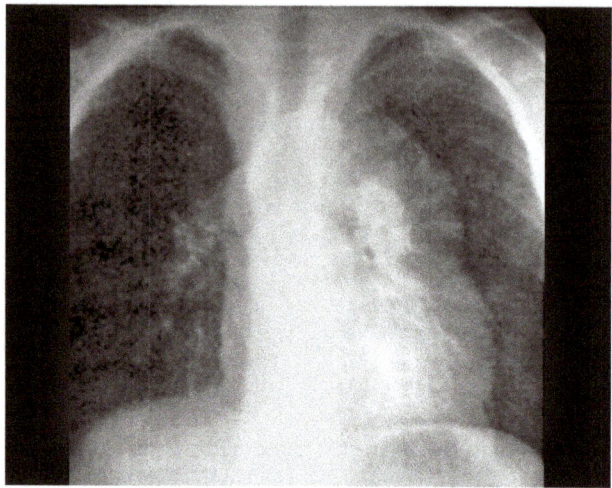

Fig. 9: X-ray of chest in congenitally corrected transposition of the great arteries, ventricular septal defect, and pulmonary stenosis: Left-anterior ascending aorta. Aorta anterior and left to pulmonary artery produces a typical bulge in left upper heart border; an indentation on left heart border just above the left hemidiaphragm, indicating the apical position of interventricular groove.

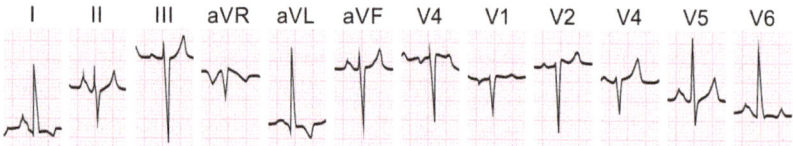

Fig. 10: ECG in tricuspid atresia, ventricular septal defect, pulmonary stenosis: Left axis deviation, counterclockwise; depolarization; tall, notched *p* wave in lead I and II; and left ventricular dominance.

- Apical impulse is typical left ventricular type, along with absent right ventricular impulse.
- First heart sound is exclusively contributed by mitral component. Restrictive subpulmonic obstruction gives origin of pansystolic murmur, best heard at 3rd and 4th left intercostal space, radiating to 2nd left intercostal space. Here, flow is from left ventricle through subpulmonic obstruction zone of VSD into RVOT. Second heart sound is usually single, which is A2. However, in presence of nontransposed great artery, pulmonary component may be subdued but audible, because obstruction is mostly at the level of restrictive VSD. A strong right atrial contraction can be transmitted through interatrial communication and may be palpable as presystolic wave and audible as S4 at the apex.
- ECG shows left axis deviation and counterclockwise depolarization. *p* wave of right atrial origin is very tall. All the typical features of left ventricular dominance are present (**Fig. 10**).

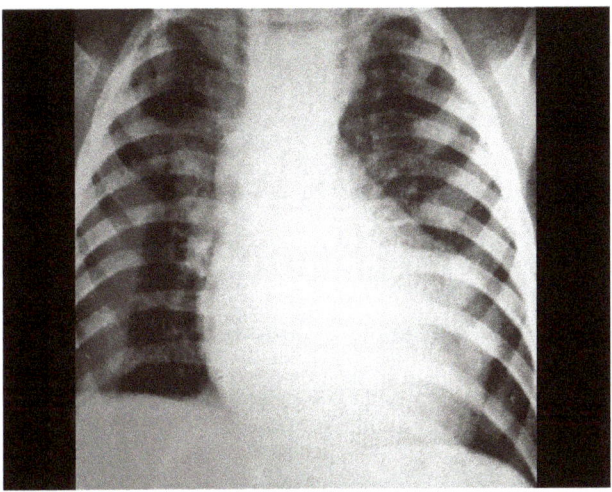

Fig. 11: X-ray of chest in tricuspid atresia, ventricular septal defect, and pulmonary stenosis: Square appearance of cardiac silhouette.

- X-ray of chest shows prominent right atrium, convex left ventricle, absent right ventricle, and concave pulmonary segment. The most striking differential feature in the frontal projection appears to be the shape of the left heart border. Concavity of the pulmonary segment, together with prominence in the upper part of the left lower segment and a vertical border below this, can give a square shape to the heart (**Fig. 11**).

CONCLUSION

The steps, those we follow to make anatomical diagnosis in tetralogy physiology, are like the steps to solve a complex algebraic mathematics! We may be wrong in the final answer, but we will get full credit for doing the right steps!

REFERENCES

1. Vogelpoel L, Schrire V. Auscultatory and phonocardiographic assessment of Fallot's tetralogy. Circulation. 1960;22:73.
2. Mccord M, Van Elk J, Blount S. Tetralogy of Fallot: Clinical and hemodynamic spectrum of combined pulmonary stenosis and ventricular septal defect. Circulation. 1957;16;736-49.
3. Wood P. Diseases of the Heart and Circulation, 2nd edition. London: Eyre and Spottiswoode; 1956.
4. Neufeld HN, DuShane JW, Edwards JE. Origin of both the great vessels from the right ventricle II. With pulmonary stenosis Circulation. 1961;23:399-412.
5. Krongard E, Ritter DG, Weidman WH, et al. Hemodynamic and anatomic correlation of electrocardiogram in double outlet right ventricle. Circulation. 1972;46:995.
6. Mirowski M, Mehrlizi A, Taussig HB. The Electrocardiogram in patients with both great vessels arising from the right ventricle combined with pulmonary stenosis. Circulation. 1963;28:1116.

CHAPTER 29

Clinical Approach: Left-to-Right Shunt and Eisenmenger Physiology

PREAMBLE

Dr Victor Eisenmenger published his paper[1] on "congenital defects of the ventricular septum" in 1897 that had since become known as Eisenmenger's complex till 1958. In 1958, Paul Wood delivered Croonian Lectures[2] before the Royal College of Physicians of London on May 13. Paul Wood first defined Eisenmenger's complex as—"*pulmonary hypertension at systemic level, due to a high pulmonary vascular resistance (PVR) (over 800 dynes sec/cm^3), with reversed or bidirectional shunt through a large ventricular septal defect (VSD) (1.5-3 cm across).*" In the same lecture, he suggested extending the meaning of the expression "Eisenmenger's syndrome" to embrace other conditions when behaving physiologically like "Eisenmenger's complex" proper, i.e., pulmonary arterial hypertension (PAH) due to PVR at systemic level results in reversed or bidirectional shunt at atrial, ventricular or great artery level. Paul Wood studied a series of 127 cases over 11 years. Cardiac catheterization was done in every patient and necropsy was obtained in 15 patients.

PREVALENCE

Exact prevalence is not known. Historically, Eisenmenger syndrome was accounted for 8% of Paul Wood's first 1,000 cases of congenital heart disease. It is accounted for 11% of all congenital shunt lesions. Eisenmenger syndrome is the most common cause of congenital cyanotic heart disease encountered in adults.[3]

WHO ARE CLINICALLY SUSCEPTIBLE?

- Large defect
- Down syndrome
- Shunt at multiple levels
- Transposition physiology
- Truncus arteriosus

INCIDENCE OF EISENMENGER SYNDROME IN LARGE SHUNT

- *Great artery level:* 53%
- *Ventricular level:* 52%
- *Atrial level:* 9%

PULMONARY ARTERIAL HYPERTENSION LEADING TO PULMONARY VASCULAR DISEASE

Pulmonary Arterial Hypertension due to Left-to-Right Shunt[4]

Eisenmenger Syndrome
Eisenmenger syndrome includes all large intra- or extracardiac defects which begin as systemic-to-pulmonary shunts and progress with time to a severe elevation in PVR and to reversal (pulmonary-to-systemic) or bidirectional shunting.

Pulmonary Arterial Hypertension Associated with Prevalent Systemic-to-Pulmonary Shunts
It includes moderate to large defects; PVR is mildly to moderately increased, systemic-to-pulmonary shunting is still prevalent.

Pulmonary Arterial Hypertension with Small Defects
Marked elevation in PVR in the presence of small cardiac defects [usually VSDs <1 cm and atrial septal defects (ASDs) <2 cm of effective diameter assessed by echo], which themselves do not account for the development of elevated PVR; the clinical picture is very similar to idiopathic PAH.

When the defects are not large, such as VSD <10 mm and ASD <20 mm, increased PVR cannot be explained by the shunt effect only; the clinical course follows that of idiopathic PAH.

Pulmonary Arterial Hypertension after Corrective Cardiac Surgery
In these cases, congenital heart disease has been corrected but PAH is either still present immediately after surgery or has recurred several months or years after surgery in the absence of significant postoperative residual congenital lesions or defects that originate as a sequela to previous surgery.

Pulmonary Hypertension with Unclear and/or Multifactorial Mechanism
There are certain complex congenital cardiac anomalies with differential pulmonary blood flow, leading to pulmonary hypertension (PH). They have included as cause of PH under the heading of segmental PH.

LIST OF DISEASES LEADING TO EISENMENGER SYNDROME

Tables 1 and **2** show the list of diseases leading to Eisenmenger syndrome.

TABLE 1: Paul Wood's series.[2]

Disease	Total cases	Number with Eisenmenger reaction	Frequency (%)
PDA	180	29	16
AP window	10	6	60
Truncus arteriosus	4	4	100
TGA (with VSD)	12	7	58
CC-TGA (with VSD)	3	3	100
Single ventricle	6	6	100
VSD	136	21	16
AVSD	21	9	43
ASD	324	19	6
TAPVD	6	1	17
Site uncertain	22	22	

(AP: aortopulmonary; ASD: atrial septal defect; AVSD: atrioventricular septal defect; CC-TGA: congenitally corrected transposition of great arteries; PDA: patent ductus arteriosus; TAPVD: total anomalous pulmonary venous drainage; VSD: ventricular septal defect)

TABLE 2: Physiology-wise diseases causing Eisenmenger syndrome.

Simple Eisenmenger	
Physiology	Disease
Left-to-right shunt: • Great artery level • Ventricular level • Atrial level • Both atrial and ventricular level	• PDA, AP window • VSD • All types of ASD • AVSD
Complex Eisenmenger	
Mixing physiology	Univentricular connection, Tricuspid atresia with large VSD, truncus arteriosus, TAPVC, and common atrium DORV
Transposition physiology	TGA, CC-TGA, large VSD, DORV, transposed great arteries, and subpulmonic VSD

(AP: aortopulmonary; ASD: atrial septal defect; AVSD: atrioventricular septal defect; CC-TGA: congenitally corrected transposition of great arteries; DORV: double outlet right ventricle; PDA: patent ductus arteriosus; TAPVC: totally anomalous pulmonary venous connection; VSD: ventricular septal defect)

PATHOPHYSIOLOGY OF EISENMENGER SYNDROME

Pulmonary vascular disease (PVD) accompanied by PH in Eisenmenger syndrome stems from the reduction in cross-sectional area of pulmonary arteries due to combined effect of vasoconstriction, thrombosis, inflammation, and proliferative and obstructive remodeling of the pulmonary arterial wall. In 1958, Heath and Edwards[5] proposed a grade of pulmonary arteriopathy in PAH.

Pulmonary Arteriopathy

Pulmonary arteriopathy, more precisely plexogenic arteriopathy, is the six-graded pathophysiological hallmark of any form of PAH, as described by Heath and Edwards.[5] The arteriopathy involve small pulmonary arteries, <500 μm to arterioles as small as 30 μm.

- *Grade 1—stage of muscularization*: There is increased muscularization of muscular arteries, and extension of muscularization to normally nonmuscularized arterioles. Even the small arterioles as small as 30 μm become muscular.
- *Grade 2—stage of medial hypertrophy with cellular intimal reaction*: There is cellular intimal proliferation in the smaller muscular pulmonary arteries and arterioles, leading to occlusion of these vessels.
- *Grade 3—stage of progressive fibrous vascular occlusion*: (A) Intimal proliferation is changed from cellular proliferation to fibrous tissue proliferation. There is widespread occlusion of small pulmonary arteries and arterioles by acellular fibrous tissue admixed with fine elastic fibrils. (B) Some thinning and dilatation of media start in the later part of this stage.
- *Grade 4—plexogenic arteriopathy*: This stage is characterized by plexogenic form of dilatation of the media. There is generalized thinning and dilatation of the small arteries and arterioles. In addition, there is excessive dilatation of some part of those arteries and arterioles to form distended sacs. In those microaneurysms, intimal thickening and in situ thrombosis occur. This dilatation lesion is seen in four forms:
    1. Plexiform lesion
    2. Vein-like branches of hypertrophied muscular pulmonary arteries
    3. Angiomatoid lesions
    4. Cavernous lesions
- Grade 5—stage of chronic dilatation with formation of numerous dilatation lesions.
- Grade 6—necrotizing arteritis.

This form of arteriopathy is more often observed in patients with PAH harboring a bone morphogenetic protein receptor type II (BMPR2) mutation (**Box 1**).[6]

BOX 1   Pulmonary arteriopathy in pulmonary arterial hypertension.

- Muscularization
- Intimal cellular proliferation
- Intimal fibrotic proliferation
- Plexogenic arteriopathy
- Further dilatation
- Necrotizing arteritis

Difference between Pretricuspid and Post-tricuspid Shunt

The hemodynamic burden of both increased flow as well as pressure is more detrimental on pulmonary circulation. This pattern occurs in cases of large left-to-right shunt at post-tricuspid level, such as large VSD, atrioventricular septal defect (AVSD), patent ductus arteriosus (PDA), and aortopulmonary (AP) window. They develop progressive and irreversible PVDs in >50% of cases by first year of life.[7] In contrast, the hemodynamic burden of only increased flow is less detrimental on pulmonary circulation. Only one-tenth to one-fifth of patients with large shunt at pretricuspid level, such as ASD, develop significant PAH and PVD in their third or fourth decade.[8]

The grade 1 change as describe above is present only in those pulmonary vasculature, which is exposed to high pulmonary artery pressure from birth, i.e., post-tricuspid shunt such as VSD, PDA or AP window. As Heath and Edward[5] mentioned grade 1 change—"*refer to changes seen in patients having congenital heart disease associated with pulmonary hypertension from birth.*" In ASD and other congenital heart diseases, characterized by high pulmonary blood flow over a long period of time, the grade 1 change is different. There is no muscularization of small pulmonary arteriole. Grade 1 arteriopathy is different in pretricuspid shunt. First, there is intense endothelial cellular reaction to increased pulmonary blood flow, leading to intimal proliferation and occlusion of small pulmonary arteries and arterioles. Another change occurs in the pulmonary veins, which shows pronounced intimal acellular fibrosis. This venous intimal change remains characteristic of ASD in all grade of PH. When PH sets in, subsequent grades 2–6 are same as changes as in post-tricuspid shunt. Onset of Eisenmenger syndrome also differs in pre- and post-tricuspid shunt (**Table 3**).

PATHOBIOLOGY

In a simplest form, the sheer force of PH and the pulsatile flow lead to endothelial dysfunction. There are three pathways, which control vasomotor tone of arterial wall. Endothelial dysfunction enhances endothelial pathway and reduces nitric oxide and prostacyclin pathways, leading to vasoconstriction, proliferation, inflammation, apoptosis, and eventually pulmonary arteriopathy (**Fig. 1**).

Beyond this simplest and conventional factor, there are diverse cellular processes and signaling pathways contribute to the pathogenesis of PAH. These processes and pathways include vascular stiffness, endothelial-to-mesenchymal

TABLE 3: Onset of Eisenmenger syndrome.

	Infancy	Childhood	Adult
PDA	80%	5%	15%
VSD	83%	15%	2%
ASD	8%		92%

(ASD: atrial septal defect; PDA: patent ductus arteriosus; VSD: ventricular septal defect)

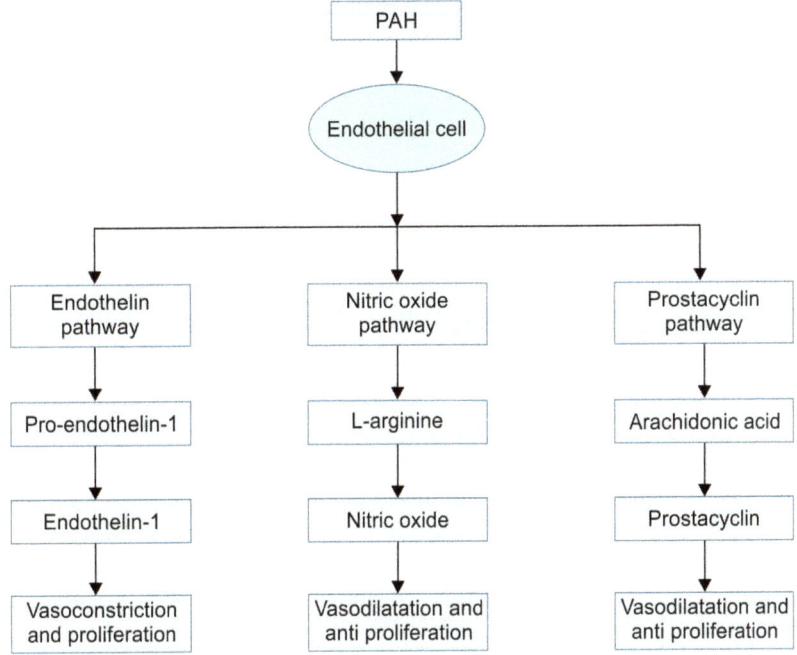

Fig. 1: Basic pathobiology for pulmonary arterial hypertension.

| BOX 2 | Signaling factors in pathobiology of pulmonary arterial hypertension. |

- TGF-β: Transforming growth factor-β
- BMP: Bone morphogenetic protein
- IL-6: Interleukin-6
- FGF-2: Fibroblast growth factor-2
- PDGF: Platelet-derived growth factor
- E2: Estradiol
- ER: Estrogen receptor
- YAP/TAZ: Yes-associated protein/transcriptional coactivator with PDZ-binding motif

transition, pericyte-mediated vascular remodeling, growth factor signaling [transforming growth factor-beta (TGF-β) signaling platelet-derived growth factor and fibroblast growth factor (FGF) signaling], inflammation and immunity, resting membrane potential, estrogen signaling, and iron homeostasis (**Box 2**).

Bone Morphogenetic Protein

Patients with PAH may carry mutation in genes encoding receptors of the TGF-β superfamily. The most common gene is bone morphogenetic protein 2 (BMP-2), which encodes the cell surface receptor type II (BMPR2). The mutation of BMP-2 is present in 80% of patients with heritable PAH and 11–40% of idiopathic PAH.[9]

The mutation leads to suppression of BMPR-II signaling, resulting in increased proliferation and decreased apoptosis in vascular cells. Inflammatory mediators, like TNF-α, may play a role in pathobiology of PAH in the context of BMPR2 mutations.

CLINICAL PRESENTATION OF EISENMENGER SYNDROME

Sex Distribution

Male:Female ratio both in uncomplicated PDA and PDA with Eisenmenger syndrome is 1:2, whereas the ratio both in uncomplicated VSD and VSD with Eisenmenger syndrome is 1:1. However, in uncomplicated ASD, this ratio is 2:3, whereas in ASD with Eisenmenger syndrome, male:female ratio is 1:4.

Symptom

- *Dyspnea on effort*: This is a common symptom in Eisenmenger physiology with VSD or ASD, but of lesser grade in patient with PDA. As in PDA with reversal of shunt, saturation in upper half of body is higher than lower half, carotid-cerebral circulation sends less signal to the cortical center and patient feels lesser dyspnea on effort.
- *Hemoptysis*: Overall incidence is around 33%. Incidence is uncommon before 20 years and almost 100% over 40 years. Neither the high pulmonary arterial pressure, nor the initial high pulmonary flow is responsible for hemoptysis. This is evidenced from the fact that incidence of hemoptysis in idiopathic hypertension is just 4% and in uncomplicated ASD is around 3%. A combination of PAH and cyanosis is probably the causative factor.
- *Squatting*: Though squatting is hallmark of tetralogy of Fallot (TOF), very uncommonly it may present in patient with Eisenmenger syndrome. Incidence of squatting in VSD, ASD, and PDA is 15%, 5%, and 3% of cases, respectively.[2]

Angina, syncope, hyperviscosity syndrome, and heart failure symptoms have been discussed previously.

Triad

The triad of any cyanotic heart disease is very obvious in Eisenmenger physiology: Cyanosis, clubbing, and polycythemia. Out of the three, cyanosis and clubbing are more consistent and severe in VSD, intermediate in ASD, and less severe and less consistent in PDA.

JVP and Pulse

- *Neck veins*: A prominent *a* wave may be present in 20–25% cases irrespective of level of shunt; a large *a* wave is present in ASD in around 18% cases.
- *Pulse*: Water hammer pulse may be found in 10% cases in PDA with Eisenmenger syndrome.

Palpation

Apical impulse is always diffuse, i.e., right ventricular (RV) type. Left parasternal pulsation in ASD grade 2/3 in 50–60% cases. In other groups, insignificant and not more than 1/2. P2 is palpable in almost 90% cases in both VSD and PDA and not >55% in ASD. Pulmonary artery pulsation can be felt in 65% cases.

Auscultation

Auscultatory features have been discussed in previous section; some additional features have been described here (**Box 3**).

Eisenmenger Syndrome: ASD

- Adult presentation
- Female
- Prominent/large *a* wave in jugular venous pressure (JVP)
- Parasternal pulsation grade 2
- *ECG:* RV preponderance or hypertrophy in 80% cases
- *X-ray chest:* Cardiomegaly is found consistently; dilatation of both the proximal pulmonary arteries and/or dilatation of right lower descending branch of pulmonary artery is characteristic (**Fig. 2**).

Eisenmenger Syndrome: VSD

- Presentation in infancy or early childhood.
- Squatting may be there.
- X-ray chest may be unimpressive (**Fig. 3**).

BOX 3   **Auscultatory features in Eisenmenger syndrome.**

- Pulmonary ejection click can be found in 65% cases. It diminishes in intensity with inspiration. Occasionally, it can be transmitted to the apex. Higher the pulmonary artery diastolic pressure, more delayed will be the click in relation to S1

Typical S2
- RV S4, S3: RV S4 is found near 40% cases in ASD, but <3% cases in VSD or PDA. RV S3 is rare
- Midsystolic pulmonary flow murmur may be found in 85% cases. In 25% cases, it is grade 3 and in 5% cases, grade 4, thus associated with thrill. This murmur is brief, symmetric, not very rough, follows the click and delayed in onset

TR murmur
- Graham Steell murmur may be found in 55% cases and in 10% cases it is even grade 4 with accompanying thrill
- Mid-diastolic murmur may be found occasionally. Someone has described it as right-sided Austin Flint murmur

(ASD: atrial septal defect; PDA: patent ductus arteriosus; RV: right ventricualr; S1: first heart sound; S2: second heart sound; S3: third heart sound; S4: fourth heart sound; TR: tricuspid regurgitation; VSD: ventricular septal defect)

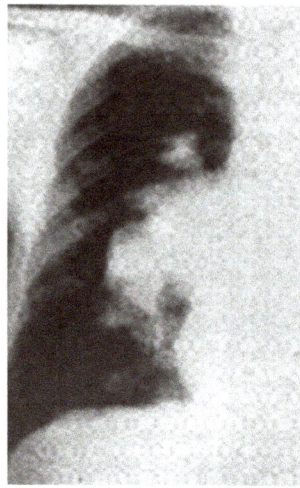
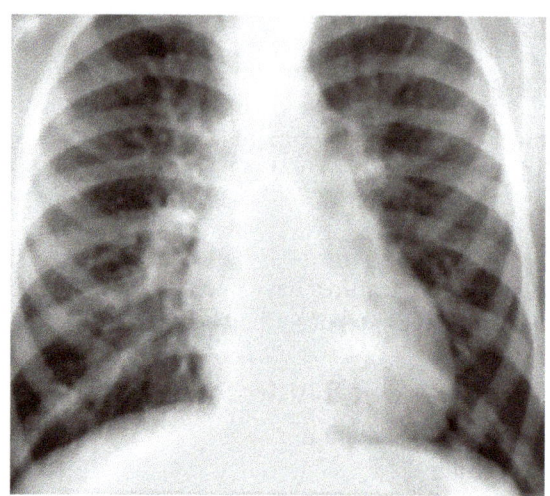

Fig. 2: Atrial septal defect: Dilated right pulmonary artery.

Fig. 3: Ventricular septal defect: Can be passed as normal.

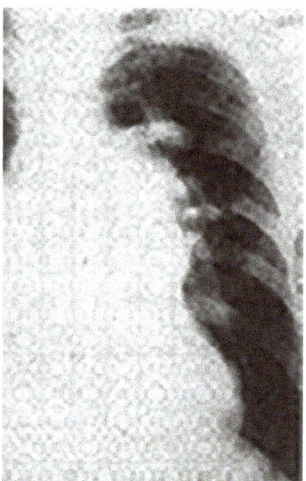

Fig. 4: Patent ductus arteriosus: Dilated aortic knuckle and main pulmonary artery.

Eisenmenger Syndrome: PDA

- Less symptomatic
- Less cyanotic
- Differential cyanosis and clubbing
- *ECG:* Prominent q waves may be preserved in V_5 and V_6.
- *X-ray chest*: A prominent AP complex or a rounded shadow above the aortic knuckle with or without calcification (**Fig. 4**).

SECOND HEART SOUND

Second heart sound (S2) is the most important clinical hallmark in differentiating the shunt at three different level. A loud P2 at pulmonary area can obscure the preceding A2 and makes it difficult to appreciate the split. Hence, split is better appreciated at lower space or at the apex. Grading of splitting helps to appreciate narrow or wide splitting (**Box 4**). S2 is single in VSD in 55% cases, around 5% in PDA and unusual in ASD. Similarly, significant splitting is unusual in VSD, found in 50% cases of PDA and in 85% cases of ASD.

Atrial Septal Defect

- *Splitting*: S2 remains fixed in ASD, irrespective of PAH.
- *Intensity*: As Sutton and Leatham[10] described—"*P2 was almost always heard and recorded in the mitral area in atrial septal defect, irrespective of the presence or absence of pulmonary hypertension, and was probably related both to the increased size of the right ventricle which forms the cardiac apex and to increased intensity of P2. Although the simple A2-P2 intensity ratio was not helpful in diagnosing pulmonary hypertension in atrial septal defect, a great broadening of P2, together with dwarfing of A2, made pulmonary hypertension likely.*"

Ventricular Septal Defect

- *Splitting*: Sutton and Leatham further described,[10] "*In ventricular septal defect with hyperkinetic pulmonary hypertension, the splitting of S2 remains the same as in ventricular septal defect without pulmonary hypertension, except that in expiration S2 tends to be single, which may be explained by greater overloading of the left ventricle and delay of A2 from the bigger shunt. In an Eisenmenger ventricular septal defect, however, the two components of S2 become very close and indistinguishable, both to auscultation and phonocardiography, in all phases of respiration, giving rise to the impression of "slurring." This is associated with identical systemic and pulmonary vascular resistance, for we have noticed that A2 and P2 may be asynchronous even in a patient with a single ventricle if systemic and pulmonary vascular resistance are different.*"
- *Intensity*: In VSD with hyperkinetic PAH, P2 is loud and occasionally transmitted to apex. In Eisenmenger VSD, P2 should be loud, but it is difficult to appreciate as A2 and P2 are inseparable. Apical transmission of P2 also cannot be appreciated due to same reason.

BOX 4   Grading of splitting.

- Grade 1: 30–60 ms
- Grade 2: 60–80 ms
- Grade 3: 80–110 ms
- Grade 4: >110 ms

Patent Ductus Arteriosus
- *Splitting*: In hyperkinetic PDA, splitting is physiological or reversed, like PDA without PAH. In an Eisenmenger PDA, splitting is physiological.
- *Intensity*: The intensity of P2 is loud in hyperkinetic PAH. It is loud and is transmitted to the apex in an Eisenmenger PDA.

NATURAL HISTORY OF EISENMENGER SYNDROME
Survival
Long-term prognosis in Eisenmenger syndrome is substantially better than that of idiopathic PAH. 10 years, 15 years, and 25 years survival are 80%, 77%, and 42%, respectively.[11] How the survival better in Eisenmenger syndrome has been explained by comparing Eisenmenger heart with fetal heart.[12] Eisenmenger right ventricle preserves the fetal pattern with a flat ventricular septum throughout the cardiac cycle and equal thickness of the right and left ventricular free walls. This morphology is same in patient independent of age and defect type. Eisenmenger syndrome develops in third to fourth decade in patients with pretricuspid shunt, when right ventricle already has lost its fetal pattern. This is the reason, why the right ventricle in ASD Eisenmenger cannot tolerate the pressure overload and fails early.[13] This, in turn translates into a worse prognosis in patients with pretricuspid defects after the fourth decade of life.

Poor Prognostic Markers
In a retrospective medical record review[14] of Eisenmenger syndrome patients in a tertiary center from 1980 to August, 2017, only two prognostic determinants for survival were found as:
1. SpO_2 <85%
2. *A low platelet count:* <100 × 109/L.

The conventional poor prognostic markers are severe pulmonary vascular obstructive disease, significant RV dysfunction, decreased cardiac output, syncope, and SaO_2 <85% (**Box 5**). Causes of death in Eisenmenger syndrome are described in **Box 6**.

BOX 5 | **Prognostic factors.[15]**

- Right ventricular failure
- Raid deterioration
- Syncope
- WHO functional class II–IV
- 6-minute walk test <300 meter
- Cardiopulmonary exercise testing: Predicted peak O_2 consumption <31%
- BNP plasma level >30 pmol/L
- Echocardiographic parameters:
  - TAPSE <1.5 cm
  - Right atrial area ≥25 cm²
  - Right atrium/left atrium ≥1.5
- Cardiac catheterization data:
  - Right atrial pressure >15 mm Hg
  - Cardiac index ≤2.0 L/min/m²

(BNP: brain-type natriuretic peptide; TAPSE: tricuspid annular plane systolic excursion; WHO: World Health Organisation)

BOX 6	Causes of death.
• Sudden cardiac death (30%)	• Thromboembolism
• Congestive heart failure (25%)	• Pregnancy
• Hemoptysis (15%)	• Noncardiac surgery
• Brain abscess	

HOW TO ASSESS THAT PAH IS HYPERKINETIC (REVERSIBLE) OR OBSTRUCTIVE (IRREVERSIBLE)

Assessment of reversibility of PAH is very crucial. Shunt closure when PAH is irreversible is more detrimental than natural history of Eisenmenger's syndrome. Every step, clinical examination, ECG, X-ray chest, echocardiogram, and invasive hemodynamics, is important.

Clinical Examination

There are some hard points: Presence of ejection click, single S2 in VSD, Graham Steell murmur, and desaturation appearing or increasing on exercise indicate irreversible PAH. Other clinical indices are relative (**Table 4**).

TABLE 4: Clinical indices of irreversibility of pulmonary arterial hypertension.

	Reversible PAH	Fixed PAH
Cardiomegaly	Present	Absent
Right ventricular impulse	Hyperkinetic	Grade 1 to silent
P2 intensity	Loud	Louder, apical transmission
Splitting:		
• ASD	• Wide, fixed	• Still wide, fixed
• VSD	• Normal, wide or narrow, variable	• Single
• PDA	• Normal to paradoxical	• Normal or narrow physiological
Pulmonary vascular click	Absent	Present
Murmur across shunt	Present	Absent/brief
Flow murmur	Present	Absent
TR murmur	May be present	Present
Graham Steell murmur	Absent	Present (not in all cases)
Resting saturation	<95%	<90–95%
Saturation on exercise	No significant change	Further fall

(ASD: atrial septal defect; PAH: pulmonary arterial hypertension; PDA: patent ductus arteriosus; TR: tricuspid regurgitation; VSD: ventricular septal defect)

ECG and X-ray Chest

Preservation of left ventricular force in lateral chest leads (like taller r wave and q wave) indicates a significant left-to-right shunt and hyperkinetic PAH, whereas absence of these features along with RV hypertrophy and strain pattern in right chest leads indicates fixed PAH. Cardiomegaly and increased vascularity in X-ray chest are suggestive that left-to-right shunt is still dominant, whereas normal heart size and reduced vascularity, peripheral pruning, and blotchy shadow >3 in lung field (plexogenic arteriopathy) indicate predominant right-to-left shunt.

Cardiac Catheterization

Acute Vasodilator Testing[16]

Acute vasodilator testing (AVT) is commonly done to see the acute vasodilatory response of PAH in idiopathic PAH to see the therapeutic response of calcium entry blocker. This test has been standardized long back. This test has been extrapolated in case of Eisenmenger syndrome to decide reversibility of PAH and thus potential operability.[17,18] Oxygen has been used for a longtime as vasodilator, but its role is questionable.[19] Inhaled nitric oxide at 10–100 ppm is the preferred agent.[20] Alternate agents are intravenous epoprostenol or adenosine and inhaled iloprost may be used as alternatives. Combined oxygen and nitric oxide have been tried. PAH is irreversible in patients with PVR:SVR (systemic vascular resistance) >0.41 on oxygen and nitric oxide, whereas PAH is reversible in patients with PVR:SVR <0.16.[18]

Balloon-occlusion Study

Balloon occlusion of the defect can reduce pulmonary pressure immediately, when PAH is hyperkinetic. Fixed PAH does not show much change. Balloon occlusion of PDA is feasible. VSD, due to its complex shape and ASD due to its size cannot be occluded effectively by balloon. However, they can be effectively occluded by device itself. There is no protocol or guideline to decide who are responders? In one study[21] on balloon occlusion of PDA, a fall in pulmonary artery pressure >20 mm Hg was taken as responder. In a large trial,[22] balloon occlusion of PDA was done in 137 patients with PDA and PAH. A post-trial systolic pulmonary artery pressure/systemic pressure ratio >0.5 indicates nonresponders, in whom PAH will persists after PDA closure. A different criterion was proposed[23] by another group, where responder was in whom there was ≥25% fall in pulmonary artery pressures on balloon occlusion or a 50% fall in the ratio between pulmonary and aortic diastolic pressures.

Operability and Pulmonary Vascular Resistance

Pulmonary vascular resistance is determined from cardiac catheterization data and operability is guided by the range of PVR (**Table 5**).[18]

TABLE 5: Operability and pulmonary vascular resistance in shunt lesion.[18]

Indexed PVR (Wood unit-m^2)	PVR (Wood unit)	Operability
<4	<2.3	Yes
4–8	2.3–4.6	Individual patient evaluation in tertiary care centre
>8	>4.6	No

(PVR: pulmonary vascular resistance)

CONCLUSION

Large shunt must be intervened before the onset of Eisenmenger process. PAH due to shunt lesion has a better prognosis than idiopathic PAH or PH due to other cause. Post-tricuspid shunt, in compare to pretricuspid shunt, is more susceptible to develop Eisenmenger syndrome. However, in long run, pretricuspid shunt shows poorer prognosis. A thorough clinical, noninvasive, and hemodynamic assessment can establish the issue of reversibility of PAH.

REFERENCES

1. Eisenmenger V. Die angeborenens Defect der Kammerschiei-dewand des Herzen. Z Klin Med Suppl. 1897;32:1-28.
2. Wood P. The Eisenmenger syndrome or pulmonary hypertension with reversed central shunt. I. Br Med J. 1958;2(5098):701-9.
3. Kaplan S. Eisenmenger syndrome. In: Third Annual Congenital Heart Disease in the Adult. ACC. San Diego, California, January 19–21, 1992.
4. Simonneau G, Gatzoulis MA, Adatia I, et al. Updated clinical classification of pulmonary hypertension. J Am Coll Cardiol. 2013;62:D34-41.
5. Heath D, Edwards JE. The Pathology of Hypertensive Pulmonary Vascular Disease. A Description of Six Grades of Structural Changes in the Pulmonary Arteries with Special Reference to Congenital Cardiac Septal Defects. Circulation. 1958;18:533-47.
6. Ghigna MR, Guignabert C, Montani D, et al. BMPR2 mutation status influences bronchial vascular changes in pulmonary arterial hypertension. Eur Respir J. 2016;48:1668-821.
7. Hornberger LK, Sahn DJ, Krabill KA, et al. Elucidation of the natural history of ventricular septal defects by serial Doppler color flow mapping studies. J Am Coll Cardiol. 1989;13:1111-8.
8. Craig RJ, Selzer A. Natural history and prognosis of atrial septal defect. Circulation. 1968;37:805-15.
9. Fessel JP, Loyd JE, Austin ED. The genetics of pulmonary arterial hypertension in the post-BMPR2 era. Pulm Circ. 2011;1:305-19.
10. Sutton G, Harris A, Leatham A. Second heart sound in pulmonary hypertension. Brit Heart J. 1968;30:743.
11. Saha A, Balakrishnan KG, Jaiswal PK, et al. Prognosis for patients with Eisenmenger syndrome of various aetiology. Int J Cardiol. 1994;45:199-207.
12. Hopkins WE, Waggoner AD. Severe pulmonary hypertension without right ventricular failure: the unique hearts of patients with Eisenmenger syndrome. Am J Cardiol. 2002;89:34-8.
13. Moceri P, Kempny A, Liodakis E, et al. Physiological differences between various types of Eisenmenger syndrome and relation to outcome. Int J Cardiol. 2015;179:455-60.

14. An HS, Kim GB, Song MK, et al. Eisenmenger Syndrome in Adults: Treatment Pattern and Prognostic Factors in the Advanced Pulmonary Vasodilator Era. Ped Cardiol. 2019;40(1):23-8.
15. Gatzoulis MA, Beghetti M, Landzberg MJ, et al. Pulmonary arterial hypertension associated with congenital heart disease: recent advance and future direction. Int J Cardiol. 2014;177(2):340-7.
16. Douwes JM, Humpl T, Bonnet D, et al. Acute vasodilator response in pediatric pulmonary arterial hypertension: current clinical practice from the TOPP Registry. J Am Coll Cardiol. 2016;67:1312-23.
17. Apitz C, Hansmann G, Schranz D. Hemodynamic assessment and acute pulmonary vasoreactivity testing in the evaluation of children with pulmonary vascular disease. Expert consensus statement on the diagnosis and treatment of paediatric pulmonary hypertension. The European Paediatric Pulmonary Vascular Disease Network, endorsed by ISHLT and DGPK. Heart. 2016;102 Suppl 2:ii23-9.
18. Rosenzweig EB, Abman SH, Adatia I, et al. Paediatric pulmonary arterial hypertension: updates on definition, classification, diagnostics and management. Eur Respir J. 2019;53(1).
19. Keane JF, Lock E. Hemodynamic evaluation of congenital heart disease. In: Lock JE, Keane JF, Perry SB (Eds). Diagnostic and Interventional Catheterization in Congenital Heart Disease, 2nd edition. Amsterdam: Kluwer Academic Publishers; 2000. pp. 37-2.
20. Balzer DT, Kort HW, Day RW ET, et al. Inhaled nitric oxide as a preoperative test (INOP Test I): The INOP test study Group. Circulation. 2002;106 (Suppl 12):176-8.
21. Roy A, Juneja R, Saxena A. Use of Amplatzer duct occluder to close severely hypertensive ducts: utility of transient balloon occlusion. Indian Heart J. 2005;57(4):332-6.
22. Zhang DZ, Zhu XY, Lv B, et al. Trial Occlusion to Assess the Risk of Persistent Pulmonary Arterial Hypertension After Closure of a Large Patent Ductus Arteriosus in Adolescents and Adults With Elevated Pulmonary Artery Pressure. Circ Cardiovasc Interv. 2014;7:473-81.
23. Viswanathan S, Kumar RK. Assessment of operability of congenital cardiac shunts with increased pulmonary vascular resistance. Catheter Cardiovasc Interv. 2008;71(5):665-70.

Index

Page numbers followed by *b* refer to box, *f* refer to figure, *t* refer to table.

A

A wave
  absent 97
  prominent 97*f*, 98*b*, 307
Abdominovisceral situs 283
Abundant neck skin 54
Acrocyanosis 78
Acro-pectoral-renal-field defect 63
Acute aortic syndrome 31
Acute coronary syndrome 1, 29, 30
Airways 19
Alae nasi 42
Ambulatory blood pressure
  monitoring 134, 137
American College of Cardiology 136
American Heart Association 129, 136
Anacrotic notch 107*f*, 108
Anacrotic pulse 111, 112*f*, 113
Anatomically corrected malposition 299, 300*f*
Anemia 80, 188
Aneroid manometer 72
Angina 276
  types of 29*t*
Angiotensin receptor blocker 39
Angiotensin-converting enzyme 39
Anomalous pulmonary venous connection,
  totally 332
Anoxia 47
Antianginal medications 32
Aorta 165, 295, 296, 301
  ascending 79, 108, 300, 301*b*
  crossover of 175
  palpation, abdominal 125
Aortic aneurysm 24
  abdominal 125
Aortic arch, right 320*f*
Aortic atresia 298
Aortic ball valve 208
Aortic bodies 17
Aortic click, mechanism of 198*b*
Aortic component 165, 216, 220, 221, 228, 230, 231
Aortic dilation
  ascending 24
  mild 51

Aortic dissection 55
Aortic distensibility 133
Aortic ejection 170
Aortic knuckle, dilated 338*f*
Aortic pressure 107, 197*f*, 255*f*
  central 108, 255*f*
  fall of 255*f*
  transient rise of 255*f*
Aortic pulse, central 109
Aortic regurgitation 71, 112, 112*f*, 114*f*, 120,
    121, 132, 181, 189, 213, 218, 228, 241*f*,
    252, 317
  acute 230
    severe 169
  mild 229
  mild-to-moderate 236
  moderate-to-severe 128
  murmur 214, 229, 230*f*, 237
  presence of 125
  severe 169, 229
Aortic stenosis 112, 146, 181*f*, 182, 193, 213,
    218, 218*f*, 252
  severe 112*f*, 128
  syndrome, supravalvular 58
  to-and-fro murmur of 241*f*
Aortic valve
  closure 113
  opening 106, 145*f*
  sclerosis 220
Aortic valvular click 197, 197*f*, 198
Aorticomitral discontinuity 297
Aortopulmonary collateral arteries 158, 317, 321*f*
Aortopulmonary window 241, 334
Apex
  cardiogram 145*f*, 158*f*, 191
  phonocardiogram 165*f*
Apical impulse 3, 142, 145, 146, 156, 308
  abnormal 146
  normal 145
  palpation for 145
Arachnodactyly 51*f*
Arm
  circumference 75*f*
  pressure 130
Arrhythmia 25, 100, 133

Arterial blood gas 80
Arterial bruit 125
Arterial pressure 237
   response, square wave 266*f*
Arterial pulsation 88*f*, 142, 152
Arterial pulse 106
   wave 106
Arterial wall 108, 110
   condition of 119
Arterioles, pulmonary 274
Artery
   brachial 124*f*
   hypertensive pulmonary 42
   hypertrophied bronchial 276
Aspirin 39
Asplenia 284, 287
Atherosclerosis 142
   multi-ethnic study of 36
Atresia 287
   pulmonary 298, 320, 321*f*
Atrial contraction 233
Atrial depolarization 27
Atrial events 153
Atrial fibrillation 2, 14, 97, 98, 102*f*, 110, 133, 170, 179, 203*f*, 233*f*
   postexercise 28
   potentiation 217
   scale, severity of 12
Atrial flutter 110
Atrial impulse 153
Atrial pressure, mean 191*f*
Atrial septal defect 23, 38, 41, 53, 140, 166, 178*f*, 179, 198, 205, 205*f*, 206*f*, 255*f*, 306, 331, 332, 334, 337, 338*f*, 339, 341
   large 203
Atrial septum 24
Atrial situs 284
Atrial tachycardia, multifocal 110
Atriogenic valve 166
Atrioventricular alignment 289-291, 291*b*, 291*f*, 292, 292*f*
Atrioventricular block 193
   first degree 101*f*
Atrioventricular concordance 296*f*
Atrioventricular connection 287, 287*b*, 290
   absence of
      left 290*f*
      right 290*f*
Atrioventricular discordance 295*f*
Atrioventricular dissociation 109
Atrioventricular hemodynamic, right 87
Atrioventricular nodal reentrant tachycardia 28
Atrioventricular pressure
   gradient, higher 191*f*
   pulse crossover 223*f*

Atrioventricular septal defect 332, 334
Atrioventricular valve
   atresia
      left 290*f*
      right 290*f*
   regurgitation 189
Atrium, identify right and left 285*t*
Auscultation 337
Auscultatory electronic manometer 72
Auscultatory gap 130
Austin Flint murmur 228, 235
Automated nonauscultatory electronic manometer 72
Autonomic dysfunction 138
Autopsy, sketch of 63
Autosomal dominant 55
Axillary artery aneurysm 85
Azygos veins, accessory 37
Azygos-hemiazygos venous system 37

B

Baby's muscles 54
Balloon-occlusion study 342
Bedside cardiology 1, 4*b*
Bell 69, 135
   transmits 69
Bendopnea 24, 264, 265, 276
Beta blockers 39
Bicuspid aortic valve 198
Bilobed lungs, bilateral 284
Biochemical theory 115
Bioprosthesis 210
Bisferiens pulse 111
Biventricular impulses 152*f*
Bladder 74, 74*f*
   central point of 75*f*
   dimensions, acceptable 74*t*
   length 75*f*
Bleeding parameters 48
Blood
   flow, normal 212
   pressure 45, 127, 130, 132, 133, 136, 137
      auscultatory 133
      diastolic 133
      level of 133
      measure 128*b*, 138
      measurement 133, 135
   pushes 164
   rushes 213
   volume of 87
Bone morphogenetic protein 335
Borg scale, modified 21, 21*t*
Brachial atrioventricular malformation 85
Bradyarrhythmia 109
   causes of 110*b*

Bradycardia 203
  presence of 134
Brain natriuretic peptide 188
Breast
  euphemism for 68
  hypoplastic 140
Breathing, difficult 42
Bronchial asthma, acute 118
Bronchial hyperemia, chronic 37
Bronchial mucosa 37
Bronchial veins 37
Bronchiectasis 42, 286
Brotmacher theory 46
Bulboventricular loop 294

C

Calf-leg pressure 133
Calibration 73
Canadian Cardiovascular Society 12
  functional classification of angina pectoris 8, 9*t*
  severity of atrial fibrillation scale 13*b*
  system 6
Cannon wave 97
  causes of 98*b*
  regular 98, 102*f*
Capillary pulsation 121
Cardiac abnormalities 53, 55, 56, 58
  incidence of 56
Cardiac anomalies, congenital 331
Cardiac auscultation 173
Cardiac catheterization 184, 342
Cardiac defect 51, 59, 61, 62
Cardiac disease 32
  severity of 261
Cardiac drugs 39
Cardiac filing pressure 251
Cardiac hemodynamics 266
Cardiac index 34, 267
Cardiac malposition 282
Cardiac motion 190
  theory 191*f*
Cardiac percussion 160
Cardiac position 282
Cardiac pulsation 141
Cardiac silhouette, square appearance of 329*f*
Cardiac syndrome 200
Cardiac tamponade 103, 117
Cardiohemic system 173
Cardiohepatic angle 162*f*
Cardiomyopathy
  dilated 23
  hypertrophic 146, 157, 157*f*, 193, 219
Cardiorenal rescue study 264

Cardiorenal syndrome 14, 267
Cardiovascular system 34, 212
  cardinal symptoms in 17
Carditis 237
Carey Coombs murmur 228, 237
Carotid
  artery 94, 123*f*, 215*f*
  bodies 17
  bruit 3
  pulse 96*f*, 107
Catecholamine excess 28
Cellular intimal reaction 333
Central venous pressure 87
Chaotic atrial tachycardia 110
Chemoreceptors 18
Chest
  in single ventricle, X-ray of 324*f*
  in tricuspid atresia, X-ray of 329*f*
  pain 1, 28
    cardiac 28, 32
    causes of 29*t*
    score, emergency department assessment of 30
  radiography 287
  wall 142
    anterior 240*f*
    deformity 63
    muscles 18
    pain 31
    posterior 240*f*
    structures 19
  X-ray of 309, 319, 323, 327
Cheyne-Stokes respiration 23
Chromosome 60
Chronic fatigue syndrome 34
Circular fasciculi 144*f*
Clubbed finger 82, 84*f*
Clubbing
  congenital 85
  grading of 82*b*
  unilateral 85
Coarctation of aorta 122, 123*f*, 133
Cold extremity 265
Collagen fibers accompanies 133
Collapsing pulse 114*b*
Compression, abdominal 94
Concomitant cardiovascular disease 14
Congestion 262, 263, 267
  hemodynamic 262
  pulmonary 36, 41, 262
  systemic 262
Conotruncal face 60*b*, 61*f*
Conus 298, 299*f*
Co-oximeter 80
Corneal arcus 142

Coronary arteriovenous fistula 242
   continuous murmur of 242f
Coronary artery
   anomalous left 306
   disease 2, 29
      pretest probability of 29t
Coronary sinus 285
Corpuscular hemoglobin, mean 81
Corpuscular volume, mean 81
Corrective cardiac surgery 331
Corrigan's sign 120
Cortical function 17
Cough 37-39
   cardiac causes of 39b
   chronic 38
Counterclockwise depolarization 313f, 322f
Crescendo-Decrescendo
   murmur 214, 248, 249
   nature 215, 235
Crown-top baldness 142
Cuff 74
   leg pressure, systolic 132
Cutis marmorata 78
Cyanosis 77, 77b, 78, 79, 79f, 85, 306f, 317
   absence of 44
   differential 307
   onset of 305t
   reverse differential 79, 307
Cyanotic burdens, grading 81t
Cyanotic heart disease 140, 157, 212, 304
   cardinal symptoms in congenital 44
   complex 304
   congenital 77, 77b, 82, 104, 244, 245f, 303

D

de Musset's head 122
Death, causes of 341b
Deep vein thrombosis 31, 32
Dennison's sign 121
Deoxyribonucleic acid 61
Depolarization, clockwise 314f
Dextrocardia 282, 282f, 284, 286f, 293, 301
   cardiac abnormalities in 283t
Dextrorotation 283
Dextroversion 283, 293
Diabetes mellitus 137
Diaphragm 69, 135
Diastolic augmentation 113
Diastolic pressure gradient 202f, 274
Dicrotic notch 108
Dicrotic pulse 111, 112
Dicrotic wave 108
Distal phalangeal depth 84f
Dizziness 27
Dock murmur 228, 232

Dorsalis pedis 131
Double-inlet ventricle 289, 289f
Down's syndrome 53, 53f, 54, 54t
Duke Activity Status Index 10, 11t
Duroziez's murmur 122
Dynamic auscultation 214, 251
   role of 251
Dysplasia, acromelic 51
Dysplastic ear 54
Dysplastic pulmonary valve 182
Dyspnea 1, 17, 19, 27, 32, 41, 42, 263, 275
   assessment of 20, 21
   Borg scale of 21t
   circuit of 17, 18f
   feeling of 18
   formal measurement of 20
   mechanism of 18, 275
   on effort 336
   physiologic components of 17
   severity scale of 20t

E

Ear
   low set 64, 64f
   normal 64f
Ebstein's anomaly 104, 159, 169, 307
Echocardiogram 303
Echocardiographic diastolic dysfunction 194
Echocardiography 266
Ectopia cordis 287
Edema 35, 82, 264
   grading of 35, 35t, 36t
   interstitial 42
Eisenmenger complex 46, 330, 332
Eisenmenger physiology 303, 304, 307, 330
Eisenmenger syndrome 38, 38b, 278, 330, 331, 337, 343
   atrial septal defect 312f, 337
   auscultatory features in 337b
   clinical presentation of 336
   diseases leading to 332
   in large shunt, incidence of 331
   natural history of 340
   onset of 334t
   patent ductus arteriosus 338
   pathobiology of 334
   pathophysiology of 333
   physiology-wise diseases causing 332t
   ventricular septal defect 337
Ejection click 171, 220, 308
Ejection murmur 218
Ejection sound 195
Ejection systolic murmur 215, 220, 318
   causes of 216b
   physiology 215

Elastic fibrils 333
Electrocardiogram 30, 191
Electronic manometer 72
Elevated jugular venous pressure 93*b*
Emphysema 24
  infantile lobar 42
End-diastolic pressure 230
  normal 94
  raised 193
  ventricular 188
Endocardial cushion defect 53
Endocarditis, infective 82
Endothelial dysfunction 334
End-systolic volume 103
Eosinophil 82
Epicanthic eye-fold 54
Erythrocytosis 48
Esophageal spasm 32
European Heart Rhythm Association 26
  functional classification of atrial
    fibrillation 14
  modified 14, 14*t*
European Society of Cardiology 136
European Society of Hypertension 136
Eustachian valve 24, 285
Exercise testing 266
Exertional dyspnea, mechanism of 276*b*
Extra-alveolar vessel resistance 117

F

Failure to thrive 42
Fatigue 34, 138, 265, 276
  measure 34
  mechanism of 34
  signs of 34
  symptom inventory 34
Feeding difficulty 42
Femoral artery, simultaneous palpation
  of 124*f*
Femoral bruit 3
Femoral pulse 109
Femoral venous return 94
Fibroblast 82
  proliferation 82
Fibrous vascular occlusion, stage of
  progressive 333
First heart sound 164, 169, 171, 174, 192,
  197*t*, 200, 214-218, 220, 221, 223, 225,
  226, 228, 230, 231, 233, 234, 253, 337
  components of 164
  factors determining intensity of 167*b*
  loud 167*b*
  soft 170*b*
Fistula
  arteriovenous 127, 188

  atrioventricular 85
  pulmonary arteriovenous 243
Flat face 54
Flip-flopping, feeling of 27
Fluctuation test 82, 83*f*
Forceful impulse 149
Forearm pressure 131*f*
Fourth heart sound 171, 190-194, 226, 253,
  337
  causes of 192*b*
Frequent ventricular premature beats 110
Frog sign 27
Frontoparietal baldness 142

G

Gallavardin phenomenon 218
Gallbladder disease 32
Gallop rhythm, systolic 200
Gallop sound 185, 187
Gastrointestinal diseases 32
Geneva Score for Pulmonary Embolism,
  revised 32*t*
Gerhardt's sign 121
Ghent diagnostic criteria, revised 52*b*
Giddiness 138
Goldman-specific activity scales 9*t*
  determination of 9*t*
Graham Steell murmur 278
Great artery 281, 286
  classical transposition of 326*f*
  congenitally corrected transposition of
    294, 325, 332
  D-transposition of 159, 182
  malposed 182, 297
  nontransposed 328
  normally related 297
  spatial relations 299, 299*b*, 300*f*
  transposition of 79, 160, 294, 297, 305, 306
Great vessel
  complete transposition of 324
  situs 284
Gross scoliosis, X-ray feature of 141*f*

H

Hall's criteria 54*t*
Hamman sign 207
Handgrip dynamometer 259*f*
Handheld echocardiogram 70*f*
Hang-out interval theory 178
Harsh murmur 213
Headache, coat-hanger 138
Heart 30
  block, complete 101*f*, 127
  boot-shaped 320*f*
  classification of right-sided 282*b*

disease 7, 303
  congenital 56, 305t, 306t, 331, 334
  functional class, congenital 12, 12b
  ischemic 23, 157
  left 273b, 274
  segmental approach in congenital 281
  valvular 23
  failure 15, 19, 20, 24, 34, 35, 262, 263t, 266f, 267, 268
    acute decompensated 264
    acute hypertensive 36
    boston criteria of 268, 269t
    clinical features of 262b
    congestive 22, 29, 41, 94, 100, 263, 266, 307
    diagnosis of 43
    Framingham criteria of 268, 268f
    functional classification of 14, 14t
    grade of 269
    index, pediatric 269, 270t
    management of 262
    mild 266
    predictor of 1
    right-sided 267
    ross criteria of 268, 269, 269t
    signs of 263t
    symptoms of 263t
    three symptoms of 24t
  rate 237
  score 30
  sound 3, 95, 96f, 152, 308
  surface anatomy of 161f
Hemiazygos connection 284
Hemiplegia 85
Hemithorax, right 282
Hemodynamic classification 273
Hemodynamic correlation 165, 186
Hemoglobin 78
Hemoptysis 37, 38b, 336
  cardiac causes of 39b
Hepatic pulsation 120
Hepatic pulse 104
Hepatojugular reflex 93, 94, 225, 264
  positive 264
Heterotaxy syndrome 284, 287
High amplitude 111
Hill's sign 2, 122, 132, 132t
Holt-Oram syndrome 57, 585f
Horse's left ventricle, level of 127
Hypercalcemia 59
  idiopathic infantile 58
Hypercapnia 18
Hyperdynamic apical impulse 146
Hyperemia 37
Hyperkinetic impulse 146, 149

Hyperkinetic pulse 111
Hyperoxia test 80
Hyperplasia, vascular 82
Hypertelorism 63, 64f
  ocular 64, 64f
Hypertension 59, 120, 136, 137t, 248
  diastolic 134
  exercise pulmonary 275
  grade of 136
  hyperkinetic pulmonary 241
  isolated systolic 137
  masked 137
  precapillary pulmonary 273
  supine 138
  sustained 136
Hypertrophic obstructive cardiomyopathy 112, 112f, 122, 252, 253
  murmur of 257f
Hypertrophy, biventricular 151
Hyperventilation 45
Hyperviscosity syndrome 47
  grading 48t
  symptoms of 48b
Hypokinetic apical impulse 146
Hypokinetic pulse 111
Hyponychial angle 83f
Hypoplasia 63
Hypotension
  orthostatic 138
  postprandial 138
Hypotonia, general 54
Hypoxemia 81, 82
Hypoxia 17, 18, 47, 273b
Hypoxic spell 44

I

Ileus, cirrhosis of 24
Immotile cilia syndrome 286
Immune status, abnormal 286
Imperceptible apical impulse 148b
Incident pressure pulse 108
Incisura 107, 175
Inflammatory bowel disease 82
Infundibular obstruction, development of 43
Innocent murmur 248
  and sound 247, 248b
  prevalence of 247
Inspiration 103, 195
Intensity 167, 183, 195, 213, 339
Interatrial septum, part of 24
Intercanthal distance, inner 64
Intercostal space 89, 279
Internal jugular pulsation 87
Interphalangeal depth 84f

Interpupillary distance 64
Intra-abdominal pressure 94
Intra-aortic balloon pump 113
Intra-arterial femoral artery pressure 133
Intra-arterial pressure 72
  measurement 132
Intrathoracic pressure 87, 103, 117, 118
Iron binding capacity, total 81
Irregular cannon waves 98, 101, 101f
Irritant receptors 18
Ischemic pain, symptoms of acute 29t
Isometric handgrip 256
Isovolumetric contraction 197f
Ivemark syndrome 286

J

J-receptor 18
Jugular pulse pressure 315
Jugular venous pressure 2, 24, 87, 88, 92f, 93, 93f, 96, 105f, 263, 267, 337
  mean 93
Jugular venous pulse 87, 95, 100, 102, 104, 204f, 276, 307, 317
Junctional rhythm 101, 102f
Juxtacapillary receptors 18

K

Kartagener syndrome 286
Kidney disease, chronic 137
Korotkoff sound 118, 128, 128b, 129, 130, 134, 135
  mechanism of 129
Kussmaul's sign 103

L

Landolfi's sign 120
Left atrial
  appendage 285
  impulse 153
  pressure gradient 117
Left atrium 223, 233, 234, 240, 242, 285
  pressure curve of 165f
Left axis deviation 328f
Left bundle branch block 180, 181
Left lower sternal border 219
Left parasternal cardiogram 154f
Left ventricle 223, 230, 231, 233, 234, 240, 242, 295
  double outlet 297, 298
  pressure curve of 165f, 168f
Left ventricular
  angiographic morphology 288f
  apical impulse 160t
  apical segment 150

dysfunction 3, 113, 189
end-diastolic pressure 41
enlargement 3, 147, 148b
hypertrophy 135, 147f
inflow obstruction, common causes of 235b
left atrial pressure 223
muscle 186f
outflow tract 181, 325
  obstruction 324
pressure pulse 202
systole 143
volume overload 41
Leg
  pressure 130, 131, 131f
  raising, passive 259
Length-tension inappropriateness 19
Leopard syndrome 61
Lesion, common mixing 304b
Levocardia 286f, 301
  isolated 287
Levoversion 293
Limbus, superior 285
Liver
  cirrhosis of 24
  midline 286f
Lovibond angle 83, 83f
Low pressure
  chamber 113
  tricuspid regurgitation 227b
Lower limb 133
  pressure, measure 131
  pulsations, absent 307
  saturation 47
Luetic aorta 229
Lung 19
  carcinoma 82
  disease 273b
  hypothesis 19
  parenchyma 42
Lutembacher's syndrome 233
Lymphatic system 22
Lymphocytes 82

M

Mammary soufflé 245
Marfan syndrome 50, 50f, 51f, 52, 52b, 140
  inheritance 50
Maxillary molar teeth 66f
Means–Lerman sign 207
Mechanical alternans 115
Mechanical theory 115
Mechanoreceptors 17, 18
Mediastinal crunch 207
Medullary center 17

Mercury manometer 71, 73f
Mesocardia 287
Metacarpal index 51f
Methemoglobinemia 78
Midsystolic click 200
Midsystolic murmur, physiology of 217f
Minervini's sign 120
Mitochondrial oxidative phosphorylation 20
Mitral ball valve 210
Mitral leaflets 164
  posterior 169
Mitral opening snap 202, 204t
  causes of 204b
Mitral regurgitation 51, 71, 177, 182, 203, 213, 223, 226, 252, 278
  acute 38, 193f, 226
  chronic severe 226
  congenital 224b
  functional 227
  ischemic 227
  murmur 218, 224
    physiology of 223f
  severe 154f, 177
  systolic murmur of 252
Mitral stenosis 23, 37, 156, 156f, 168, 168f, 188, 194, 204b, 205, 205t, 206f, 213, 228, 232, 233f, 257, 278
  cases of 233
  dominant 156
  murmur 3, 214, 237
  severity of 202, 202f, 232, 234f
  silent 234
Mitral valve 51, 166, 168f
  closure 165f, 169, 169f, 171
  opening 202
  premature 185
  prolapse 51, 140, 168, 169, 200, 201, 227, 253, 254, 258f
    nonejection click of 200f
    syndrome 168
Modern cardiology 104
Monosomy X 53
Morris sign 162f
Motor cortex 17
Motor innervation 68
Mucous membrane 77
Muller's maneuver 256
Muller's sign 120
Multifactorial mechanism 331
Murmur 3, 212, 213, 224, 228, 309
  causes of continuous 245f
  classification of continuous 240t
  continuous 239, 243f, 244, 254, 309
  decrescendo diastolic 241f
  determinant of 213

diamond-shaped 214
  midsystolic 241f
diastolic 3, 129, 134, 140, 210, 228, 228b, 229, 232, 249, 260, 309
  flow 225
different
  diastolic 228f
  shapes of 214f
  systolic 216f
early
  diastolic 228
  systolic 215, 226
features of innocent 248b
functional 248
grade of 222
hemodynamic classification of continuous 239b
high-frequency 240
intensity of mid-diastolic 233
late systolic 215, 227
late-crescendo 243
Levine grading system of systolic 214b
loud 155, 228
mid-diastolic 278
mid-late systolic 219
mid-systolic 215
mitral diastolic flow 241
pansystolic 215, 223
presystolic 233
pulmonary branch 249
shape of 222
supraclavicular 249, 249f
systolic 200, 207, 213, 215, 239, 309
timing of 215f
Muscle hypothesis 19
Muscularization, stage of 333
Myopia 51

N

Nail fold 83
Narrow physiological splitting 182, 182b
Natriuretic peptide 266
  brain-type 340
Neck
  short 65
  veins 336
Negative predictive value 263
New York Heart Association 6, 10, 12, 14
  classification 12b
    system, uniqueness of 8
  functional classification 6, 7t
    limitation of 8
Nocturnal dyspnea, paroxysmal 1, 22
Nonejection click, causes of 201b
Nonejection sound 200

Noonan syndrome 55, 56, 56f
  diagnostic criteria for 57b
Norepinephrine blood levels 266
Normotension, true 136

O

O'Donnell theory 47
Obstruction, severe 219
Obstructive pulmonary disease
  acute exacerbation of chronic 118
  chronic 1
Opening snap 202, 205, 233, 234
Operability and pulmonary vascular
    resistance 342
Orthodema 264
  score 264t
Orthopnea 21, 22, 263
Orthostasis 265
Oscillometric manometer 72
Osler's sign 134
Outer intercanthal distance 64
Oximeter 77
Oxygen
  consumption 45
  saturation 81

P

Packed-cell volume 81
Pain
  esophageal 32
  pericardial 30
Palate
  height 66f
  high-arched 66
  width 66f
Palfrey's sign 121, 121f
Palmar arch aneurysm 85
Palpation 142, 276, 308, 337
  abdominal 125
  tool 142
Palpitation 2, 25, 27, 28
  causes of 25
  clinical
    classification of 26b
    evaluation 27
    types of 26
  etiological classification of 25t
  etiology 25
  pathophysiology 25
Pancreatitis 32
Pansystolic prolapse 169f
Parasternal impulse 148
  grading 150b
Parasympathetic pathway 25

Parenteral vasoconstrictor 260
Paroxysmal hypoxic spell 44
Patent ductus arteriosus 127, 181, 239, 254,
    305, 306, 332, 334, 337, 338f, 340, 341
  continuous murmur of 241f
Patent foramen ovale 23, 305, 307
Paul Wood's series 332t
Peak systolic arterial pressure 134
Pectus
  carinatum 50f, 140, 141f
  excavatum 50f, 141f
Peptic ulcer disease 32
Percussion
  method 160
  wave 107, 111
Perfusion 262
Pericardial constriction 103
Pericardial disease 102
Pericardial effusion 23f, 162, 162f, 163
Pericardial knock 103f, 155f, 206
Pericardial rub 207
Pericardial sound 206
Pericarditis
  adhesive 201
  constrictive 94, 103f, 155, 155f, 207
Pericardium, part of 30
Peripheral artery, major 258
Peripheral sign 120
Peripheral transmission 108, 108f
Phalangeal depth ratio 84, 84f
Phenotype 51, 53, 55, 57-59, 61-63
Physiological zero point 89
Physiology
  common mixing 303, 304
  transposition 303
Pivotal dextrocardia 283
Platypnea-orthodeoxia syndrome 23
Plexiform lesion 333
Plexogenic arteriopathy 333
Pneumectomy 24
Pneumonia 42
Pneumothorax, left-sided 201
Poland syndrome 62
Polycythemia 82
Polysplenia 284, 286, 287
  syndrome 286
Polyuria 28
Popliteal artery 124f
  pulse 124f
Popliteal fossa 124f
Positive predictive value 263
Precordial impulse 154f
Precordium 140, 315
Pregnancy 188
Premature beat 259

Premature closure theory 186f
Premature ovarian failure 56
Pressure
  difference 133
  overload 192
  volume
    relation 190
    theory 191f
Presyncope 27
Pretricuspid and post-tricuspid shunt 334
Proinflammatory cytokines 20
Prosthetic valve 208
  different 209f
  types of 208b
Provocative dyspnea assessment scale 20, 21b
Proximal aortic pulse 107, 107f
Pseudocyanosis 78
Pseudoejection sound 201
Pseudohypertension 134
Pulmonary and aortic diastolic pressures 342
Pulmonary arterial hypertension 12, 12b, 38, 273, 273b, 274, 330, 331, 333b, 335b, 341
  hyperkinetic 341
  irreversibility of 341t
  obstructive 341
  pathobiology for 335f
  with small defects 331
Pulmonary arterial pressure 279
  mean 274
Pulmonary arterial pulsation 152
Pulmonary arterial wall 333
Pulmonary arteriopathy, pulmonary 333, 333b
Pulmonary artery 79, 177, 179, 197, 222, 231, 240-242, 242f, 244, 295, 296, 305, 306, 338f
  catheterization effectiveness 1, 22, 263
  dilated right 338f
  distension of 38
  ipsilateral main 286
  left 42, 284
  left and anterior to 301b
  lower 196f
  pressure 2
    systolic 3
  right 42
  stenosis, peripheral 222
Pulmonary capillary wedge pressure 1, 22, 273, 274
  tracing 154f
Pulmonary circulation 303
Pulmonary component 216, 220, 221, 228, 230, 231, 328
Pulmonary edema, acute 23

Pulmonary ejection
  click 277
  murmur 277
Pulmonary embolism 31, 32
  well model for 31t
Pulmonary hypertension 3, 15, 43, 156, 180, 203, 232, 272, 273b, 274, 276b, 279, 330, 331, 334
  auscultatory features of 277b
  borderline 275
  clinical
    classification of 272, 272b
    grading of 279, 279t
  pattern 274
  postcapillary 273, 274
  primary 272
Pulmonary interstitial space 41
Pulmonary outflow
  resistance, total 315
  tract, transposed 323
Pulmonary overcirculation 41
Pulmonary regurgitation 228, 231, 277
  murmur of 231f
  normal pressure 232
  severe 317
Pulmonary stenosis 160, 182, 195, 198, 213, 220, 220f, 221, 221f, 252, 287, 305, 316, 322, 322f, 323, 325, 326f, 327, 328f, 329f
  mild 195
  severe 158, 196
Pulmonary stretch receptors, stimulation of 18
Pulmonary valve 196, 279, 285, 294
  absent 182
  aortic to 296
  syndrome 232
Pulmonary valvular
  click 195-197, 199, 277t
  disease 274, 331, 333
  ejection click 196f
  resistance 42, 45, 274, 315, 330, 343, 343t
  stenosis 177, 322
Pulmonary vascularity, reduced 320f
Pulmonary venous system 177
Pulmonary ventricle decompresses 303
Pulsation and obstruction scale 109b
Pulse 2, 110, 120, 122, 307, 336
  double-beating 111, 112f
  origin of 106
  oximeter 80
  peripheral 108
  pressure 108, 111, 114f, 122, 127, 230f
    normal 111
    proportional 128, 265
  wave contour 108

Pulsus
    alternans 115
        causes of 115b
    bigeminy 109
    bisferiens 112f, 114
    magnus 120
    paradoxus 116, 116b, 118
        amount of 118
        reverse 119, 119b
    parvus et tardus 113
Pump failure 3

Q
Quincke's sign 121

R
Radial arteries, simultaneous palpation of 124f
Radial pulse 109
Radionuclide ventriculography 266
Recoil theory 143
Recumbent posture, squatting in 46
Red blood cell 47
Reflective wave augments 108
Reflux, abdominojugular 93
Regurgitant systolic murmur 215, 222
    characteristic 223
    physiology 222
Regurgitation, hypertensive pulmonary 231
Renal disease, end-stage 14
Renal failure, chronic 207, 228, 237
Renal insufficiency 248
Renal replacement therapy 14
Respiration 260
    effect of 90
    on pulse volume 116
Respiratory center 23
Respiratory discomfort, sensation of 19
Respiratory muscle 17
    activity 18
Respiratory pressure 19
Respiratory symptoms 43
Respiratory tract infection 43
Respiratory variation 195
Rheumatic fever, acute 237
Right and left atrium, morphology of 285f
Right atrial
    appendage 285
    impulse 153
    pressure 95, 103, 267
        curves 97f
Right atrium 103, 240, 242, 285
    center of 91f
    contracts 96
    prominent 329
Right axis deviation 322f
Right bundle branch block 166, 176, 177
Right ventricle 231, 240, 242, 295
    double outlet 160, 298, 303, 322, 332
    forming apex 151f
Right ventricular
    angiographic morphology 288f
    apical impulse 160t
    cavity 143f
    dysfunction, severe 180
    end-diastolic pressure 195, 196f
    hypertrophy 314f, 320, 322f
    impulse 148
        abnormal 149
        normal 148
    inflow obstruction, common causes of 235b
    obstruction 45
    outflow tract 28, 318
    pressure curves 97f
    systole 94
Rosenbach's sign 120
Rotch sign 162f
Rule of thumb 250
Rytand murmur 228, 237

S
Schamroth's sign 84, 84f
Schizophrenia 61
Second heart sound 144, 165, 171, 173, 174, 177b, 191, 193, 214-218, 221, 223, 225, 226, 228, 230, 233, 234, 256, 278, 318, 337, 339
    production, mechanism of 173
    single 182b
    wide splitting of 177b
Semilunar valves 173
Sensory cortex 17
Serum ferritin 81
Serum transferrin 81
Sex distribution 336
Shock, septic 113
Short stature 55
Shoulder pain 138
SHOX gene 54
Shunt
    bidirectional 330
    cardinal symptoms in left-to-right 41
    left-to-right 42, 43, 189, 330, 331
    lesion 77, 343t
        congenital 330
    prevalent systemic-to-pulmonary 331
    right-to-left 24

Simplified Emergency Department
    Assessment of Chest Pain Score 30
Single arterial trunk 298
Single inlet ventricle 290f
Sinus
    ambiguous 286
    bradycardia 127, 266
Sinus of Valsalva, ruptured 243, 243f
Sinus tachycardia 110, 266
    inappropriate 28
    mild 187
Sinusitis, chronic 286
Situs 283
    ambiguous 282, 286f
    inversus 282, 285, 286f, 293, 295f, 296f, 301
    solitus 282, 284, 293, 301
        D-loop with 294
Six-minute walk test 15
Skeletal muscle 19
Skin
    bluish 78
    discoloration of 77
Sleep 28
Slows down pulse wave 113
Small amplitude pulse 113
Small pulmonary arteries 333
Smaller ring finger 58f
Snowman sign 311f
Specific activity scale 10
Sphygmomanometer 71
    auscultatory 256
Sphygmomanometric artifact 2
Sphygmomanometric pressure 134
Spiral fibers 147f
Splenic nodules, two 286f
Splitting 339
    grading of 339b
    reverse 180, 181b
Squatting 45, 336
    diseases associated with 46
Stable angina 28
Stenosis, severe 221f, 234
Stethoscope 68
    acoustic 69
    advantage of 140
    diaphragm of 125
    digital 70
    electronic 70
    ideal 69
    modern 68
    ultrasound 70
Stiff skin syndrome 51
Stiffness, vascular 134
Still's murmur 247
Stomach 286f

Straight back syndrome 140, 141f, 248
Stroke 213
    index 34
Subclavian artery, right 62
Subxiphoid palpation 192
Summation gallop 187
Supraclavicular fossa 249f
Supravalvular stenosis 219
Supraventricular tachycardia,
    paroxysmal 110
Sympathetic nervous system 256
Sympathetic pathway 25
Synchrony 120, 130
Syncope 27, 276
Systemic arterial pressure 46
Systemic vascular resistance 315, 342
Systemic venous congestion 267
Systolic fall 98
Systolic murmur, types of 215b
Systolic pressure 108, 118, 127, 135, 256
Systolic wave 108
    rest of 107f
Systolo-diastolic murmur 244

T

Tabatznik's syndrome 57
Tachyarrhythmia 110, 115
    causes of 110b
Tachycardia 28
    re-entry 27
    ventricular 101, 110
Tachypnea 41
Tamponade, presence of 116
Telecanthus 63, 64, 64f
Tension 19
Tetralogy of Fallot 53, 157, 158f, 198, 198b,
    221, 307, 316, 317, 319f, 336
    X-ray in typical 320f
Tetralogy physiology 303, 304, 315, 316
    extremely severe 317
    mild 316
    moderate 316
    severe 317
    under umbrella of 317
Third heart sound 185, 187, 188, 193, 204t,
    225, 226, 337
    ventricular theory of 186f
Thoracic aorta 125
Thoracic structural deformity 140
Thoracovisceral situs 284
Thumb sign 50f
Thyrotoxicosis 188
Tibial artery, posterior 131
Tidal wave 108
Tilting-disk valve 210

Tissue oxygenation 48
To-and-fro murmur 244
  causes of 244b
Total anomalous pulmonary venous 286
  connection 305, 306
    Snowman sign of 311f
  drainage 332
Tracheal tug 152
Tracheobronchial situs 284f
Tracheobronchial tree 37
Transcatheter aortic prosthetic valve,
    different 211f
Transient arterial occlusion 258
Transpulmonary pressure gradient 274
Traube's sign 121
Trepopnea 23
Tricuspid annular plane systolic
    excursion 340
Tricuspid atresia 158, 327, 328f
Tricuspid opening snap 203, 204f
Tricuspid regurgitation 71, 155, 156, 224,
    253, 276, 337, 341
  murmur 71, 224, 259, 277
  primary 227
  severe 99f, 141, 155, 204f
Tricuspid stenosis 169, 213, 228, 235
Tricuspid valve 24, 98
  closure 169, 171
  disease 94
Trigeminal nerve modulate dyspnea 18
Trilogy of Fallot's 158
Triple apical impulse-presystolic
    wave 157f
Trisomy 21 53
Truncus arteriosus 160, 182, 312f
Turner's syndrome 53, 54, 55f, 140
  diagnostic criteria for 56b
  phenotype of 54

U

Upper arm veins 104
Upper lobe bronchus, carcinoma right 85
Upper-to-lower segment ratio 65
Urate metabolism 48

V

V wave, abnormal 99
Valsalva
  effect of 255f
  maneuver 255, 256, 266, 266f
Valve 208
  ventriculogenic 166
Van Praagh classification double inlet
    ventricle 289b

Vasodilator 260
  testing, acute 342
Veins 87
  bronchopulmonary 37
  pulmonary 117
  systemic 37
Velo-cardio-facial syndrome 59
Vena cava
  inferior 24, 79, 283, 285
  superior 47, 242, 285, 295
Vena caval connection 160
Venous pressure 98
  normal 89
Venous pulsation 88, 88t, 102f
Venous pulse 104
  abnormal 96
  normal 94
Venous tone 87
Ventricular dysfunction 27, 188
Ventricular filling pressure 263
Ventricular loop 293f
Ventricular premature beat 38
Ventricular septal defect 44, 53, 104, 140,
    160, 177, 182, 221, 221f, 222, 225, 225f,
    241, 252, 288, 303, 305, 315, 320, 321f,
    322, 322f, 326f, 328f, 329f, 332, 334, 337,
    338f, 339, 341
  murmur of 241f
Ventriculoarterial connection 294, 296b,
    297b, 298f
  normal 294
Ventriculoarterial junction 281
Venturi effect 112
Vertigo 138
Vision, blurring of 138
Visual analog scale 21, 22f
Vortex shedding 212

W

Water hammer
  pulse 114
  theory 129
Weight gain 35, 36
Weill-Marchesani syndrome 51
Wheeze, pulmonary 265
White coat
  hypertension 137
  reverse 137
Wide fixed splitting 177
Williams syndrome, diagnostic criteria
    for 60t
Williams-Beuren syndrome 58, 59f
Wolff-Parkinson-White syndrome 176, 177
World Health Organization 12, 340
  classification 12b

X

X descent
  abnormal 98
  reduced 99*b*
  systolic 94
X monosomy
  complete 56
  partial 56
Xanthelasmata 142
X-chromosomal materials 54

Y

Y descent
  abnormal 99
  prominent 100*b*
Yellow sputum 39

Z

Z-score 52

EU GSPR Authorised Reprsentative
Logos Europe, 9 rue Nicolas Poussin
1700, La Rochelle, France
Phone: +33 (0) 6 67 93 73 78
E-mail: contact@logoseurope.eu

www.ingramcontent.com/pod-product-compliance
Ingram Content Group UK Ltd.
Pitfield, Milton Keynes, MK11 3LW, UK
UKHW051237180426
11947UKWH00013B/826